Thyroiditis

Mahmoud Sakr

Thyroiditis

Diagnosis and Therapeutic Management

Springer

Mahmoud Sakr
Department of Surgery
Alexandria University, Faculty of Medicine
Alexandria, Egypt

ISBN 978-3-032-19512-8 ISBN 978-3-032-19513-5 (eBook)
https://doi.org/10.1007/978-3-032-19513-5

This Springer imprint is published by the registered company Springer Nature Switzerland AG
The registered company address is: Gewerbestrasse 11, 6330 Cham, Switzerland

To my dear students and colleagues

Preface

Thyroiditis comprises a group of diseases that can present with strikingly similar symptoms. This frequently poses a diagnostic dilemma to uncover the exact etiology. These patients may present with hyper or hypothyroid symptoms with subtle differences depending on the etiology. A thorough history-taking and physical examination is the key to uncover these subtle differences. Thyroiditis represents about 20% of all thyroid diseases and is caused by several factors, most commonly autoimmune diseases.

This authored book, in 16 chapters with 31 figures, and 36 tables, will provide a valuable source of knowledge and reference for all specialists and trainees entrusted with the care of patients suffering from thyroid disease. It addresses a wide range of topics including the anatomy, physiology, and investigations of the thyroid gland. It also discusses the etiology, pathophysiology, diagnosis, and treatment strategy of the different forms of thyroiditis, which may be "autoimmune" such as Hashimoto's disease, de Quervain's subacute thyroiditis, Riedel's fibrosing thyroiditis, or "non-autoimmune" such as acute suppurative thyroiditis, drug-induced thyroiditis, post-operative necrotizing thyroiditis, or radiation thyroiditis. Finally, this book includes also a chapter summarizing the studies published recently related to surgical management of the different types (variants) of thyroiditis, including indications of surgical intervention, type of surgery performed, and postoperative complications encountered.

It is my collective hope that head and neck surgeons, maxillofacial surgeons, endocrinologists, oncologists, otolaryngologists, and clinicians of other specialties will find this book to be a useful and indispensable resource as they face the most challenging of thyroid gland disorders to help provide individual patients with the best possible outcome.

Alexandria, Egypt
Mahmoud F. Sakr

Acknowledgments

I would like to thank all those who helped and encouraged me during the writing, editing, and revision of this book. Specifically, I would like to thank Dr. Fatima Soufan, Beirut Arab University, Lebanon, for performing the art work and providing the illustrations of thyroid anatomy for this book. I would like also to express my appreciation and gratitude to my wife and children for their continuous support and unconditioned love.

Contents

Thyroid Gland: Anatomy, Physiology, and Investigations

1

1.1 Surgical Anatomy

1.1.1 Anatomical Position and Physiological Variants

The thyroid gland is a highly vascular, brownish-red endocrine gland located anteriorly in the lower neck, inferior to the laryngeal thyroid cartilage and posterior to the sterno-thyroid and sterno-hyoid muscles, wrapping around the cricoid cartilage and tracheal rings. It typically extends from the level of the fifth cervical vertebra (C5) down to the first thoracic (T1). The normal thyroid gland weighs between 20 and 35 g in adults, and consists of two elongated lateral lobes with superior and inferior poles connected by a median isthmus overlying the second to fourth tracheal rings. The superior poles extend toward the oblique line of the thyroid cartilage, lying deep to the sternothyroid muscle and superficial to the cricothyroid muscle [1]. Two pairs of parathyroid glands (PTGs) usually lie in proximity to the thyroid gland, each on either side. The position of the thyroid gland and its close relationship with various important structures in the neck such as the recurrent laryngeal nerve (RLN) brings about several surgical considerations with clinical relevance.

A conical "pyramidal lobe" often ascends from the isthmus or the adjacent part of either lobe (more often the left) toward the thyroid cartilage, to which it may be attached by a fibrous or fibro-muscular band, the levator of the thyroid gland. It occurs in only 28–55% of individuals. Typically, the presence of a pyramidal lobe is asymptomatic. It can be separated entirely from the main thyroid gland and has also been documented to occur bilaterally.

"Ectopic thyroid tissue" can be found anywhere along the migratory pathway of the thyroid gland and has been documented in locations ranging from the tongue to the diaphragm. The prevalence of an ectopic thyroid gland is between 1 per 100,000 and 1 per 300,000. The most common site for ectopic thyroid tissue is the ectopic lingual thyroid at the base of the tongue [2]. Ectopic thyroid tissue can present with varying symptomatology depending on its location. Lingual ectopic thyroid tissue

M. Sakr, *Thyroiditis*, https://doi.org/10.1007/978-3-032-19513-5_1

may present with dysphagia, bleeding, and dyspnea. Supra-hyoid and infra-hyoid thyroid tissue may present as a midline neck swelling, similar to a thyroglossal duct cyst. Intra-tracheal or intra-laryngeal thyroid tissue may present with respiratory obstruction, while intra-esophageal thyroid tissue may present with dysphagia.

Remnants of the thyroglossal duct may persist as accessory nodules or cysts of thyroid tissue between the isthmus and the foramen cecum of the tongue base. In addition, a wide variety of morphological variations exists. The isthmus may be large, narrowed, or entirely absent, and the lateral lobes of the thyroid may vary in size and symmetry when comparing right to left.

1.1.2 Fascia and Ligaments

The thyroid gland (along with the esophagus, pharynx, and trachea) is found within the visceral compartment of the neck, which is bound by pre-tracheal fascia. The thyroid gland is thus enveloped by a fibrous "capsule" condensed from the pre-tracheal fascia. The "anterior suspensory ligament" extends from the superior-medial aspect of each thyroid lobe to the cricoid and thyroid cartilage. The postero-medial aspect of the gland is attached to the side of the cricoid cartilage, first and second tracheal rings, by the "posterior suspensory ligament" (Berry's ligament), which is responsible for movement of the thyroid gland and related structures during swallowing. On its way to the larynx, the recurrent laryngeal nerve (RLN) usually passes deep to Berry's ligament or between the main ligament and its lateral leaf [3]. Modern surgical resection of the thyroid gland involves a "capsular dissection." Maintenance of the capsule helps reduce damage to the plexus of veins that lie on its surface and its highly vascular parenchyma. Additionally, it reduces the chance of injury to the adjacent neuro-vascular structures.

1.1.3 Relation with the Platysma and Infra-Hyoid (Strap) Muscles

The "platysma" is the first muscle encountered during thyroidectomy and neck dissection and is enveloped by the superficial cervical fascia. It sits in the anterior neck and extends from the superficial fascia of the deltoid over the clavicle, reaching the mandible and superficial fascia of the face superiorly.

The "infra-hyoid muscles" (also referred to as "strap muscles") include four paired muscles on the antero-lateral surface of the thyroid gland. The strap muscles result in gross movement of the larynx during swallowing and also adjust the positioning of the larynx during vocalization. The lateral surface of the thyroid is covered by the sterno-thyroid muscle, and its attachment to the oblique line of the thyroid cartilage prevents the superior pole of the thyroid gland from extending superiorly under the thyro-hyoid muscle. The thyro-hyoid muscle extends from the oblique line of the thyroid cartilage to the hyoid bone superiorly. More anteriorly are the sterno-hyoid and superior belly of omohyoid muscle, overlapped inferiorly by the anterior border of the sterno-cleidomastoid (SCM) muscle. The sterno-hyoid and sterno-thyroid muscles are joined in the midline by an avascular deep cervical fascia that must be incised to retract the strap muscles laterally in order to access the thyroid gland during thyroidectomy. Transection of strap muscles, if necessary for better exposure, should be done high in the neck to avoid injury of their motor nerve supply, the "ansa cervicalis," which enters these muscles inferiorly. The anterior jugular vein is covered by the platysma and skin and lies superficial to these muscles.

1.1.4 Arterial Supply

The thyroid gland has an extremely rich blood supply and is estimated to be 6 times as vascular as the kidney and relatively 3–4 times more vascular than the brain. The arterial supply to the thyroid gland comes from the superior and inferior thyroid arteries and, occasionally, the thyroidea ima (Fig. 1.1). These arteries have abundant collateral anastomoses with each other, both ipsilaterally and contralaterally.

1.1.4.1 Superior Thyroid Artery (STA)

The superior thyroid artery (STA) arises as the first branch of the external carotid artery (ECA) near the level of the superior horn of the thyroid cartilage and passes in a caudal direction toward the midline behind the sterno-thyroid muscle to the superior pole of the thyroid gland lobe. It has close relations to the external branch of the superior laryngeal nerve (EB-SLN), which lies deep to the artery before turning medially to supply the crico-thyroid muscle. High ligation of the STA during thyroidectomy places this nerve at risk of inadvertent injury, which would produce dysphonia by altering pitch regulation. Thus, during thyroidectomy, the STA should be ligated as close as possible to the thyroid gland to avoid injury of the EB-SLN [4].

Branches of the STA include the following [4]:

- *Infra-hyoid branch:* It runs along the inferior border of the hyoid bone.
- *Superior laryngeal branch:* It pierces the thyrohyoid membrane to enter the larynx.
- *Sternomastoid branch:* It runs backwards across the common carotid artery (CCA) to supply the SCM muscle.
- *Cricothyroid branch:* It runs across the cricothyroid membrane to anastomose with the artery of the opposite side.
- *Anterior terminal branch:* It runs downwards in front of the upper pole of thyroid gland.
- *Posterior terminal branch:* It runs downwards behind the upper pole of the thyroid gland.
- *Parathyroid branch:* It arises from the posterior terminal branch and passes to the superior parathyroid gland.

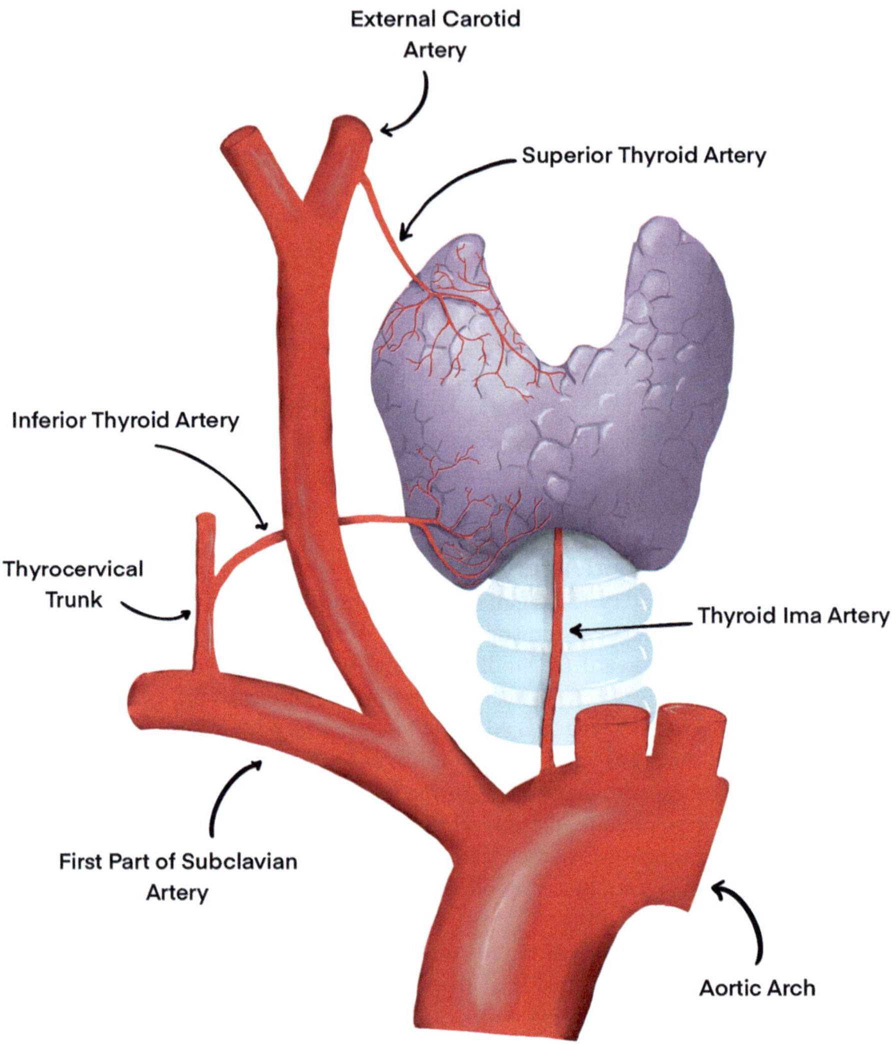

Fig. 1.1 Diagrammatic representation of the arterial supply of the thyroid gland (With prior permissions from the illustrator Dr. Fatima Soufan)

1.1.4.2 Inferior Thyroid Artery (ITA)

The inferior thyroid artery (ITA) arises, at the inner border of the anterior scalene muscle, from the thyro-cervical trunk, a branch of the first part of the subclavian artery, and passes in the trachea-esophageal groove (TEG) to reach the postero-lateral aspect of each lobe at the level of the junction of the upper two-thirds and lower third of the outer border. It has a variable branching pattern and a variable relationship with the RLN, most commonly passing in front of the nerve and less commonly behind the nerve. The largest branch of the ITA is the "ascending cervical branch," and it is important not to mistake this branch for the inferior thyroid artery itself [5].

To avoid injury to the RLN during thyroidectomy, the ITA has been recommended to be ligated *away* from the gland. However, this may jeopardize the vascular supply to the parathyroid glands, which are all supplied mainly by the ITA. Thus, it is preferable that during thyroidectomy, the secondary and tertiary branches of the ITA (not the main trunk) are ligated under vision in order to preserve both, the RLN and the blood supply to the parathyroid glands.

1.1.4.3 Thyroidea Ima Artery

The "thyroidea ima" is a single artery that most commonly originates from the brachio-cephalic trunk or the arch of the aorta and supplies the isthmus and anterior thyroid gland. It is present in <10% of the population, most commonly 3%. This artery has a variable origin, including not only the brachio-cephalic trunk and aortic arch but also the right common carotid, the subclavian, the pericardio-phrenic artery, the thyro-cervical trunk, the transverse scapular, or internal thoracic artery.

1.1.4.4 Small Esophageal and Tracheal Branches

Small esophageal and tracheal branches supply also the thyroid gland. They supply the thyroid remnant after partial or subtotal thyroidectomy.

1.1.5 Venous Drainage

Veins of the thyroid gland form a plexus of vessels lying in the substance and on the surface of the gland. This plexus is drained by three pairs of veins. The superior and middle thyroid veins drain into the internal jugular vein (IJV), while the inferior thyroid veins follow different paths on each side (Fig. 1.2). The right passes anterior to the innominate artery to the right brachio-cephalic vein or anterior to the trachea to the left brachio-cephalic vein. On the left side, drainage is to the left brachio-cephalic vein. Occasionally, both right and left inferior thyroid veins form a common trunk called the "thyroid ima vein," which empties into the left brachio-cephalic vein.

1.1.6 Lymphatic Drainage

Lymphatic drainage of the thyroid gland is extensive and flows multi-directionally with intra-glandular and sub-capsular lymphatic drainage into the IJV. Immediate lymphatic drainage flows to the peri-glandular lower deep cervical lymph nodes (LNs), to the pre-laryngeal (Delphian), pre-tracheal, and para-tracheal nodes along the RLN, and then to mediastinal LNs. The para-tracheal and lower deep cervical nodes, specifically, receive lymphatic drainage from the isthmus and the inferior lateral lobes. The superior portions of the thyroid gland drain into the superior pre-tracheal and cervical nodes.

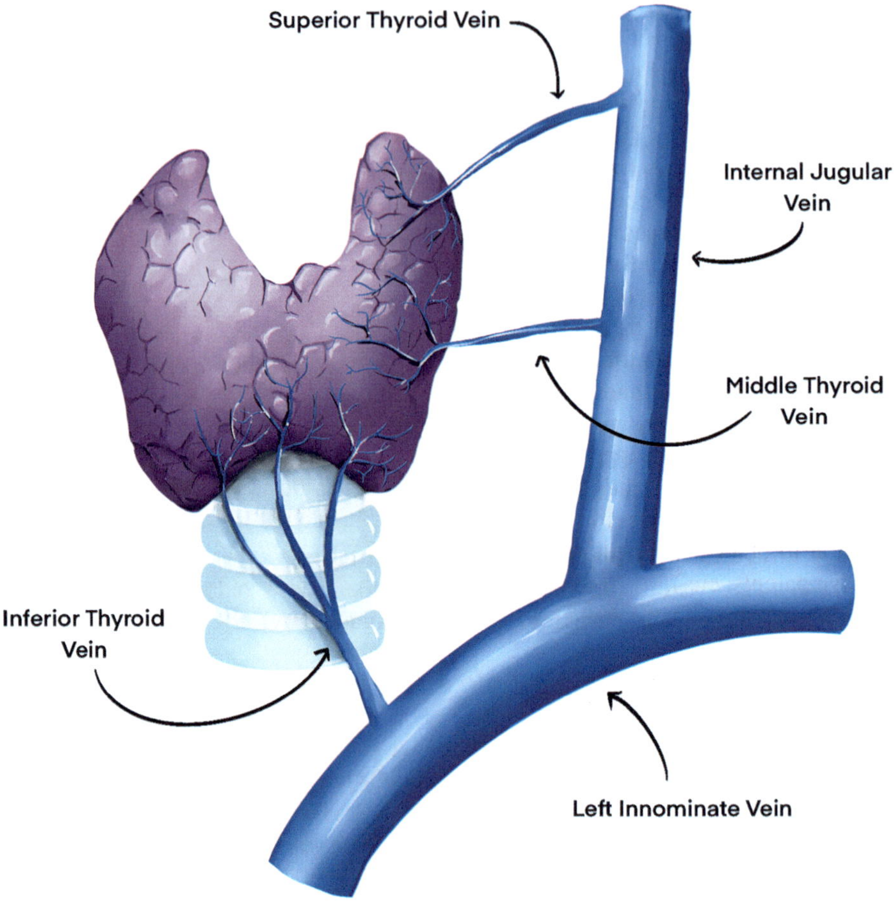

Fig. 1.2 Diagrammatic representation of the venous drainage of the thyroid gland (With prior permissions from the illustrator Dr. Fatima Soufan)

Regional metastases of thyroid carcinoma can also be found laterally, higher in the neck along the IJV. This can be explained by tumor invasion of the pre-tracheal and para-tracheal nodes causing an obstruction of normal lymph flow. Often the first LN involved in papillary thyroid carcinoma (PTC) is the Delphian LN, which is a pre-laryngeal node that lies just above the isthmus.

1.1.7 Innervation and Related Nerves

1.1.7.1 Innervation

Principal innervation of the thyroid gland derives from the autonomic nervous system. Parasympathetic fibers come from the vagus nerves, and sympathetic fibers are distributed from the superior, middle, and inferior ganglia of the sympathetic trunk

[6]. These small nerves enter the gland along with the blood vessels. Autonomic nervous regulation of the glandular secretion is not clearly understood. It does not play a role in the control of hormonal production or secretion, but mostly influences vasculature, and thus most of its effect is postulated to be on the perfusion rates of the glands [6].

The relationship of the thyroid gland to the RLN and to the external branch of the superior laryngeal nerve (EB-SLN) is of major surgical significance because damage to these nerves leads to disability in phonation or to difficulty in breathing. Both nerves are branches of the vagus nerve.

1.1.7.2 Recurrent Laryngeal Nerve (RLN)

The right RLN arises from the vagus nerve, loops posteriorly around the subclavian artery, and ascends behind the right lobe of the thyroid. It enters the larynx behind the cricothyroid muscle and the inferior cornu of the thyroid cartilage and innervates all the intrinsic laryngeal muscles except the cricothyroid. The left RLN comes from the left vagus, loops posteriorly around the arch of the aorta, and ascends in the trachea-esophageal groove (TEG) posterior to the left lobe of the thyroid, where it enters the larynx and innervates the musculature in a similar fashion as the right nerve.

Several factors make the RLN vulnerable to injury, especially in the hands of inexperienced surgeons. The nerve is *not* always in the TEG where it is expected to be. It can often be posterior or anterior to this position, or may even be surrounded by thyroid parenchyma. Thus, the nerve is vulnerable to injury during thyroidectomy if it is not visualized and traced up to the larynx. The variable relationship of the RLN to the ITA is another factor. The nerve often passes anterior, posterior, or through the branches of the ITA as reported by Sturinoli [7] in 1999. Medial traction of the lobe often lifts the nerve anteriorly, thereby making it more vulnerable. Likewise, ligation of this artery, practiced by many surgeons, may be dangerous if the nerve is not identified first. Moreover, in the presence of large nodules, the RLNs may not be in their "regular" anatomical location, but may be found even anterior to the thyroid gland. Finally, there may be a "non-recurrent laryngeal nerve," which occurs more on the right side (0.6%) than on the left side (0.04%) and is associated with vascular anomalies.

There is no substitute for identification of the nerve in a gentle and careful manner. Hints for Identification (landmarks) of the RLN include the following:

- The RLN can be found after it emerges from the superior thoracic outlet, in "Beahr's triangle" bounded laterally by the common carotid artery (CCA), medially by the trachea, and superiorly by the ITA [8].
- Another hint to the location of the RLN is the parathyroid gland location and Zuckerkandl tubercle, an extension of the thyroid, close to Berry's ligament.
- On rare occasions, the nerve may pass directly from the vagus to the larynx, close to the superior thyroid vessels [9].

1.1.7.3 External Branch of the Superior Laryngeal Nerve (EB-SLN)

The external branch of the superior laryngeal nerve (EB-SLN) (also known as the external laryngeal nerve—ELN) innervates the crico-thyroid muscle. It is important to the pitch of voice as the cricothyroid muscle is tensor of the vocal cords. In most cases, this nerve lies close to the vascular pedicle of the superior pole of the thyroid lobes descending on the fascia of the inferior pharyngeal constrictor. In some patients, it lies on the anterior surface of the thyroid lobe, making the possibility of damage during thyroidectomy even greater [10].

In about 50% of cases, there is enough length (> 2 cm) from the upper pole so that the STA can be ligated safely with sparing of the EB-SLN. However, in only 15% of patients is the SLN sufficiently distant from the superior pole vessels to be protected from manipulation by the surgeon. Unfortunately, many surgeons do not even attempt to identify this nerve before ligation of the upper pole vessels of the thyroid [10, 11].

"Joll's triangle" is used to identify the location of EB-SLN during thyroid surgery as it lies within this triangle. "Joll's triangle," also known as "sterno-thyro-laryngeal triangle," is bounded laterally by the upper pole of the thyroid gland and superior thyroid vessels, superiorly by the attachment of the strap muscles and deep investing layer of fascia to the hyoid bone, and medially by the midline. The floor of the triangle is formed by the crico-thyroid muscle.

1.1.8 Parathyroid Glands (PTGs)

The parathyroid glands (PTGs) are small glands that secrete parathormone (parathyroid hormone—PTH) that controls serum calcium (Ca) homeostasis. In about 80% of cases, four glands are present; two on each side, but three to six glands have been reported. Because of their small size, their delicate blood supply, and their usual anatomical position adjacent to the thyroid gland, these glands are at risk of being accidently removed, traumatized, or devascularized during thyroidectomy. Disruption of the PTGs may result in transient or permanent hypo-parathyroidism and consequential hypocalcemia. However, auto-transplantation to a "dry" pocket in the sterno-cleidomastoid (SCM) muscle, a subcutaneous (SC) area, or forearm (e.g. brachio-radialis muscle of the non-dominant arm) can be performed if end-artery damage does occur.

The "superior" PTGs arise embryologically from the fourth pharyngeal pouch. They descend only slightly during embryological development, and their position remains quite constant, being adjacent to the posterior surface of the middle part of the thyroid lobe, often just anterior to the RLN as it enters the larynx. On the other hand, the "inferior" PTGs arise from the third pharyngeal pouch, along with the thymus; hence, they often descend with the thymus, and have a wide range of distribution in adults, from just beneath the mandible to the anterior mediastinum [12]. With experience, one becomes much more capable of recognizing the PTGs by their tan appearance and small vascular pedicle, and of differentiating them from either lymph nodes (LNs) or adipose tissue [13].

1.1.9 Micro-anatomy (Histology)

The thyroid gland is formed of connective tissue stroma and parenchyma of endocrine cells. The connective tissue (true) capsule of the thyroid gives off multiple fibrous septa (trabeculae) passing into the gland, carrying blood vessels, nerves, and lymphatics, to form lobules. The gland is further divided into 20–40 much smaller functional subunits called follicles which store a colloid substance which functions as a hormone store. The colloid is maintained by a single layer of follicular epithelial cells sitting on a basal lamina. These follicles are surrounded by fenestrated capillaries, lymphatics, and so-called para-follicular or C-cells.

Microscopically, each lobe or lobule is made of two types of secretory cells: "follicular cells" that secrete thyroxin (T4) and tri-iodothyronine (T3), and in smaller numbers the "para-follicular" or "clear" cells (C-cells), which secrete "thyrocalcitonin" (also known as calcitonin). The follicles are separated from each other by a highly vascular connective tissue, and each follicle is lined with a single layer of flattened to low columnar epithelial cells depending on their degree of activity.

Oncocytes (Hürthle cells, oxyphilic cells, Ashkenazy cells) are large follicular cells with abundant deeply eosinophilic granular cytoplasm and numerous mitochondria. They are commonly seen in long-standing Graves' disease, chronic lymphatic thyroiditis (Hashimoto's thyroiditis), radiation-induced thyroiditis, follicular-derived neoplasms, and some adenomatoid goiters [14–16].

1.2 Physiology

1.2.1 Synthesis and Release of Thyroid Hormones

The function of the thyroid gland is to synthesize, store, and secrete thyroxin (T4) and tri-iodothyronine (T3). Mono-iodotyrosine (MIT) and di-iodotyrosine (DIT) are also found in thyroid venous blood.

Inorganic iodide (I^-) is *absorbed* from gastrointestinal tract and actively *trapped* by the acinar cells of the thyroid gland via a transport mechanism that is frequently called the "I^- trapping mechanism" or "I^- pump." A transporter named "pendrin" is located on the luminal surface of the follicular cell and is responsible for allowing passage of I^- into the follicle. In the acinar cells, I^- is *oxidized* to iodine (I_2), which passes through the follicle cell membrane into the colloid, where it is *bound* to the 3-position of tyrosine molecules with the aid of the enzyme thyroid peroxidase (TPO) to form MIT, and then to the 5-position to form DIT. Two DIT molecules then undergo an oxidative *condensation* with the release of an alanine residue and the formation of thyroxin (T4). Condensation of MIT with DIT results in tri-iodothyronine (T3) formation. These reactions occur while the tyrosine molecules are attached to thyroglobulin (Tg). The peptide bonds between the iodinated residues and Tg are broken by proteases in lysosomes, and so T4, T3, DIT, and MIT are *liberated* into the cytoplasm. The iodinated tyrosines are de-iodinated by a microsomal iodotyrosine dehalogenase. Then, T3 and T4 are *released* into the circulation by diffusion across the follicle cell membrane [17].

Most circulating T3 derives from peripheral conversion of T4, which is really a pro-hormone and is significantly less potent than the more metabolically active hormone T3. Many cells convert T4 to T3 through the removal of an iodine atom. In the bloodstream, <1% of the circulating T3 and T4 remains unbound. This free T3 and T4 can cross the lipid bilayer of cell membranes and be taken up by target cells. The remaining 99% of circulating T3 and T4 is bound to the plasma proteins, mainly thyroxin-binding globulin (TBG) and pre-albumin. This "packaging" prevents their free diffusion into body cells. It is only the "free" unbound forms of hormones that are metabolically active, and T3 is quick-acting within a few hours, while T4 acts more slowly from 4 to 14 days.

1.2.2 Regulation of Thyroid Hormone Synthesis

Production of T3 and T4 is regulated by the "hypothalamic-pituitary-thyroid axis," which is a multi-loop feedback circuit. The production of T3 and T4 from the thyroid is stimulated directly by the thyroid-stimulating hormone (TSH), produced by the anterior pituitary. Levels of T3 and T4 are also increased indirectly by thyrotropin-releasing hormone (TRH), which is produced by the hypothalamus in response to low levels of T3/T4 and acts on the pituitary to increase TSH production. Conversely, TRH and TSH production are suppressed by high levels of T3 and T4. Additionally, TRH production is also suppressed by high levels of TSH. Thus, the circulating levels of active thyroid hormones are normally self-regulating [18].

1.2.3 Functions of Thyroid Hormones

The thyroid hormones, T3 and T4, are often referred to as "metabolic" hormones because their levels influence the body's basal metabolic rate, the amount of energy used by the body at rest. When T3 and T4 bind to intra-cellular receptors located on the mitochondria, they cause an increase in nutrient breakdown and the use of oxygen to produce ATP. In addition, T3 and T4 initiate the transcription of genes involved in glucose oxidation. Although these mechanisms prompt cells to produce more ATP, the process is inefficient, and an abnormally increased level of heat is released as a byproduct of these reactions. This so-called calorigenic effect (calor- = "heat") raises body temperature.

Adequate levels of thyroid hormones are also required for protein synthesis and for fetal and childhood tissue development and growth. They are especially critical for normal development of the nervous system both in utero and in early childhood, and they continue to support neurological function in adults. These thyroid hormones have a complex inter-relationship with reproductive hormones, and deficiencies can influence libido, fertility, and other aspects of reproductive function. Finally, thyroid hormones increase the body's sensitivity to catecholamines from the adrenal medulla by up-regulation of receptors in the blood vessels. When levels of T3 and T4 hormones are excessive, this effect accelerates the heart rate, strengthens the heartbeat, and increases blood pressure. Because thyroid hormones regulate metabolism, heat production, protein synthesis, and many other body functions, thyroid disorders can have severe and widespread consequences.

1.2.4 Secretion of Calcitonin

The thyroid also contains "para-follicular or C-cells," which produce a hormone called "calcitonin," which is released in response to a rise in blood calcium levels (hypercalcemia). It appears to have a function in decreasing blood calcium (Ca) concentrations by:

- Inhibiting the activity of osteoclasts that release Ca into the circulation by degrading bone matrix
- Increasing osteoblastic activity
- Decreasing calcium absorption in the intestines
- Inhibiting renal resorption of Ca and hence increasing Ca loss in the urine

Blood levels of PTH are far more clinically relevant to Ca homeostasis than calcitonin, and no exogenous replacement for calcitonin is required following thyroidectomy. However, pharmaceutical preparations of calcitonin are sometimes prescribed to reduce osteoclast activity in people with "osteoporosis" and to reduce the degradation of cartilage in people with osteo-arthritis.

1.3 Investigations

1.3.1 Serological Studies/Thyroid Function Tests

The serum level of TSH should be routinely measured, while T3 and T4 levels are required if TSH level was abnormal (Table 1.1). When hypothyroidism is confirmed,

Table 1.1 Serological tests in thyroid disease

TSH	Additional testing	Diagnosis
Normal	Not needed	Euthyroid
Decreased	Free T4 ↑	Hyperthyroid
	Free T4 normal	T3 thyrotoxicosis
	Free T4 ↓	Non-thyroid disease or drugs
Increased	Free T4 ↑	Thyroid resistance or pituitary tumor
	Free T4 normal	Subclinical hypothyroid
	Free T4 ↓	Hypothyroid

T4 thyroxin, *T3* tri-iodothyronine

thyroid peroxidase (TPO) antibodies should be requested to check for autoimmune thyroid disease such as chronic lymphocytic thyroiditis (Hashimoto's thyroiditis).

Serum thyroglobulin (Tg) level does *not* help in the initial management of thyroid nodule and is *not* routinely recommended. Serum Tg levels may be elevated in patients with cancer, but are not diagnostic, since similar increases are seen in benign thyroid disorders. However, serum Tg is useful in the follow-up of patients after total thyroidectomy (TT) for well-differentiated thyroid cancer (WDTC). A level >10 ng/ml is a reliable indicator of locally recurrent or metastatic disease and predicts the need for an ablative dose of radioactive iodine (^{131}I) [19, 20].

Basal plasma calcitonin levels may be useful if medullary thyroid carcinoma (MTC) is suspected. In addition, pheochromocytoma is associated with MTC in multiple endocrine neoplasia (MEN) Type II, presenting with signs and symptoms of sympathetic nervous system hyper-activity [21].

1.3.2 Imaging Studies

1.3.3 Ultrasonography (US)

Ultrasonography (US) is the imaging study of choice for thyroid nodules. It can identify nodules too small to be palpated, the presence of multiple nodules, central or lateral neck lymphadenopathy, and provides accurate measurements of nodule diameter, allowing serial scans and better assessment of growth. Additionally, it allows characterization of nodules by sonographic features that suggest malignancy. *Comet-tail sign* and *coarse calcification* suggest very low risk of malignancy. Hypoechoicity and absent halo with indistinct margin are associated with moderate risk of malignancy. The presence of micro-calcification is highly suggestive of malignancy, especially papillary thyroid carcinoma (PTC) (Fig. 1.3) [22].

Color flow patterns are categorized as: (a) Type 1: no blood flow, (b) Type 2: peri-nodular flow, and (c) Type 3: intra-nodular blood flow (peri-nodular vessels may or may not be present). Although non-specific, thyroid cancers may have internal hyper-vascularity, whereas benign nodules may have peripheral vascularization. However, type 3 vascularization can be found in both benign and malignant nodules [23]. Completely avascular nodules are more likely to be benign.

There is certainly some subjectivity to sonographic features, which cannot, alone, reliably distinguish malignant from benign lesions, but are very useful in selecting the site within a nodule for fine-needle aspirate biopsy (FNAB) in order to improve diagnostic yield, or to select appropriate nodules to aspirate within a multinodular goiter (MNG) [24, 25].

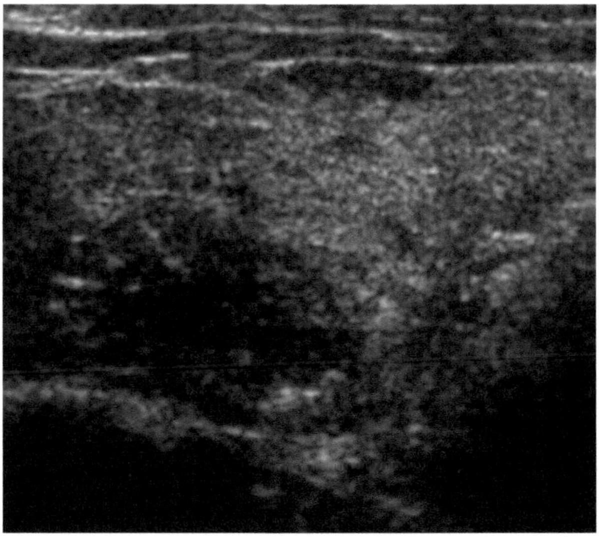

Fig. 1.3 Ultrasonography showing hypoechoic, ill-defined margin and micro-calcifications. Biopsy proved to be a papillary thyroid carcinoma (PTC)

1.3.3.1 Magnetic Resonance Imaging (MRI) and Computed Tomography (CT) Scan

Magnetic resonance imaging (MRI) is superior to scintigraphy in evaluating retrosternal goiters (RSGs). It is non-invasive, easily tolerated, and unlike contrast media used with computed tomography (CT) scan, contrast media used in MRI does *not* influence thyroid function. CT scan gives structural information about the gland and its relationship to adjacent structures. Both CT scan and MRI are relatively expensive and have a limited ability in distinguishing benign from malignant lesions. However, they are necessary in some cases for staging of the disease and for planning surgery.

Indications of CT scan and/or MRI include (1) the presence of a fixed thyroid mass, (2) hemoptysis indicating pulmonary metastasis, (3) cervical lymphadenopathy, and (4) RSGs (Fig. 1.4). They can also show involvement of the larynx, pharynx, trachea, esophagus, or major blood vessels [26].

1.3.3.2 Thyroid Scintigraphy

The use of radionuclide agents is helpful in delineating the presence, size, and function of thyroid nodules. Scanning with ^{123}I has the advantages of low-dose radiation (30 mrad) and a short half-life (12–14 h). This compares favorably with the use of ^{131}I with a higher dose (500 mrad) and a longer half-life (8–10 days). ^{123}I scanning is usually used for patients with a suspected lingual thyroid or RSG, whereas ^{131}I is used in patients with WDTC to screen for distant metastasis. Malignancy occurs in 15–20% of "cold" nodules and, additionally, in 5–9% of nodules with uptake that is "warm" or "hot," mandating a continued aggressive approach to clinically suspicious nodules even if they are *not* "cold" [27].

Technetium-pertechnetate-99 m (^{99m}Tc) is also used for the evaluation of thyroid nodules. It is trapped by the thyroid, but not organified, and has a short half-life and

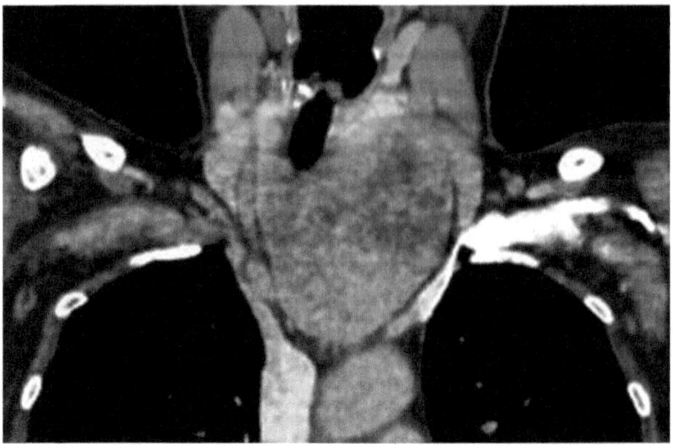

Fig. 1.4 Computed tomography (CT) scan showing retro-sternal goiter (arrow) in a 47-year-old gentleman

a low radiation dose. Screening with ^{99m}Tc also shows uptake in the salivary glands and major vascular structures, and therefore, requires a higher sophistication of interpretation [20].

1.3.4 Biopsy

1.3.4.1 Fine-Needle Aspiration Cytology (FNAC)—Free-Hand or US-Guided

The most important step (cornerstone) in the management of thyroid nodules is FNAC. Free-hand or palpation-guided FNAC has a sensitivity of 65–98% and a specificity of 72–100% [28]. The US-guided FNAC improves the accuracy of FNAC. The acellular or non-diagnostic (Thy 1) aspirate is reduced from 14% to 8% with US guidance [28], sensitivity increases from 92% to 98%, and specificity from 69% to 71% [29]. It can also be used to help localize impalpable nodules, lesions <1 cm, or when initial FNAC was non-diagnostic.

The indications of FNA are all thyroid nodules with a maximal diameter >1 cm and smaller nodules with suspicious features on US. A lower limit for the maximal diameter does *not* exist; however, there are technical difficulties in the sampling procedure in tiny lesions (<0.5 cm), even under US guidance [30]. The aims of the FNAB include the following [30]:

- To confirm the benign diagnosis of a nodule justifying the clinicians for a conservative approach avoiding an unnecessary surgery.
- To confirm the clinical diagnosis of a diffuse goiter like Hashimoto's thyroiditis or subacute de Quervain's thyroiditis.
- To recognize an aggressive thyroid tumor and to recognize or at least to suspect a clinically relevant low-grade tumor among all nodular enlargements of thyroid.
- To classify or to suspect some tumor types demanding a special therapeutic approach such as medullary thyroid carcinoma (MTC), lymphoma, anaplastic thyroid carcinoma (ATC), or metastatic carcinoma.

- To clarify eventual post-operative enlargements in the thyroid region, differentiating mainly between residual or recurrent disease versus granulomas or lymph node (LN) enlargements.
- To explore various neck enlargements outside the thyroid gland, mainly cystic lesions of the neck, and differentiating between ectopic thyroid cysts, thyroglossal cyst, branchial cyst, and cystic degenerated LN metastases of PTC.
- To confirm the presence of cervical LN enlargement suspicious of metastases.

Fine-needle aspiration cytology (FNAC) is *not* successful in the (1) detection of a microscopic focus of PTC, (2) differentiation of follicular adenoma from follicular carcinoma, (3) determination of the extent of a thyroid tumor, (4) exclusion of LN metastases, and (5) the safe recognition of a parathyroidal lesion [31].

Cytology results can be placed in five diagnostic categories (Thy 1-Thy 5) as indicated by the British Thyroid Association (BTA) Guidelines [32] (Table 1.2).

The probability of a benign thyroid nodule being accurately diagnosed as benign from a single FNAC is 90%. However, the accuracy of diagnosis increases significantly to 98% if two separate aspirates were performed on separate occasions [33].

The recently issued (2023) *Bethesda System for Reporting Thyroid Cytopathology* (BSRTC) [34] is currently considered to be the most suitable for communicating findings from thyroid smears (Table 1.3).

A positive finding of a metastasis is principally a safe diagnosis, whereas a negative smear does *not* exclude the presence of a metastasis since it might be missed by sampling. Cervical LN metastases frequently undergo extensive cystic degeneration, resulting in "acellular smears." Cystic foci in LNs remain highly suspicious, even with negative FNA results. The measurement of thyroglobulin (Tg) in the

Table 1.2 Diagnostic FNA categories and recommended actions

Category	Description	Recommended action
Thy 1	Non-diagnostic, insufficient sample. Cyst containing colloid or histiocytes only, in absence of epithelial cells	To repeat FNAC (US guidance may help). If the cyst is aspirated to dryness with no residual swelling, clinical/US follow-up alone may be sufficient
Thy 2	Benign, non-neoplastic Cyst containing benign epithelial cells	Repeat FNAC in 3–6 months. Two non-neoplastic results 3–6 months apart should exclude neoplasia
Thy 3	Follicular or Hürthle cell lesion/suspected follicular, or Hürthle cell tumor	MDT discussion—diagnostic lobectomy
Thy 4	Suspicious of malignancy	MDT discussion—total thyroidectomy
Thy 5	Diagnostic of malignancy	MDT discussion—total thyroidectomy

MDT Multidisciplinary team

Table 1.3 TBSRTC 2023: Categories, risk of malignancy, and recommended management

Diagnostic category	ROM mean % (range)	Recommended management
I—Non-diagnostic	13% (5–20)	Repeat FNA with US guidance
II—Benign	4% (2–7)	Clinical and US follow-up
III—Atypia of unknown significance (AUS)	22% (13–30)	Repeat FNA, molecular testing, diagnostic lobectomy, or surveillance
IV—Follicular neoplasm	30% (23–34)	Molecular testing, diagnostic lobectomy
V—Suspicious for malignancy	74% (67–83)	Molecular testing, lobectomy, or near-total/total thyroidectomy (TT)
VI—Malignant	97% (97–100)	Lobectomy or near-total/TT

AUS Atypia of unknown significance, *ROM* risk of malignancy, *FNA* fine-needle aspiration, *US* ultrasound, *TT* total thyroidectomy.

cystic fluid would be a helpful option to confirm a suspicion if the amount of cancer cells is not sufficient for the diagnosis [30].

1.3.4.2 Core-Biopsy (with or Without US Guidance)

A core-biopsy, preferably under US guidance, should be considered after two aspiration procedures showing non-diagnostic specimen (Thy 1) or when a thyroid lymphoma is suspected, typically in an elderly woman or on a background of autoimmune thyroiditis.

1.3.5 Flexible Laryngoscopy

Indirect laryngoscopy is important to assess vocal cord movements. Patients with difficult breathing (increased respiratory rate or diminished oxygen saturation) or stridor should be referred as an "emergency."

References

1. Policeni BA, Smoker WRK, Reede DL. Anatomy and embryology of the thyroid and parathyroid glands. Semin Ultrasound CT MRI. 2012;33:104–14.
2. Patel S, Bhatt AA. Thyroglossal duct pathology and mimics. Insights Imaging. 2019;10(1):12.
3. Naidoo D, Boon JM, Mieny CJ, Becker PJ, van Schoor AN. Relation of the external branch of the superior laryngeal nerve to the superior pole of the thyroid gland: an anatomical study. Clin Anat. 2007;20(5):516–20.
4. Gupta P, Bhalla AS, Thulkar S, Kumar A, Mohanti BK, Thakar A, et al. Variations in superior thyroid artery: a selective angiographic study. Indian J Radiol Imaging. 2014;24(1):66–71.
5. Roman BR, Randolph GW, Kamani D. Conventional thyroidectomy in the treatment of primary thyroid cancer. Endocrinol Metab Clin N Am. 2019;48(1):125–41.
6. Shindo ML. Considerations in surgery of the thyroid gland. Otolaryngol Clin N Am. 1996;29(4):629–35.
7. Sturinoli G. The recurrent laryngeal nerve related to thyroid surgery. AJS. 1999;177:485–8.

8. Zada B, Anwar K, Malik SA, Niamatullah KN, Salam F. Anatomical relationship between recurrent laryngeal nerve and inferior thyroid artery in thyroidectomy patients. J Ayub Med Coll Abbottabad. 2014;26(3):380–3.
9. Gravante G, Delogu D, Rizzello A, Filingeri V. The Zuckerkandl tubercle. Am J Surg. 2007;193(4):484–5.
10. Droulias C, Tzinas S, Harlaftis N, Akin JT Jr, Gray SW, Skandalakis JE. The superior laryngeal nerve. Am Surg. 1976;42(9):635–8.
11. Jonas J, Bahr R. Neuromonitoring of EBSLN during thyroid surgery. Am J Surg. 2000;179:234–6.
12. Gray SW, Skandalakis JE, Akin JT Jr, Droulias C, Vohman MD. Parathyroid glands. Am Surg. 1976;42(9):653–6.
13. Dozois RR, Beahrs OH. Surgical anatomy and technique of thyroid and parathyroid surgery. Surg Clin North Am. 1977;57(4):647–61.
14. Baloch ZW, LiVolsi VA. Oncocytic lesions of the neuroendocrine system. Semin Diagn Pathol. 1999;16(2):190–9.
15. Weiss ML, Deckart H, Pilz R, Deckart E, Kleinau E. Oncocytes in thyroid gland aspirates–differential diagnostic problem: tumor/thyroiditis. Radiobiol Radiother (Berl). 1984;25(5):765–8.
16. Mikhailov IG, Vasil'ev NB, Smirnova EA. Comparative quantitative electron-microscopic study of the nucleoli of human thyroid oncocytes and follicular cells. Arkh Patol. 1980;42(4):32–6.
17. Portulano C, Paroder-Belenitsky M, Carrasco N. The Na+/I- symporter (NIS): mechanism and medical impact. Endocr Rev. 2014;35(1):106–49.
18. Mullur R, Liu Y-Y, Brent GA. Thyroid hormone regulation of metabolism. Physiol Rev. 2014;94:355–82.
19. Cooper DS, Doherty GM, Haugen BR, Kloos RT, Lee SL, Mandel SJ, et al. Revised American Thyroid Association management guidelines for patients with thyroid nodules and differentiated thyroid cancer. Thyroid. 2009;19(11):1167–214.
20. Gharib H, Papini E, Paschke R, Duick DS, Valcavi R, Hegedus L, et al. American Association of Clinical Endocrinologists, Associazione Medici Endocrinologi, and European Thyroid Association medical guidelines for clinical practice for the diagnosis and management of thyroid nodules: executive summary of recommendations. J Endocrinol Invest. 2010;3(5 Suppl):1–6.
21. Elisei R, Bottici V, Luchetti F, Di Coscio G, Romei C, Grasso L, et al. Impact of routine measurement of serum calcitonin on the diagnosis and outcome of medullary thyroid cancer: experience in 10,864 patients with nodular thyroid disorders. J Clin Endocrinol Metab. 2004;89(1):163–8.
22. Mehanna HM, Jain A, Morton RP, Watkinson J, Shaha A. Investigating the thyroid nodule. BMJ. 2009;338:705–9.
23. Cantisani V, Catania A, De Antoni E, Greco R, Caruso R, Di Segni M, et al. Is pattern III as evidenced by US color-Doppler useful in predicting thyroid nodule malignancy? Large-scale retrospective analysis. Clin Ter. 2010;161(2):e49–52.
24. Papini E, Guglielmi R, Bianchini A, Crescenzi A, Taccogna S, Nardi F, et al. Risk of malignancy in non-palpable thyroid nodules: predictive value of ultrasound and color-Doppler features. J Clin Endocrinol Metab. 2002;87(5):1941–6.
25. Fish SA, Langer JE, Mandel SJ. Sonographic imaging of thyroid nodules and cervical lymph nodes. Endocrinol Metab Clin N Am. 2008;37(2):401–17.
26. Tan GH, Gharib H. Thyroid incidentalomas: management approaches to nonpalpable nodules discovered incidentally on thyroid imaging. Ann Intern Med. 1997;126(3):226–31.
27. Price DC. Radioisotopic evaluation of the thyroid and the parathyroids. Radiol Clin North Am. 1993;31(5):991–1015.
28. Gharib H, Goellner JR. Fine needle aspiration biopsy of the thyroid gland. In: Randolph surgery of the thyroid and parathyroid glands. Philadelphia: Saunders WB; 2003.
29. Regina Castro M, Gharib H. Continuing controversies in the management of thyroid nodules. Ann Intern Med. 2005;142:926–31.

30. Linos D, Chung WY. SpringerLink (Online service). Minimally invasive thyroidectomy. Berlin/Heidelberg: Springer Berlin Heidelberg; 2012. p. 37–58.
31. Gharib H. Fine-needle aspiration biopsy of thyroid nodules: advantages, limitations, and effect. Mayo Clin Proc. 1994;69(1):44–9.
32. British Thyroid Association, Royal College of Physicians. British Thyroid Association Guidelines for the management of thyroid cancer. 2nd ed. British Thyroid Association, Royal College of Physicians; 2007.
33. Baloch ZW, LiVolsi VA, Asa SL, Rosai J, Merino MJ, Randolph G, et al. Diagnostic terminology and morphologic criteria for cytologic diagnosis of thyroid lesions: a synopsis of the National Cancer Institute Thyroid Fine-Needle Aspiration State of the Science Conference. Diagn Cytopathol. 2008;36(6):425–37.
34. Ali SZ, Baloch ZW, Cochand-Priollet B, Schmitt FC, Vielh P, VanderLann PA. The 2023 Bethesda system for reporting thyroid cytopathology. Thyroid. 2023;23(9):1039–44.

2 Thyroiditis: Overview and Classification

2.1 Introduction

The term “thyroiditis” reflects inflammation of the thyroid gland. It represents about 20% of all thyroid diseases [1] and is caused by several factors, most commonly autoimmune diseases. Thyroid autoantibodies are mainly directed against thyroid peroxidase (TPO) or thyroglobulin (Tg) and have an association with defined HLA haplotypes implying a genetic predisposition [2]. Iodine therapy, viral infections, pregnancy, menopause, stress [3], and immune-modulating drugs such as interferon-alpha (IFN-α) have also been linked to autoimmune thyroiditis. Except for Graves’ disease, most cases of autoimmune thyroiditis present initially with hyperthyroidism that returns to euthyroidism or falls to permanent hypothyroidism (subclinical or overt).

Patients with thyroiditis may present with pain (painful thyroiditis) or without pain (painless thyroiditis), but with enlarged thyroid gland (goiter) and/or thyroid dysfunction in the form of transient or permanent hypo- or hyperthyroidism. Symptomatic thyroiditis should be differentiated from acute hemorrhage into thyroid cyst, thyroid nodule, thyroid cancer, tonsillitis, and acute pharyngitis.

2.2 Epidemiology

In the United States of America (USA), Hashimoto’s thyroiditis (chronic lymphocytic thyroiditis) is the most common cause of hypothyroidism, while Graves’ disease is the most common cause of autoimmune hyperthyroidism [4]. High intake of iodine can increase the incidence of Graves’ disease, whereas iodine insufficiency can be protective against autoimmune thyroiditis [5].

M. Sakr, *Thyroiditis*, https://doi.org/10.1007/978-3-032-19513-5_2

2.3 Classification/Etiology

Thyroiditis can be classified based on the onset of symptoms, underlying etiology, and clinical symptoms as follows.

2.3.1 According to the Onset of Symptoms

According to the onset of symptoms, thyroiditis is classified into acute, subacute, and chronic forms [6]. Acute thyroiditis is caused by bacterial infection of the gland, subacute thyroiditis (also known as granulomatous thyroiditis) is caused by viruses, while chronic thyroiditis includes autoimmune thyroiditis (e.g., Hashimoto's thyroiditis and post-partum thyroiditis), and other painless thyroiditis, including iatrogenic and drug-induced thyroiditis.

2.3.2 According to Clinical Presentation

According to clinical symptoms, patients may present either with severe thyroid pain (e.g., infectious or acute suppurative thyroiditis, subacute de Quervain's thyroiditis, radiation-induced thyroiditis, trauma-induced thyroiditis) or without evident inflammation or pain, but with goiter or thyroid dysfunction (e.g., Hashimoto's thyroiditis, Riedel's thyroiditis, silent thyroiditis, post-partum, and drug-induced thyroiditis).

2.3.3 According to the Underlying Etiology

According to the underlying etiology, thyroiditis can occur due to (1) autoimmune disease (e.g., Hashimoto's thyroiditis, Graves' disease, post-partum thyroiditis or painless sporadic thyroiditis), (2) infection (e.g., viral infection as in painful subacute thyroiditis or bacterial infection as in suppurative thyroiditis), (3) drugs (e.g., amiodarone, lithium, interferons and interleukin-2; and checkpoint inhibitors) or (4) fibrosis (Riedel's thyroiditis).

For the sake of simplification, thyroiditis can be classified by the underlying etiology into two main groups: auto-immune thyroiditis and non-immune thyroiditis as summarized in Table 2.1.

2.4 Pathophysiology

2.4.1 Acute Thyroiditis

Infectious thyroiditis is caused by gram-positive bacteria such as *Streptococcus*, *Staphylococcus*, fungi, or mycoparasitic infection [7]. Destruction of the thyroid

Table 2.1 Classification of thyroiditis by the underlying etiology

Autoimmune thyroiditis	Non-immune thyroiditis
Hashimoto's thyroiditis	Acute infectious thyroiditis
Fibrotic variant of Hashimoto's thyroiditis	Radiation-induced thyroiditis
Atrophic thyroiditis (primary myxedema)	Palpation/trauma-induced thyroiditis
Variants of autoimmune thyroiditis	Sarcoidosis
Post-partum thyroiditis	Amyloidosis
Silent or painless thyroiditis	Vasculitis-associated thyroiditis
Subacute de Quervain's thyroiditis	Post-operative necrotizing thyroiditis
Fibrotic Riedel's thyroiditis	Drug-induced thyroiditis
	Carcinoma-associated thyroiditis

parenchyma results from radiation-induced thyroiditis after exposure to radioactive iodine (RAI) for treatment of Graves' disease or thyroid cancer, and high-dose radiation to the neck for the treatment of lymphoma or other head and neck cancers.

2.4.2 Subacute Thyroiditis

Subacute thyroiditis (de Quervain's thyroiditis) is caused by viruses such as coxsackie A, B, echovirus. Granulomas are formed in the thyroid gland (hence named "granulomatous"), which becomes fibrotic, but can return to normal after treatment. Other causes of subacute thyroiditis include subacute lymphocytic thyroiditis (also known as painless or silent thyroiditis).

2.4.3 Chronic Thyroiditis

Hashimoto's thyroiditis (chronic lymphocytic thyroiditis) is an autoimmune phenomenon characterized by lymphocytic infiltration of the gland presumed to be due to similarities between thyroid protein and the viral structure resulting in cross-reacting antibodies. Anti-TPO antibodies that are present in approximately 90% of patients with Hashimoto's thyroiditis fix complement and are hence capable of inducing antibody-dependent cell-mediated cytotoxicity, causing the death of thyrocytes and eventually hypothyroidism [8].

Post-partum thyroiditis is a destructive thyroiditis characterized by lymphocytic infiltration of the thyroid gland. Fetal cells that migrate to the maternal thyroid gland tend to survive the immuno-compromised pregnancy state, and when the maternal immune system rebounds post-partum, it activates the autoimmune phenomenon and causes post-partum thyroiditis [8, 9].

Drug-induced thyroiditis causing hyperthyroidism is usually caused by either an increase in the release and synthesis of thyroid hormone or by destructive thyroiditis caused by the release of preformed hormones. On the other hand, hypothyroidism is caused by a decrease in the synthesis and release of thyroid hormone or from hypophysitis causing secondary hypothyroidism. The iodine content of the drugs also causes thyroid dysfunction.

The pathophysiology of Riedel's thyroiditis is not completely understood, but chronic inflammation by the mononuclear cells seems to play a role. It has also been claimed to belong to IgG4 thyroid diseases, which include Riedel's thyroiditis, autoimmune pancreatitis, interstitial pneumonia, and orbital pseudo-tumors [10].

2.5 Evaluation/Work-Up

2.5.1 Serological Tests

Thyroid-stimulating hormone (TSH) should be checked to see if the patient has hyperthyroidism or hypothyroidism. If TSH level is abnormal, serum levels of thyroxin (T4) and tri-iodothyronine (T3) should be checked. Thyroid microsomal antibodies and thyroid receptor antibodies can be checked for confirmation of autoimmune thyroid disease. Erythrocyte sedimentation rate (ESR) and C-reactive protein (CRP) are significantly elevated in infectious bacterial thyroiditis [7].

2.5.2 Imaging Studies

2.5.2.1 Ultrasonography

Thyroid ultrasound is the most important and most commonly used imaging modality for evaluation of the thyroid gland. Heterogenous thyroid parenchyma indicates inflammation of the thyroid gland, but it does not differentiate between production versus destruction thyroiditis. Thyroid ultrasound can also detect nodules in the thyroid gland. Characteristics of the nodules can help to differentiate between benign and suspiciously malignant nodules and guide fine-needle aspiration (FNA).

2.5.2.2 Scintigraphy

A thyroid uptake and scan can be done to differentiate production thyroiditis or destruction thyroiditis in patients who present with thyrotoxicosis characterized by low TSH with or without elevated T4 and T3. Low uptake on thyroid scan would indicate destruction thyroiditis (e.g., Hashimoto's thyroiditis, infectious thyroiditis), while increased or normal uptake indicates production thyroiditis (Graves' disease) [8]. A thyroid scan can help to further differentiate between Graves' disease, which will show increased uptake throughout the thyroid gland and toxic adenoma, which will show increased uptake in the nodule (hot nodule) with suppression of the rest of the thyroid gland.

2.5.3 Biopsy

Fine-needle aspiration (FNA) is done to evaluate suspicious thyroid nodules to rule out malignancy. In general, any thyroid nodule, which is less than 10 mm, can be monitored without fine-needle aspiration.

2.6 Prognosis

2.6.1 Outcome

Thyroiditis, with or without thyroid dysfunction, has a good prognosis, but long-standing hypothyroidism can predispose to myxedema coma, which occurs more commonly in the elderly population and has a high mortality rate. Many patients with hypothyroidism may suffer from ongoing symptoms even with appropriate treatment, which may have a negative impact on the quality of life.

2.6.2 Complications

2.6.2.1 Myxedema Coma

Myxedema coma is considered a medical emergency and is characterized by severe hypothyroidism with clinical features of hypothermia, hyponatremia, and bradycardia. It is mostly seen in older patients. Treatment should be initiated on clinical suspicion without awaiting lab results. Steroids are given first, followed by thyroxin replacement to prevent an adrenal crisis in the scenario of underlying adrenal insufficiency [11, 12].

2.6.2.2 Thyroid Storm

Thyroid storm is a life-threatening endocrine emergency often triggered by a metabolically stressful event in a patient with long-standing hyperthyroidism like Graves' disease. It can present with hyperpyrexia, tachycardia, agitation, and psychosis with laboratory evidence of low TSH, high free T4, and T3. Prompt recognition and treatment of the condition are necessary as this condition is associated with high mortality. The Burch-Wartofsky diagnostic criteria can help with the timely detection of thyroid storm [13]. The standard of care is immediate initiation of beta-blockers, thionamides, and glucocorticoids. Additionally, iodine and cholestyramine can also be used [14].

2.6.2.3 Abscess Formation/Septicemia

Infectious bacterial thyroiditis can lead to acute abscess formation and septicemia if not promptly and adequately treated [7].

2.6.2.4 Thyroid Cancer (Lymphoma—Carcinoma)

Patients with Hashimoto's thyroiditis are at risk of developing thyroid lymphoma and carcinoma; thus, a rapidly progressing thyroid nodule enlargement or development of new nodules should raise suspicion and provoke further evaluation.

2.6.2.5 Other Complications of Hypothyroidism

Several complications can occur in case of untreated hypothyroidism caused by thyroiditis, including cardiac problems, goiter with its pressure effects, and pregnancy problems (e.g., pre-eclampsia, anemia, congenital hypothyroidism, birth defects, bleeding after birth, retarded baby's physical and mental development, premature birth or a low- birth weight, and stillbirth or miscarriage).

References

1. Vanderpump MPJ. The epidemiology of thyroid disease. Br Med Bull. 2011;99(1):39–51.
2. Weetman AP. Chronic autoimmune thyroiditis. In: Braverman LE, Utiger RD, editors. The thyroid. Philadelphia: Williams & Wilkins, Lippincott; 2000. p. 721–32.
3. Mizokami T, Wu Li A, El-Kaissi S, Wall JR. Stress and thyroid autoimmunity. Thyroid. 2004;14:1047–55.
4. Hollowell JG, Staehling NW, Flanders WD, Hannon WH, Gunter EW, Spencer CA, et al. Serum TSH, T(4), and thyroid antibodies in the United States population (1988 to 1994): National Health and Nutrition Examination Survey (NHANES III). J Clin Endocrinol Metab. 2002;87(2):489–99.
5. Burikhanov RB, Matsuzaki S. Excess iodine induces apoptosis in the thyroid of goitrogen-pretreated rats in vivo. Thyroid. 2000;10(2):123–9.
6. Khan A, Nosé V. Pathology of the thyroid gland. In: Lloyd RV, editor. Endocrine pathology. Totowa: Humana; 2004. p. 153–89.
7. Paes JE, Burman KD, Cohen J, Franklyn J, McHenry CR, Shoham S, et al. Acute bacterial suppurative thyroiditis: a clinical review and expert opinion. Thyroid. 2010;20(3):247–55.
8. Peng CC, Huai-En Chang R, Pennant M, Huang HK, Munir KM. A literature review of painful Hashimoto thyroiditis: 70 published cases in the past 70 years. J Endocr Soc. 2020;4(2):bvz008.
9. Keely EJ. Postpartum thyroiditis: an autoimmune thyroid disorder which predicts future thyroid health. Obstet Med. 2011;4(1):7–11.
10. Umehara H, Okazaki K, Masaki Y, Kawano M, Yamamoto M, Saeki T, et al. Comprehensive diagnostic criteria for IgG4-related disease (IgG4-RD), 2011. Mod Rheumatol. 2012;22(1):21–30.
11. Ono Y, Ono S, Yasunaga H, Matsui H, Fushimi K, Tanaka Y. Clinical characteristics and outcomes of myxedema coma: analysis of a national inpatient database in Japan. J Epidemiol. 2017;27(3):117–22.
12. Popoveniuc G, Chandra T, Sud A, Sharma M, Blackman MR, Burman KD, et al. A diagnostic scoring system for myxedema coma. Endocr Pract. 2014;20(8):808–17.
13. Idrose AM. Acute and emergency care for thyrotoxicosis and thyroid storm. Acute Med Surg. 2015;2(3):147–57.
14. Akamizu T, Satoh T, Isozaki O, Suzuki A, Wakino S, Iburi T, et al. Diagnostic criteria, clinical features, and incidence of thyroid storm based on nationwide surveys. Thyroid. 2012;22(7):661–79.

Acute Suppurative (Infectious) Thyroiditis

3

3.1 Overview

Infectious thyroiditis may be non-suppurative, suppurative, or septic thyroiditis. Infection of the thyroid gland is rare as the gland is remarkably resistant to infection. This has been attributed to (1) its rich blood supply, (2) its extensive lymphatic drainage, (3) the high iodine content of the gland, which may have bactericidal effect, (4) the fact that hydrogen peroxide (H_2O_2) is generated within the gland as a requirement for the synthesis of thyroid hormone, and (5) its normal encapsulated position and fascial planes that anatomically separate the thyroid from other cervical structures.

Acute suppurative thyroiditis (AST) is a rare condition, reported to account for less than 1% of thyroid disease [1, 2], which may result in up to 12% or higher mortality if left untreated [1, 3, 4]. In the pre-antimicrobial era, the case fatality rate of AST was as high as 22% [5], which makes early recognition of AST crucial in order to prevent life-threatening complications.

Infectious thyroiditis is usually seen in the elderly, chronically ill, and immuno-compromised patients [6]. It may follow upper respiratory tract infection (e.g., tonsillitis), or thyroidectomy (in the remnant), and includes all forms of infection; other than viral, it is caused by invasion of the thyroid by bacteria, mycobacteria, fungi, protozoa, or flatworms. Most commonly, infectious thyroiditis is caused by gram-positive bacteria such as *Staphylococcus* or *Streptococcus*. Mycobacteria and fungi, including pneumocystis, can be the culprit in immuno-compromised patients.

3.2 Demographics

It is widely reported in the literature that the incidence of AST lies between 0.1% and 0.7% of all thyroid disease [1, 2]; however, this is largely derived from retrospective studies of surgical specimens [3, 7]; its true incidence is thus likely to be

M. Sakr, *Thyroiditis*, https://doi.org/10.1007/978-3-032-19513-5_3

much lower. It can occur at any age with a median age of 40 years for bacterial AST [4, 6, 8, 9].

Tuberculous AST should be considered in countries with high incidence of tuberculosis (TB). Two previous reviews found that AST occurs equally in both sexes [4, 6]; however, Lafontaine et al. [9] reported a slight female predominance, which has also been described by several authors [8, 10].

3.3 Source of Infection

The source of infection is usually hematogenous from a primary focus, congenital abnormalities like pyriform sinus, which is usually seen in children, or by direct extension from adjacent neck structures, especially in children. Other less common sources of infection include neck trauma or lymphatic spread, or rarely, surgical site infections [6].

3.4 Predisposing Factors

Acute thyroiditis may involve a normal gland and arise in a multinodular goiter (MNG) [11] or even Hashimoto's thyroiditis (chronic lymphocytic thyroiditis). As shown in Table 3.1, the presence of certain predisposing factors such as pyriform sinus fistula, third and fourth arch anomalies, tooth abscess, and endocarditis makes the gland susceptible to infections, particularly in immuno-compromised patients.

3.4.1 Pyriform Sinus Fistula

A persistent fistula from the pyriform sinus may make the left lobe of the thyroid particularly susceptible to abscess formation, particularly in children [12–22]. In a study by Sheng et al. [23], 7 out of 48 (15%) children undergoing piriform sinus fistula surgery presented with a thyroid abscess [23]. The possibility of a persistent thyro-glossal duct should be considered for patients with midline infections [24]. Infection of the thyroid gland is a result of direct extension from an internal fistula from the pyriform sinus [15, 17, 18, 25–28]. This tract is thought to represent the

Table 3.1 Predisposing factors of acute thyroiditis

Common predisposing factors	Rare predisposing factors
Pyriform sinus fistula Third and fourth arch abnormalities Immuno-compromised states	Tooth abscess Fine-needle aspiration Endocarditis Pre-existing thyroid diseases, such as multi-nodular goiter, autoimmune thyroiditis, and cancer (e.g., thyroid metastases) Juvenile systemic lupus erythematosus

course of migration of the ultimo-branchial body from the site of its embryonic origin in the fifth pharyngeal pouch [19]. Occasional cells positive for calcitonin have been found in the fistulae, and increased numbers of C-cells were noted in the thyroid lobe at the point of termination of the tract.

The predominance of acute thyroiditis in the left lobe of the thyroid gland, particularly in infants and children, is explained by the fact that the right ultimo-branchial body is often atrophic and does *not* develop in humans. Approximately, 92% of cases involve the left thyroid lobe, 6% the right lobe, and 2% are bilateral [29]. The left-sided predominance may be due to embryological asymmetry of the transformation of the fourth branchial arch to form the aortic and innominate arteries [30] or to poor development of the ultimo-brachial body on the right side of the embryo [31].

3.4.2 Third and Fourth Arch Abnormalities

Recurrent left-sided thyroid abscess has also been reported due to a fourth branchial arch sinus fistula [32]. A review of 526 cases of congenital fourth branchial arch anomalies by Nicoucar et al. [33] noted that they presented with acute suppurative thyroiditis in 45% of cases.

3.4.3 Immuno-compromised States

The most common predisposing factor for suppurative thyroiditis is immuno-suppression associated with human immuno-deficiency virus (HIV), tuberculosis (TB), old age, or debilitating diseases. The immuno-compromised state predisposes patients to unusual bacteria such as *Nocardia* [34, 35] and *Salmonella* [36] and fungi like *Candida* [37–39], *Coccidioides immitis* [40], and *Aspergillus* [41]. Among patients >20 years old in the study by Yu et al. [4], 32/66 (49%) were immuno-compromised [4]. Occasionally, acute bacterial suppurative thyroiditis occurs in immuno-compromised children receiving cancer chemotherapy [42].

3.4.4 Other Rare Predisposing Factors

Acute thyroiditis from a “peri-apical abscess” of an inferior molar has been reported by Acocelia et al. [43]. Acute suppurative thyroiditis associated with “thyroid metastasis” from esophageal cancer has also been recently reported by Dai et al. [44].

Rarely, infection may occur in a cystic or degenerated “thyroid nodule” [45, 46] and presumed hematogenous spread in the setting of “endocarditis” [47] or due to septic emboli derived from infective endocarditis [47–49]. Acute thyroiditis has also been reported to arise as the initial presentation of “juvenile systemic lupus erythematosus” (SLE) [50].

3.5 Etiology

Virtually any bacterium can infect the thyroid, but at times no causative organism can be demonstrated. *Streptococcus, Staphylococcus, Pneumococcus, Salmonella* [51–54], *Klebsiella* [55], *Bacteroides, Treponema pallidum, Pasteurella* spp. [56, 57], *Porphyromonas* [58], *Eikenella* [54, 59–61], and *Mycobacterium tuberculosis* [62–66] have all been described. Rare cases of disseminated *Nocardia* infections with thyroiditis along with subcutaneous nodules have been reported [67–70] (Table 3.2).

In addition, certain fungi, including *Coccidioides immitis* [40], *Aspergillus* [41, 71], *Actinomyces* [72–74], *Blastomyces* [75, 76], *Candida albicans* [37–39], *Acinetobacter baumannii* [4], *Cryptococcus* [77], and *Pneumocystis* [78], have also been associated with acute thyroiditis. In a recent meta-analysis by Lafontaine et al. [9], 94% of the patients with fungal AST were immuno-compromised [9], mostly due to malignancy or acquired immuno-deficiency syndrome (AIDS) [35, 36, 79, 80]. *Coccidioides immitis* from infected donor tissue in an immuno-compromised host has also been reported [40]. Rarely acute suppurative thyroiditis is due to thyroid abscess with deep neck infection [81] and fistulous connection [82].

Thyroid abscess due to *Clostridium perfringens* has been reported [83], and *Clostridium septicum* is almost always associated with carcinoma of the colon [84]. Metastatic breast cancer has been described as presenting clinically with acute thyroiditis [85]. Hashimoto's thyroiditis [86, 87], large goiters [88], or thyroid cancer could predispose individuals to acute thyroiditis [89]. It has also been reported by several investigators that AST could arise by hematogenous or lymphatic spread or by iatrogenic infections after fine-needle aspiration biopsy (FNAB). Recently, the role of diagnostic thyroid FNA has been emphasized as a factor in the cause of acute suppurative thyroiditis [83, 90–94]. Thus, care should be taken when performing FNA in patients who may be susceptible to tracking of infection into the thyroid gland.

Table 3.2 Microbiology of acute suppurative thyroiditis (AST)

Common organisms	Rare organisms
Aerobic: *Staphylococcus aureus,* Streptococcus *pyogenes,* *Streptococcus epidermidis,* *Streptococcus pneumoniae,* *Escherichia coli* [95]	*Bacterial*: Atypical mycobacteria, *Clostridium perfringens* [83], *Eikenella corrodens*, Enterobacteriaceae, *Haemophilus influenzae, Klebsiella* spp., *Mycobacterium tuberculosis, Porphyromonas* [58], *Salmonella* spp., *Streptococcus viridans, Treponema pallidum, Brucella* [96], *Lactococcus* [97], *Citrobacter freundii* [98], *Nocardia* [67–70]
Anaerobic: *Clostridium* Septicum [84], gram-negative bacilli, Peptostreptococcus spp.	*Fungal*: *Aspergillus* spp. [41, 71], *Blastomyces, Candida* spp. [37–39], *Coccidioides immitis* [40], *Actinomyces* [72–74], Pneumocystis *jirovecii* [78].
	Parasitic: *Trypanosoma* [25], *Echinococcus* spp.

3.6 Pathology

Pathological examination of acute thyroiditis reveals the characteristic changes of acute inflammation in general. With bacterial infections, heavy polymorphonuclear and lymphocytic cellular infiltrate is found in the initial phase, often with necrosis and abscess formation. As healing occurs, fibrosis becomes prominent. In samples obtained by FNA, the infectious agent may be seen on a gram, acid-fast, or appropriate fungal stain [17], and grown out in culture for antibiotic sensitivity assessment.

3.7 Clinical Picture

3.7.1 History-Taking/Symptoms

Although acute thyroiditis is quite rare, cases of suppurative thyroiditis are increasing due to the higher incidence of immuno-compromised patients. A recent (2021) meta-analysis of about 200 patients with acute suppurative thyroiditis (AST) published in 148 articles between 2000 and 2020 noted that the median duration of symptoms prior to presentation was 6 days (range 3–12 days) in bacterial AST and 21 days in fungal AST (range 12–26 days) [9]. The most common symptoms in bacterial AST were neck pain (89%) and fever (82%), followed by dysphagia (46%). Neck pain and fever were the most common symptoms in all cases, occurring in 78% and 63% of fungal AST [9].

In 2019, another case series of six otherwise healthy adult patients without anatomical anomalies with AST was published by Falhammar et al. [99]. Of the 6 patients, 5 were female, and the median age at presentation was 51 years (28–73 years). None had third or fourth left branchial cleft anomalies or an immunocompromised state. All patients were successfully treated with antibiotics for an average of 13.5 days (10–41 days), drainage was necessary in three patients, and surgery was performed twice in the acute phase in one and at a later state in another. The length of hospital stay was 7.5 days (4–79 days).

Acute suppurative thyroiditis (AST) has been estimated to be much more common in the pediatric age group because of its relationship with pyriform sinus fistulae, where 90% of lesions develop in the left lobe of the thyroid [47] although it is still quite unusual. It has been estimated that about 8% of cases occur in adulthood [29, 47, 100–105].

The dominant clinical symptom is neck pain in the region of the thyroid gland that may subsequently enlarge and become palpably hot and tender [106]. The patient is unable to extend the neck and often sits with the neck flexed in order to avoid pressure on the thyroid gland. Swallowing is painful. There are usually signs of infection in structures adjacent to the thyroid, cervical lymphadenopathy, as well as fever and chills along with leukocytosis in about 80% of bacterial AST and 40% in fungal AST. Gas formation with AST has also been reported [107–110]. Symptoms are generally more obvious in children than in adults. Adults may present with a vague, slightly painful mass in the thyroid region without fever, which may raise the possibility of a malignancy. Immuno-suppressed patients tend to present with more chronic thyroid infections, bilateral disease, and less prominent signs and symptoms. Suppurative thyroiditis may even spread to the chest, producing necrotizing mediastinitis and pericarditis in the absence of a pyriform sinus fistula [111–113]. It may occur more commonly in the fall and winter following upper respiratory tract infections.

Previous reviews have found that thyrotoxicosis was not common in AST [4]. The recent meta-analysis by Lafontaine et al. [9] found that 42% of bacterial and 40% of fungal AST cases were thyrotoxic at presentation and at least 36% of bacterial AST cases had significant thyrotoxicosis with free thyroxin (fT4) serum level more than twice the upper limit of normal [9]. Thyrotoxicosis due to AST is plausible, given the pathogenesis of AST and the release of pre-formed thyroid hormone secondary to the destruction of thyroid follicles. It is therefore important to consider AST in patients with apparent hyperthyroidism and a painful neck, making the differentiation with subacute thyroiditis (SAT) difficult [9].

In general, there are no signs or symptoms of hyper- or hypothyroidism. However, exceptions to both have been reported, particularly if the thyroiditis is generalized, such as occurs with fungal processes [77] or mycobacterial infections. At times, even in patients with bacterial thyroiditis, destruction of the thyroid gland is extensive enough to release thyroid hormone in amounts sufficient to cause symptomatic thyrotoxicosis [57, 62]. Associated thyrotoxicosis has also been reported in both children and adults [21, 57, 90, 114]; in one study, Yu et al. [4] reported that 12% of patients presented with thyrotoxicosis while 17% were hypothyroid [4]. This variety of thyroid function findings clearly increases the difficulty of differentiating AST from SAT as both present with thyroidal pain. Unique presentations of AST have been reported where initial thyrotoxicosis has been followed by hypothyroidism and spontaneous normalization of thyroid function after treatment of the AST [58, 115].

3.7.2 Physical Examination

On physical examination, most acute thyroiditis patients have a tender, indurated, and inflamed thyroid gland with signs of acute inflammation in the skin (redness and hotness). With abscess formation, fluctuation appears, and pus may track subcutaneously low down in the midline of the neck, or into the trachea, pharynx, or mediastinum. Edema of the glottis may also occur.

3.7.3 Complications

Complications of various cases of acute infectious thyroiditis reported by Lafontaine et al. [9] in their meta-analysis included internal jugular vein (IJV) thrombophlebitis, mediastinitis and pericarditis, esophageal perforation, fistula formation and obstruction, laryngeal edema requiring tracheostomy, obstructive symptoms, Horner's syndrome, and multisystem organ failure (MSOF) [9].

3.8 Evaluation/Diagnosis

3.8.1 Clinical Evaluation and Laboratory Tests

Since the differential diagnosis will lie between acute suppurative thyroiditis (AST) and subacute thyroiditis (SAT), it is critical to compare the history, physical, and particularly laboratory data in these two conditions. In general, the patient with AST appears septic, has greater and more localized pain in the thyroid gland, may have an associated upper respiratory infection, has lymphadenopathy, and may be immuno-compromised. Localization of tenderness on palpation of the left lobe should suggest the possibility of an infection as should any erythema or apparent abscess formation. The presence of leukocytosis with a shift to the left would argue for infection; however, elevations in erythrocyte sedimentation rate (ESR) are common in both acute and subacute thyroiditis. As mentioned before, patients with bacterial thyroiditis are usually euthyroid, but a thyrotoxic presentation has been noted in 8–12% [4, 116], and hypothyroidism was noted in 17% of one series [116]. Thyrotoxicosis is clearly more common with longer duration, 52% at 7 days and 65% by 30 days of neck pain in patients with SAT [117]. The thyrotoxic presentation therefore poses a difficult differential diagnostic problem to separate AST from SAT, which may have a significant impact on the selection of initial therapy.

3.8.2 Imaging Studies

3.8.2.1 Radionuclide Scan

Discriminating tests differentiating AST from SAT have been considered; a radionuclide uptake (RAIU) and/or scanning usually shows a very low uptake value in SAT with a normal value found in the patient with localized mild AST [25] as shown in Fig. 3.1. More frequently, however, both conditions are associated with a low ^{123}I uptake at initial presentation [35, 115, 118, 119], limiting the power of iodine-based nuclear studies to effectively differentiate these two conditions.

3.8.2.2 Ultrasonography/Sono-Elastography

In the early inflammatory phase of AST, when obvious abscess formation is *not* evident, an ultrasound may show a localized hypoechoic process with an obscure border and effacement between the thyroid and surrounding peri-thyroidal tissues [120]. During the acute inflammatory stage of AST, clear-cut abscess formation is noted in the affected thyroidal tissue [120]. Peri-thyroidal unifocal hypoechoic space and effacement of the plane between the thyroid and peri-thyroidal tissues (Fig. 3.2) have been noted to be specific signs of AST [120]. In SAT, varied US findings have been reported; most commonly ill-defined hypoechoic areas that may be unilateral or bilateral [1, 121, 122].

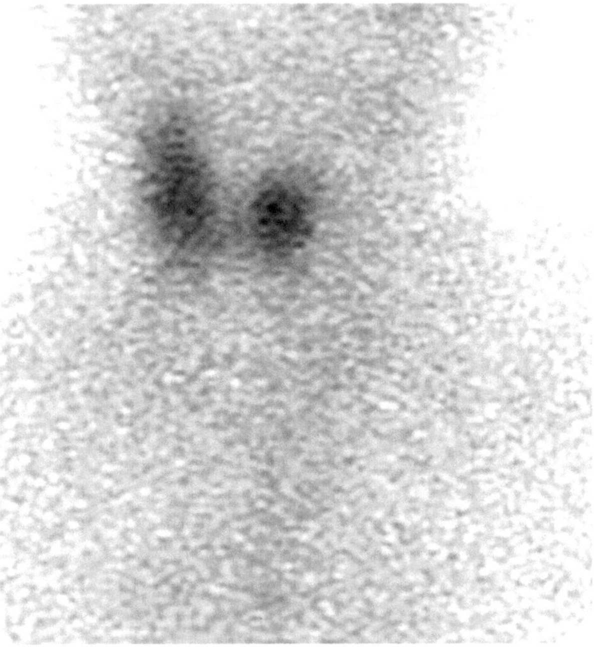

Fig. 3.1 ^{99m}Tc thyroid scintigraphy showing an asymmetrical uptake between both lobes. The left thyroid lobe has a cold area which includes the upper two-thirds reflecting an inflammatory thyroid collection in a patient with acute suppurative thyroiditis

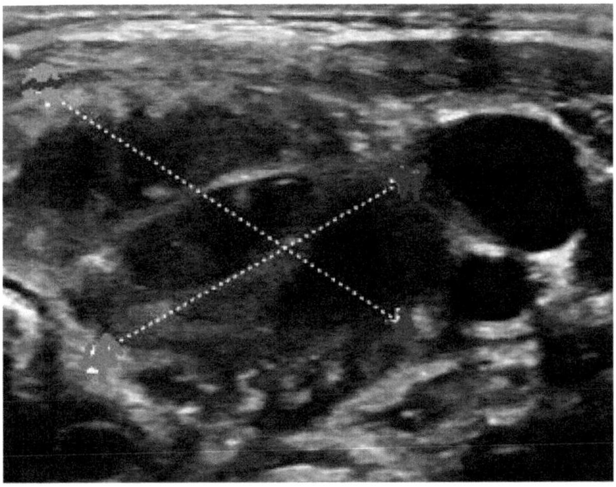

Fig. 3.2 Ultrasound of the thyroid gland showing a 3 × 2.7 cm, ovoid heterogeneous structure in the left thyroid lobe displacing the carotid artery and internal jugular vein. This picture denotes a collection in a patient with acute suppurative thyroiditis

Alternatively, the application of sono-elastography in AST may reveal very stiff lesions corresponding to the areas of the thyroid, which are especially painful [117] during acute phases of the AST episode, which soften significantly as the patient responds to treatment [123]. As AST resolves with appropriate treatment, ultrasound images may demonstrate deformity of the gland characterized by atrophy of the affected lobe, air/fluid levels in the thyroidal tissue, and scarring of the perithyroidal tissues [120].

3.8.2.3 Computed Tomography (CT) Scan

A CT scan may be useful in identifying the location of the abscess, but it is required only in unusual situations [124]. The CT findings also vary with the stage of AST. In the early inflammatory stage, non-specific low-density areas in the swollen thyroid along with potential tracheal displacement may be seen [120]. In the acute inflammatory stage, a CT scan can also demonstrate edema of the ipsilateral hypopharynx, and abscess formation. In the late inflammatory stage, deformity of the thyroid, atrophy of the affected lobe, and scarring of the peri-thyroidal tissues may be observed [120]. Recent reviews indicate a significant role of CT scan (Fig. 3.3) in the initial evaluation of those with AST [1, 120]. During the earliest stages of AST, both CT and ultrasound findings may fail to effectively differentiate between AST and SAT. In this circumstance, the use of a fine-needle aspiration (FNA) has been demonstrated to be very useful.

Occasionally, pain from an infectious process elsewhere in the neck will present as anterior neck tenderness. For example, a retro-pharyngeal abscess may present with typical symptoms of acute thyroiditis. The thyroid gland, however, will have a normal ultrasound appearance, be normal on scanning, and only on CT scan will the retro-pharyngeal abscess be recognized [120].

3.8.2.4 Barium Swallow

If an infectious process is identified, particularly of the left lobe of a younger individual, then a barium swallow should be performed with attention to the possibility of a fistulous tract located on the left side between the pyriform sinus and the thyroid gland. The barium swallow has very good sensitivity in detecting the presence of the fistula tracts as 89–97% of those examined in early and acute stages of AST have been confirmed with this technique [120]. Other methods of documenting the presence of a fistula are also utilized. On follow-up ultrasound, an "emerging

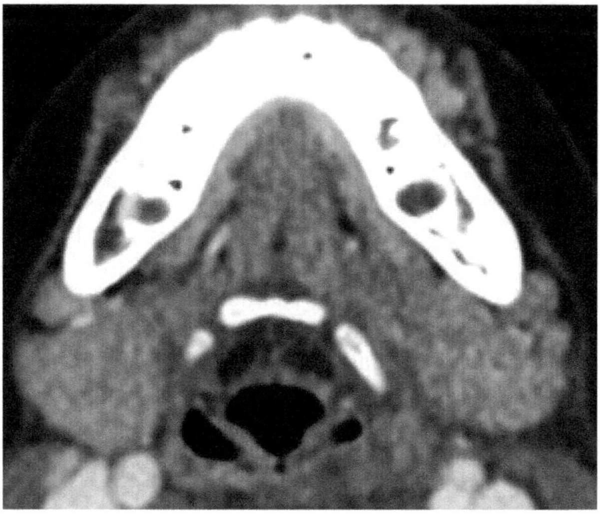

Fig. 3.3 Computed tomography scan of the thyroid gland in a 41-year-old gentleman with acute suppurative thyroiditis. It shows an inflammatory collection, 30 × 14 × 10 mm, originating in the upper pole of the left lobe and extending anteriorly to the pre-thyroid and left sternocleidomastoid muscles, and cranially through the para-laryngeal space to the level of the valleculae, while posteriorly, it extends to reach the pharynx

echogenic tract sign" suggests an associated pyriform sinus thyroid fistula [125]. During a CT scan procedure, the patient can be asked to blow into a syringe, the so-called "trumpet maneuver," which may help to identify a piriform sinus fistula [126].

3.8.3 Trans-Nasal Flexible Fiberoptic Laryngoscopy

A "light-guided procedure" to visualize the fistulous tract between the pyriform sinus and the thyroid gland may also help [127]. Trans-nasal flexible fiberoptic laryngoscopy has become increasingly utilized to identify the presence of fistula tracts [1]. This approach has been estimated to have similar sensitivity to documenting the tracts as barium swallow and CT scan methods [128–130] and can also be utilized for the instillation of chemo-cauterizing agents at an appropriate time after the resolution of the acute infection [117, 128, 130, 131].

3.8.4 Fine-Needle Aspiration (FNA)

A fine-needle aspiration (FNA) performed in the acute phase of AST is important as an aspirate has a superior ability to differentiate the patient with AST from those with SAT by cytological criteria. It also provides appropriate bacteriological specificity allowing smears and cultures providing a more accurate antibiotic selection [1] for the patient documented to have AST. In addition, trans-cutaneous drainage of the infectious material can be performed to relieve pressure on a displaced trachea in patients with a compromised airway [1]. Finally, FNA may be seen as the most accurate means of differential diagnosis when a thyrotoxic presentation is encountered [132]. Establishing a firm diagnosis of AST allows timely antibiotic therapy to be prescribed when a trial of glucocorticoids for empirically assumed SAT might result in both delay in diagnosis and initiation of a potentially inappropriate therapy [58].

3.9 Differential Diagnosis

The differential diagnosis of acute infectious (suppurative) thyroiditis includes (1) de Quervain's (granulomatous) thyroiditis, (2) hemorrhage into a thyroid nodule, (3) infected thyro-glossal or branchial cyst, (4) infected cystic hygroma, and (5) cervical lymphadenitis. In addition to FNA, US helps to establish the diagnosis, which may further be refined by CT scan.

The differential diagnoses of AST are listed in Table 3.3 [1, 121, 122]. Subacute thyroiditis (SAT) is a more common but benign condition that may confound the diagnosis of AST and results in a delayed diagnosis. Due to the similarity in clinical features of fever, neck pain, and hyperthyroidism, it can be difficult to differentiate it from AST. Helpful features include systemically unwell patient, neck erythema,

Table 3.3 Differential diagnosis of acute suppurative (infectious) thyroiditis

Causes	Examples
Inflammatory	Subacute thyroiditis Painful Hashimoto's thyroiditis Radiation-induced thyroiditis
Infective	Sternocleidomastoid abscess Para-pharyngeal abscess Lymph node suppuration Thyroglossal duct cysts infection Retro-pharyngeal deep space abscess
Malignant pseudo-thyroiditis	Thyroid carcinoma Thyroid lymphoma Metastases to thyroid Parathyroid carcinoma
Trauma	Palpation thyroiditis Blunt trauma
Infiltrative	Amyloidosis
Others	Thyroid/parathyroid nodule hemorrhage/rupture Deep vein thrombosis Branchial arches 1–4 anomalies

and greater elevation of white cell count in AST. Moreover, the response to glucocorticoids in SAT is often dramatic, while in AST, there is no response to glucocorticoids. However, fever, hyperthyroidism and an elevated ESR do *not* help differentiating between these two conditions [5, 133, 134].

3.10 Treatment

Acute suppurative thyroiditis (AST) is an urgent condition, and prompt treatment is necessary as the infection may cause destruction of the thyroid and the parathyroid glands, spread to other organs, or cause abscess rupture, descending necrotizing mediastinitis, vocal cord palsy and fistulae to the trachea or esophagus, or even tracheal compression, leading to asphyxia and death [135, 136].

In general, patients with AST can receive non-surgical management. Antibiotics are used to control infection. None-steroidal anti-inflammatory drugs (NSAIDs) are used to control severe neck pain and inflammation. When an abscess is identified, surgical incision and drainage is essential. Occasionally, complete resection of an affected lobe is required [6]. Complications of surgery include injury or damage to the parathyroid glands (PTGs) and the recurrent laryngeal nerve (RLN). As identification of anatomical structures in excessive infection often is difficult, these tissues may be impossible to find. Therefore, open surgery should be performed with caution and in selected patients.

There has been a trend toward less invasive management during active inflammation and infection [1]. A recent study by Lafontaine et al. [4] observed that 32% of the cases with bacterial AST were managed with antibiotics and a single needle aspiration, 3% required multiple needle aspirations, and 13% had a needle aspiration and antibiotics, but subsequently required surgery. In both the immediate surgery group and those with needle aspiration and antibiotics, incision and drainage was the most common procedure (57% and 53%, respectively), followed by partial thyroidectomy (30% and 40%, respectively) with or without excision of a fistula tract, and total thyroidectomy (13% and 7%, respectively). The median duration of antibiotics was 17 days (14–30 days) [9]. In contrast, only 22% of cases of fungal AST went directly to surgery (11% for incision and drainage, 11% underwent a partial thyroidectomy), 56% had a single needle aspiration and anti-fungals, and 22% failed needle aspiration and anti-fungals and subsequently required surgery. The mean duration of anti-fungal therapy was 42 days [9].

Despite a lack of randomized controlled trials (RCTs), algorithms for acute and long-term management have been suggested by several authors. Miyauchi [118] has cautioned that consideration of the basic anomaly predisposing the patient to thyroid gland infection must be duly considered. Microscopic examination and appropriate staining of a fine-needle aspirate often aid the diagnosis and choice of antibiotic therapy. The procedure is best done under ultrasound guidance so that the source of the specimen is identified. It may also serve as a mechanism for decompression of an abscess and can be repeated to facilitate healing. Some abscesses will require surgical exploration and drainage. The choice of therapy will also depend on the immune status of the patient. Systemic antibiotics are required for severe infections. *Candida albicans* thyroiditis may be treated with appropriate doses of amphotericin B and fluconazole. Successful anti-fungal combination therapy and a surgical approach for *Aspergillus* spp.-associated AST has been reported by Nicole et al. in 2017 [137].

The proper treatment of an acute thyroiditis in children generally requires the surgical removal of the fistula [15, 17, 18], although surgical treatment should be delayed until the inflammatory process is resolved [138, 139]. Combining this with partial thyroidectomy may further decrease the recurrence rate [16, 33]. Injection of 0.5% methylene blue solution through a Nélaton's catheter into the fistula usually enables the complete resection of the tract. When the origin of the fistula is difficult to identify, transection of the inferior pharyngeal constrictor muscle makes intervention easier. In addition, a lobectomy/hemi-thyroidectomy may be the safer option as it provides an adequate identification of the recurrent laryngeal nerve (RLN) in the re-operative field [140]. Alternatively, fistula tract ablation can be achieved either by surgical resection, which has been associated with recurrence-free survival [120], or less invasively obliterated with the instillation of a chemo-cauterizing agent, which has also been demonstrated to result in satisfactory outcomes [120, 122, 130, 131]. Newer, minimally invasive trans-oral video-laryngoscopic surgery (TOVS) [141] and endoscopy-assisted surgery [142] have been reported to be safe and reliable methods of pyriform sinus fistula treatment. Ultrasound-guided aspiration with or without lavage had a good treatment effect and without adverse events for the management of AST secondary to pyriform sinus fistula [143].

3.11 Prognosis

Acute infectious thyroiditis may occasionally prove fatal [112]. It has a reported mortality of 3.7%–9% [4, 6], and therefore, it is crucial to make a timely diagnosis. In some patients with thyroiditis, the destruction may be sufficiently severe that permanent hypothyroidism results [11]. Thus, patients with a particularly diffuse thyroiditis should have follow-up thyroid function studies performed to determine the need for thyroid hormone replacement. Surgical removal of a fistula or branchial pouch sinus [138, 139] is required to prevent recurrence.

References

1. Paes JE, Burman KD, Cohen J, Franklyn J, McHenry CR, Shoham S, et al. Acute bacterial suppurative thyroiditis: a clinical review and expert opinion. Thyroid. 2010;20(3):247 55.
2. Al-Dajani N, Wootton SH. Cervical lymphadenitis, suppurative parotitis, thyroiditis, and infected cysts. Infect Dis Clin N Am. 2007;21(2):523–41.
3. Hendrick JW. Diagnosis and management of thyroiditis. JAMA J Am Med Assoc. 1957;164(2):127–33.
4. Yu EH, Ko WC, Chuang YC, Wu TJ. Suppurative Acinetobacter baumanii thyroiditis with bacteremic pneumonia: case report and review. Clin Infect Dis. 1998;27(5):1286–90.
5. Pearce EN, Farwell AP, Braverman LE. Thyroiditis. N Engl J Med. 2003;348(26):2646–55.
6. Berger SA, Zonszein J, Villamena P, Mittman N. Infectious diseases of the thyroid gland. Rev Infect Dis. 1983;5(1):108–22.
7. Henderson J. Abscess of the thyroid. A discussion and report of four cases. Am J Surg. 1935;29(1):36–41.
8. Burhans EC. Acute thyroiditis. A study of sixty-seven cases. Surg Gynecol Obstet. 1928;47:478–88.
9. Lafontaine N, Learoyd D, Farrel S, Wong R. Suppurative thyroiditis: systematic review and clinical guidance. Clin Endocrinol. 2021;95(2):253–64.
10. Robertson WS. Acute inflammation of the thyroid gland. Lancet. 1911;177(4571):930–1.
11. Dugar M, da Graca BA, Bruns J Jr, Som PM. Unilateral hypopharyngitis, cellulitis, and a multinodular goiter: a triad of findings suggestive of acute suppurative thyroiditis. AJNR Am J Neuroradiol. 2009;30(10):1944–6.
12. Chi H, Lee YJ, Chiu NC, Huang FY, Huang CY, Lee KS, et al. Acute suppurative thyroiditis in children. Pediatr Infect Dis J. 2002;21(5):384–7.
13. Chang P, Tsai WY, Lee PI, Hsiao PH, Huang LM, Lee JS, et al. Clinical characteristics and management of acute suppurative thyroiditis in children. J Formos Med Assoc. 2002;101(7):468–71.
14. Brook I. Microbiology and management of acute suppurative thyroiditis in children. Int J Pediatr Otorhinolaryngol. 2003;67(5):447–51.
15. Hatabu H, Kasagi K, Yamamoto K, Iida Y, Misaki T, Hidaka A, et al. Acute suppurative thyroiditis associated with piriform sinus fistula: sonographic findings. AJR Am J Roentgenol. 1990;155(4):845–7.
16. Parida PK, Gopalakrishnan S, Saxena SK. Pediatric recurrent acute suppurative thyroiditis of third branchial arch origin - our experience in 17 cases. Int J Pediatr Otorhinolaryngol. 2014;78(11):1953–7.
17. Lucaya J, Berdon WE, Enriquez G, Regas J, Carreno JC. Congenital pyriform sinus fistula: a cause of acute left-sided suppurative thyroiditis and neck abscess in children. Pediatr Radiol. 1990;21(1):27–9.

18. Miyauchi A, Yokozawa T, Matsuzuka F, Kuma K. Acute suppurative thyroiditis; infection in thyroid nodules or infection through a piriform sinus fistula. Thyroidol Clin Exp. 1998;10:75–9.
19. Miyauchi A, Matsuzuka F, Kuma K, Katayama S. Piriform sinus fistula and the ultimobranchial body. Histopathology. 1992;20(3):221–7.
20. Shah SS, Baum SG. Diagnosis and management of infectious thyroiditis. Curr Infect Dis Rep. 2000;2(2):147–53.
21. Fukata S, Miyauchi A, Kuma K, Sugawara M. Acute suppurative thyroiditis caused by an infected piriform sinus fistula with thyrotoxicosis. Thyroid. 2002;12(2):175–8.
22. Gan YU, Lam SL. Imaging findings in acute neck infection due to pyriform sinus fistula. Ann Acad Med Singap. 2004;33(5):636–40.
23. Sheng Q, Lv Z, Xiao X, Zheng S, Huang Y, Huang X, Li H, Wu Y, Dong K, Liu J. Diagnosis and management of pyriform sinus fistula: experience in 48 cases. J Pediatr Surg. 2014;49(3):455–9.
24. Mohan PS, Chokshi RA, Moser RL, Razvi SA. Thyroglossal duct cysts: a consideration in adults. Am Surg. 2005;71(6):508–11.
25. Szabo SM, Allen DB. Thyroiditis. Differentiation of acute suppurative and subacute. Case report and review of the literature. Clin Pediatr Phila. 1989;28(4):171–4.
26. Hopwood NJ, Kelch RP. Thyroid masses: approach to diagnosis and management in childhood and adolescence. Pediatr Rev. 1993;14(12):481–7.
27. Sai Prasad TR, Chong CL, Mani A, Chui CH, Tan CE, Tee WS, et al. Acute suppurative thyroiditis in children secondary to pyriform sinus fistula. Pediatr Surg Int. 2007;23(8):779–83.
28. Wasniewska M, Vigone MC, Cappa M, Cassio A, Scognamillo R, Aversa T, et al. Acute suppurative thyroiditis in childhood: spontaneous closure of sinus pyriform fistula may occur even very early. J Pediatr Endocrinol Metab. 2007;20(1):75–7.
29. Cases JA, Wenig BM, Silver CE, Surks MI. Recurrent acute suppurative thyroiditis in an adult due to a fourth branchial pouch fistula. J Clin Endocrinol Metab. 2000;85(3):953–6.
30. Miyauchi A, Matsuzuka F, Kuma K, Takai S. Piriform sinus fistula: an underlying abnormality common in patients with acute suppurative thyroiditis. World J Surg. 1990;14(3):400–5.
31. Kingsbury BF. On the fate of the ultimobrachial body within the hyman thyroid gland. Anat Rec. 1935;61:155–67.
32. Minhas SS, Watkinson JC, Franklyn J. Fourth branchial arch fistula and suppurative thyroiditis: a life-threatening infection. J Laryngol Otol. 2001;115(12):1029–31.
33. Nicoucar K, Giger R, Pope HG Jr, Jaecklin T, Dulguerov P. Management of congenital fourth branchial arch anomalies: a review and analysis of published cases. J Pediatr Surg. 2009;44(7):1432–9.
34. Vandjme A, Pageaux GP, Bismuth M, Fabre JM, Domergue J, Perez C, et al. Nocardiosis revealed by thyroid abscess in a liver–kidney transplant recipient. Transpl Int. 2001;14(3):202–4.
35. Teckie G, Bhana SA, Tsitsi JM, Shires R. Thyrotoxicosis followed by hypothyroidism due to Suppurative thyroiditis caused by in a patient with advanced acquired immunodeficiency syndrome. Eur Thyroid J. 2014;3(1):65–8.
36. Kazi S, Liu H, Jiang N, Glick J, Teng M, LaBombardi V, Szporn AH, Chen H. Salmonella thyroid abscess in human immunodeficiency virus-positive man: a diagnostic pitfall in fine-needle aspiration biopsy of thyroid lesions. Diagn Cytopathol. 2015;43(1):36–9.
37. Massolt ET, Rijneveld AW, Vernooij MW, Kevenaar ME, van Kemenade FJ, Peeters RP. Acute Candida thyroiditis complicated by abscess formation in a severely immunocompromised patient. J Clin Endocrinol Metab. 2014;99(11):3952–3.
38. Fernandez JF, Anaissie EJ, Vassilopoulou-Sellin R, Samaan NA. Acute fungal thyroiditis in a patient with acute myelogenous leukaemia. J Intern Med. 1991;230(6):539–41.
39. Gandhi RT, Tollin SR, Seely EW. Diagnosis of Candida thyroiditis by fine needle aspiration. J Infect. 1994;28(1):77–81.

40. McAninch EA, Xu C, Lagari VS, Kim BW. Coccidiomycosis thyroiditis in an immunocompromised host post-transplant: case report and literature review. J Clin Endocrinol Metab. 2014;99(5):1537–42.
41. Alvi MM, Meyer DS, Hardin NJ, Dekay JG, Marney AM, Gilbert MP. Aspergillus thyroiditis: a complication of respiratory tract infection in an immunocompromised patient. Case Rep Endocrinol. 2013;2013:741041.
42. Imai C, Kakihara T, Watanabe A, Ikarashi Y, Hotta H, Tanaka A, et al. Acute suppurative thyroiditis as a rare complication of aggressive chemotherapy in children with acute myelogeneous leukemia. Pediatr Hematol Oncol. 2002;19(4):247–53.
43. Acocelia A, Nardi P, Sacco R, Agostini T. Acute thyroiditis of odontogenic origin. Minerva Stomatol. 2007;56:461–7.
44. Dai L, Lin S, Liu D, Wang Q. Acute suppurative thyroiditis with thyroid metastasis from oesophageal cancer. Endokrynol Pol. 2020;71(1):106–7.
45. Yildar M, Demirpolat G, Aydin M. Acute suppurative thyroiditis accompanied by thyrotoxicosis after fine-needle aspiration: treatment with catheter drainage. J Clin Diagn Res. 2014;8(11):ND12–14.
46. Unluturk U, Ceylan K, Corapcioglu D. Acute suppurative thyroiditis following fine-needle aspiration biopsy in an immunocompetent patient. J Clin Ultrasound. 2014;42(4):215–8.
47. Inoue K, Kozawa J, Funahashi T, Nakata Y, Mitsui E, Kitamura T, et al. Right-sided acute suppurative thyroiditis caused by infectious endocarditis. Intern Med. 2011;50(23):2893–7.
48. Cabizuca CA, Bulzico DA, de Almeida MH, Conceicao FL, Vaisman M. Acute thyroiditis due to septic emboli derived from infective endocarditis. Postgrad Med J. 2008;84(994):445–6.
49. Yegya-Raman N, Copeland T, Parikh P. Acute Suppurative thyroiditis in an intravenous drug user with a preexisting goiter. Case Rep Med. 2018;2018:5098712.
50. Robazzi TC, Alves C, Mendonca M. Acute suppurative thyroiditis as the initial presentation of juvenile systemic lupus erythematosus. J Pediatr Endocrinol Metab. 2009;22(4):379–83.
51. Chiovato L, Canale G, Maccherini D, Falcone V, Pacini F, Pinchera A. Salmonella Brandenburg: a novel cause of acute suppurative thyroiditis. Acta Endocrinol. 1993;128(5):439–42.
52. Dai MS, Chang H, Peng MY, Ho CL, Chao TY. Suppurative salmonella thyroiditis in a patient with chronic lymphocytic leukemia. Ann Hematol. 2003;82(10):646–8.
53. Su DH, Huang TS. Acute suppurative thyroiditis caused by salmonella typhimurium: a case report and review of the literature. Thyroid. 2002;12(11):1023–7.
54. Akhanli P, Bayir O, Bayram SM, Hepsen S, Badirshaev M, Cakal E, Saylam G, Korkmaz MH. Acute spontaneous suppurative thyroiditis caused by Eikenella corrodens presented with thyrotoxicosis. Einstein (Sao Paulo). 2020;18:eRC5273.
55. Bukvic B, Diklic A, Zivaljevic V. Acute suppurative klebsiella thyroiditis: a case report. Acta Chir Belg. 2009;109(2):253–5.
56. Fernandez Pena C, Morales Gorria MJ, Morano Amado LE, Lopez Miragalla MI, Pena GE. Pasteurella spp: a new microorganism to the cause of acute suppurative thyroiditis. An Med Interna. 1999;16:637–8.
57. McLaughlin SA, Smith SL, Meek SE. Acute suppurative thyroiditis caused by Pasteurella multocida and associated with thyrotoxicosis. Thyroid. 2006;16(3):307–10.
58. Spitzer M, Alexanian S, Farwell AP. Thyrotoxicosis with post-treatment hypothyroidism in a patient with acute Suppurative thyroiditis due to Porphyromonas. Thyroid. 2012;22(1):97–100.
59. Iniguez JL, Duyckaerts V, Badoual J. Acute thyroiditis caused by Eikenella corrodens and abnormality of the left pyriform sinus. Arch Fr Pediatr. 1989;46(10):745–7.
60. Queen JS, Clegg HW, Council JC, Morton D. Acute suppurative thyroiditis caused by Eikenella corrodens. J Pediatr Surg. 1988;23(4):359–61.
61. Yoshino Y, Inamo Y, Fuchigami T, Hashimoto K, Ishikawa T, Abe O, et al. A pediatric patient with acute suppurative thyroiditis caused by Eikenella corrodens. J Infect Chemother. 2010;16(5):353–5.
62. Nieuwland Y, Tan KY, Elte JW. Miliary tuberculosis presenting with thyrotoxicosis. Postgrad Med J. 1992;68(802):677–9.

63. Das DK, Pant CS, Chachra KL, Gupta AK. Fine needle aspiration cytology diagnosis of tuberculous thyroiditis. A report of eight cases. Acta Cytol. 1992;36(4):517–22.
64. Orlandi F, Fiorini S, Gonzatto I, Saggiorato E, Pivano G, Angeli A, Pasquali R. Tubercular involvement of the thyroid gland: a report of two cases. Horm Res. 1999;52(6):291–4.
65. Terzidis K, Tourli P, Kiapekou E, Alevizaki M. Thyroid tuberculosis. Hormones (Athens). 2007;6(1):75–9.
66. Kataria SP, Tanwar P, Singh S, Kumar S. Primary tuberculosis of the thyroid gland: a case report. Asian Pac J Trop Biomed. 2012;2(10):839–40.
67. Karabinis A, Douzinas E, Clouva P, Papanicolaou M, Kakaviatos N, Bilalis D. Acute necrotic thyroiditis caused by Candida albicans immediately after acute hemorrhagic rectocolitis. Presse Med. 1993;22(1):34.
68. Carriere C, Marchandin H, Andrieu JM, Vandome A, Perez C. Nocardia thyroiditis: unusual location of infection. J Clin Microbiol. 1999;37(7):2323–5.
69. Lewin SR, Street AC, Snider J. Suppurative thyroiditis due to Nocardia asteroides. J Infect. 1993;26(3):339–40.
70. Singer PA. Thyroiditis. Acute, subacute, and chronic. Med Clin North Am. 1991;75(1):61–77.
71. Tan J, Shen J, Fang Y, Zhu L, Liu Y, Gong Y, et al. A suppurative thyroiditis and perineal subcutaneous abscess related with aspergillus fumigatus: a case report and literature review. BMC Infect Dis. 2018;18(1):702.
72. Karatoprak N, Atay Z, Erol N, Goksugur SB, Ceran O. Actinomycotic suppurative thyroiditis in a child. J Trop Pediatr. 2005;51(6):383–5.
73. Park YH, Baik JH, Yoo J. Acute thyroiditis of actinomycosis. Thyroid. 2005;15(12):1395–6.
74. Trites J, Evans M. Actinomycotic thyroiditis in a child. J Pediatr Surg. 1998;33(5):781–2.
75. Moinuddin S, Barazi H, Moinuddin M. Acute blastomycosis thyroiditis. Thyroid. 2008;18(6):659–61.
76. Rao N, Mann SJ. Fine needle aspiration cytology of acute blastomycosis thyroiditis. Diagn Cytopathol. 2017;45(12):1119–21.
77. Avram AM, Sturm CA, Michael CW, Sisson JC, Jaffe CA. Cryptococcal thyroiditis and hyperthyroidism. Thyroid. 2004;14(6):471–4.
78. Zavascki AP, Maia AL, Goldani LZ. Pneumocystis jiroveci thyroiditis: report of 15 cases in the literature. Mycoses. 2007;50(6):443–6.
79. Orkar KS, Dakum NK, Kidmas AT, Awani KU. Pyogenic thyroiditis and HIV infection. West Afr J Med. 2001;20(2):173–5.
80. Tien KJ, Chen TC, Hsieh MC, Hsu SC, Hsiao JY, Shin SJ, et al. Acute suppurative thyroiditis with deep neck infection: a case report. Thyroid. 2007;17(5):467–9.
81. Iwama S, Kato Y, Nakayama S. Acute suppurative thyroiditis extending to descending necrotizing mediastinitis and pericarditis. Thyroid. 2007;17(3):281–2.
82. Premawardhana LD, Vora JP, Scanlon MF. Suppurative thyroiditis with oesophageal carcinoma. Postgrad Med J. 1992;68(801):592–3.
83. Valina S, Lotter O, Schaller HE, Rahmanian-Schwarz A. Abscess formation after puncture of a thyroid cyst – a case report. Zentralbl Chir (Germany). 2013;138(Suppl 2):e108–9.
84. Kale SU, Kumar A, David VC. Thyroid abscess--an acute emergency. European Archives of Oto-Rhino-Laryngology. 2004;261(8):456–8.
85. Jimenez-Heffernan JA, Perez F, Hornedo J, Perna C, Lapuente F. Massive thyroid tumoral embolism from a breast carcinoma presenting as acute thyroiditis. Arch Pathol Lab Med. 2004;128(7):804–6.
86. Robillon JF, Sadoul JL, Guerin P, Iafrate-Lacoste C, Talbodec A, Santini J, et al. Mycobacterium avium intracellulare suppurative thyroiditis in a patient with Hashimoto's thyroiditis. J Endocrinol Investig. 1994;17(2):133–4.
87. Visser R, de Mast Q, Netea-Maier RT, van der Ven AJ. Hashimoto's thyroiditis presenting as acute painful thyroiditis and as a manifestation of an immune reconstitution inflammatory syndrome in a human immunodeficiency virus-seropositive patient. Thyroid. 2012;22(8):853–5.
88. Kale SU, Kumar A, David VC. Thyroid abscess: an acute emergency. Eur Arch Otorhinolarngol. 2004;261(8):456–81.

89. Kalladi Puthanpurayil S, Francis GL, Kraft AO, Prasad U, Petersson RS. Papillary thyroid carcinoma presenting as acute suppurative thyroiditis: a case report and review of the literature. Int J Pediatr Otorhinolaryngol. 2018;105:12–5.
90. Nishihara E, Miyauchi A, Matsuzuka F, Sasaki I, Ohye H, Kubota S, Fukata S, Amino N, Kuma K. Acute suppurative thyroiditis after fine-needle aspiration causing thyrotoxicosis. Thyroid. 2005;15(10):1183–7.
91. Chen HW, Tseng FY, Su DH, Chang YL, Chang TC. Secondary infection and ischemic necrosis after fine needle aspiration for a painful papillary thyroid carcinoma: a case report. Acta Cytol. 2006;50(2):217–20.
92. Puthanpurayil SK, Francis GL, Kraft AO, Prasad U, Petersson RS. Papillary thyroid carcinoma presenting as acute suppurative thyroiditis: a case report and review of the literature. Int J Pediatr Otorhinolaryngol. 2018;105:12–5.
93. George MM, Goswamy J, Penney SE. Embolic suppurative thyroiditis with concurrent carcinoma in pregnancy: lessons in management through a case report. Thyroid Res. 2015;8:3.
94. Sicilia V, Mezitis S. A case of acute suppurative thyroiditis complicated by thyrotoxicosis. J Endocrinol Investig. 2006;29(11):997–1000.
95. Hong JT, Lee JH, Kim SH, Hong SB, Nam M, Kim YS, et al. Case of concurrent Riedel's thyroiditis, acute suppurative thyroiditis, and micropapillary carcinoma. Korean J Intern Med. 2013;28(2):236–41.
96. Akdemir Z, Karaman E, Akdeniz H, Alptekin C, Arslan H. Giant thyroid abscess related to postpartum Brucella infection. Case Rep Infect Dis. 2015;2015:646209.
97. Campos R, Perez B, Armengod L, Munez E, Ramos A. Lactococcus lactis thyroid abscess in an immunocompetent patient. Endocrinol Nutr. 2015;62(4):204–6.
98. Mohi GK, Datta P, Chander J, Das A. Citrobacter freundii as a cause of acute suppurative thyroiditis in an immunocompetent adult female. Indian J Pathol Microbiol. 2017;60(2):282–4.
99. Falhammar H, Wallin G, Calissendorff J. Acute suppurative thyroiditis with thyroid abscess in adults: clinical presentation, treatment and outcomes. BMC Endocr Disord. 2019;19(1):130.
100. Takai SI, Miyauchi A, Matsuzuka F, Kuma K, Kosaki G. Internal fistula as a route of infection in acute Suppurative thyroiditis. Lancet. 1979;1(8119):751–2.
101. Yamashita J, Ogawa M, Yamashita S, Saishoji T, Nomura K, Tsuruta J. Acute suppurative thyroiditis in an asymptomatic woman: an atypical presentation simulating thyroid carcinoma. Clin Endocrinol. 1994;40(1):145–9.
102. Miyauchi A, Matsuzuka F, Takai S, Kuma K, Kosaki G. Piriform sinus fistula. A route of infection in acute suppurative thyroiditis. Arch Surg. 1981;116(1):66–9.
103. Nonomura N, Ikarashi F, Fujisaki T, Nakano Y. Surgical approach to pyriform sinus fistula. Am J Otolaryngol. 1993;14(2):111–5.
104. Himi T, Kataura A. Distribution of C cells in the thyroid gland with pyriform sinus fistula. Otolaryngol Head Neck Surg. 1995;112(2):268–73.
105. Bar-Ziv J, Slasky BS, Sichel JY, Lieberman A, Katz R. Branchial pouch sinus tract from the piriform fossa causing acute suppurative thyroiditis, neck abscess, or both: CT appearance and the use of air as a contrast agent. AJR Am J Roentgenol. 1996;167(6):1569–72.
106. Giuffrida G, Bagnato G, Campennì A, Giovinazzo S, Keller KP, Alibrandi A, et al. Non-specific rheumatic manifestations in patients with Hashimoto's thyroiditis: a pilot cross-sectional study. J Endocrinol Investig. 2020;43(1):87–94.
107. Gaafar H, El-Garem F. Acute thyroiditis with gas formation. J Laryngol Otol. 1975;89(3):323–7.
108. Bussman YC, Wong ML, Bell MJ, Santiago JV. Suppurative thyroiditis with gas formation due to mixed anaerobic infection. J Pediatr. 1977;90(2):321–2.
109. Reksoprawiro S. Suppurative thyroiditis with gas formation. Asian J Surg. 2003;26(3):180–2.
110. Al-Kordi RS, Alenizi E, Elgazzar AH. Acute suppurative thyroiditis with abscess, gas formation, and thyrotoxic crisis. Nuklearmedizin. 2008;47(4):N44–6.
111. Lemariey, Hamelin, Muler. Acute thyroiditis complicating mediastinitis. Ann Otolaryngol. 1955;72(7):571–3.

112. Dordain ML, Coutant G, Algayres JP, Jancovici R, Pats B, Daly JP. Suppurative mediastinitis secondary to acute thyroiditis in a patient under corticotherapy. Presse Med. 1997;26(7):319–20.
113. Pereira O, Prasad DS, Bal AM, McAteer D, Abraham P. Fatal descending necrotizing mediastinitis secondary to acute suppurative thyroiditis developing in an apparently healthy woman. Thyroid. 2010;20(5):571–2.
114. Yung BC, Loke TK, Fan WC, Chan JC. Acute suppurative thyroiditis due to foreign body-induced retropharyngeal abscess presented as thyrotoxicosis. Clin Nucl Med. 2000;25(4):249–52.
115. Wu C, Zhang Y, Gong Y, Hou Y, Li S, Zou Y, Ge J. Two cases of bacterial suppurative thyroiditis caused by Streptococcus anginosus. Endocr Pathol. 2013;24(1):49–53.
116. Miyauchi A, Inoue H, Tomoda C, Amino N. Evaluation of chemocauterization treatment for obliteration of pyriform sinus fistula as a route of infection causing acute suppurative thyroiditis. Thyroid. 2009;19(7):789–93.
117. Nishihara E, Ohye H, Amino N, Takata K, Arishima T, Kudo T, et al. Clinical characteristics of 852 patients with subacute thyroiditis before treatment. Intern Med. 2008;47(8):725–9.
118. Miyauchi A. Thyroid gland: a new management algorithm for acute suppurative thyroiditis? Nat Rev Endocrinol. 2010;6(8):424–6.
119. Kim S, Park TS, Baek HS, Jin HY. Subacute painful thyroiditis accompanied by scrub typhus infection. Endocrine. 2013;44(2):546–8.
120. Masuoka H, Miyauchi A, Tomoda C, Inoue H, Takamura Y, Ito Y, et al. Imaging studies in sixty patients with acute suppurative thyroiditis. Thyroid. 2011;21(10):1075–80.
121. Ikenoue H, Okamura K, Kuroda T, Sato K, Yoshinari M, Fujishima M. Thyroid amyloidosis with recurrent subacute thyroiditis-like syndrome. J Clin Endocrinol Metab. 1988;67(1):41–5.
122. Peng CC-H, Chang RH-E, Pennant M, Huang H-K, Munir KM. A literature review of painful Hashimoto's thyroiditis: 70 published cases in the past 70 years. J Endocr Soc. 2019;4(2):bvz008.
123. Ruchala M, Szczepanek-Parulska E, Zybek A, Moczko J, Czarnywojtek A, Kaminski G, et al. The role of sonoelastography in acute, subacute and chronic thyroiditis – a novel application of the method. Eur J Endocrinol. 2012;166(3):425–32.
124. Bernard PJ, Som PM, Urken ML, Lawson W, Biller HF. The CT findings of acute thyroiditis and acute suppurative thyroiditis. Otolaryngol Head Neck Surg. 1988;99(5):489–93.
125. Park NH, Park HJ, Park CS, Kim MS, Park SI. The emerging echogenic tract sign of pyriform sinus fistula: an early indicator in the recovery stage of acute suppurative thyroiditis. AJNR Am J Neuroradiol. 2011;32(3):E44–6.
126. Miyauchi A, Tomoda C, Uruno T, Takamura Y, Ito Y, Miya A, et al. Computed tomography scan under a trumpet maneuver to demonstrate piriform sinus fistulae in patients with acute suppurative thyroiditis. Thyroid. 2005;15(12):1409–13.
127. Ukiyama E, Endo M, Yoshida F, Watanabe T. Light guided procedure for congenital pyriform sinus fistula; new and simple procedure for impalpable fistula. Pediatr Surg Int. 2007;23(12):1241–3.
128. Kim KH, Sung MW, Koh TY, Oh SH, Kim IS. Pyriform sinus fistula: management with chemocauterization of the internal opening. Ann Otol Rhinol Laryngol. 2000;109(5):452–6.
129. Smith SL, Pereira KD. Suppurative thyroiditis in children: a management algorithm. Pediatr Emerg Care. 2008;24(11):764–7.
130. Pereira KD, Smith SL. Endoscopic chemical cautery of piriform sinus tracts: a safe new technique. Int J Pediatr Otorhinolaryngol. 2008;72(2):185–8.
131. Jordan JA, Graves JE, Manning SC, McClay JE, Biavati MJ. Endoscopic cauterization for treatment of fourth branchial cleft sinuses. Arch Otolaryngol Head Neck Surg. 1998;124(9):1021–4.
132. Mordes DA, Brachtel EF. Cytopathology of subacute thyroiditis. Diagn Cytopathol. 2012;40(5):433–4.

133. Majety P, Hennessey JV. Acute and Subacute, and Riedel's Thyroiditis. 2022 Jul 25. In: Feingold KR, Anawalt B, Blackman MR, Boyce A, Chrousos G, Corpas E, et al., editors. Endotext. South Dartmouth (MA): MD Text.com, Inc; 2000. PMID: 25905408.
134. Nishihara E, Ohye H, Amino N, et al. Clinical characteristics of 852 patients with subacute thyroiditis before treatment. Intern Med. 2008;47(8):725–9.
135. Adler ME, Jordan G, Walter RM Jr. Acute suppurative thyroiditis: diagnostic, metabolic and therapeutic observations. West J Med. 1978;128(2):165–8.
136. Schweitzer VG, Olson NR. Thyroid abscess. Otolaryngol Head Neck Surg. 1981;89(2):226–9.
137. Nicole S, Lanzafame M, Cazzadori A, Vincenzi M, Mangani F, Colato C, et al. Successful antifungal combination therapy and surgical approach for aspergillus fumigatus Suppurative thyroiditis associated with thyrotoxicosis and review of published reports. Mycopathologia. 2017;182(9–10):839–45.
138. Pereira KD, Losh GG, Oliver D, Poole MD. Management of anomalies of the third and fourth branchial pouches. Int J Pediatr Otorhinolaryngol. 2004;68(1):43–50.
139. Nicoucar K, Giger R, Jaecklin T, Pope HG Jr, Dulguerov P. Management of congenital third branchial arch anomalies: a systematic review. Otolaryngol Head Neck Surg. 2010;142(1):21–28 e22.
140. Kruijff S, Sywak MS, Sidhu SB, Shun A, Novakovic D, Lee JC, et al. Thyroidal abscesses in third and fourth branchial anomalies: not only a paediatric diagnosis. ANZ J Surg. 2015;85(7–8):578–81.
141. Kamide D, Tomifuji M, Maeda M, Utsunomiya K, Yamashita T, Araki K, et al. Minimally invasive surgery for pyriform sinus fistula by transoral videolaryngoscopic surgery. Am J Otolaryngol. 2015;36(4):601–5.
142. Xiao X, Zheng S, Zheng J, Zhu L, Dong K, Shen C, et al. Endoscopic-assisted surgery for pyriform sinus fistula in children: experience of 165 cases from a single institution. J Pediatr Surg. 2014;49(4):618–21.
143. Yang H, Li Ye X, Cheng J, Jia Z, Huang X, Wang X, et al. Aspiration with or without lavage in the treatment of acute suppurative thyroiditis secondary to pyriform sinus fistula. Arch Endocrinol Metab. 2020;64(2):128–37.

Acute Radiation-Induced Thyroiditis

4

4.1 Introduction

Despite their specific functional consequences, radiotherapy-induced thyroid abnormalities remain under-estimated and underreported. These sequelae may include radiation-induced thyroiditis, primary or central hypothyroidism, Graves' disease, euthyroid Graves' ophthalmopathy, benign adenomas, multinodular goiter (MNG), and radiation-induced thyroid carcinoma [1, 2]. The pathogenesis of radiation-induced thyroid injury includes vascular damage, parenchymal cell damage, and autoimmune reactions. Total radiotherapy dose, irradiated volume of the thyroid gland, and the extent of prior thyroid resection are among the most important factors associated with the risk of hypothyroidism [1].

New radiotherapy (RT) techniques, such as stereotactic radio-surgery, three-dimensional conformal irradiation, intensity modulated RT, and proton therapy, allow generally better dose distribution with lower dose to the non-target organs. The diagnostic approach to thyroid radiation injury includes baseline thyroid function assays in all patients undergoing thyroid or parasellar irradiation. Recommended follow-up procedures include at least annual evaluation with a history of symptoms of thyroid dysfunction, physical examination, and measurement of thyroid hormones and thyroid-stimulating hormone (TSH). Further improvements in RT techniques and progress in endocrine diagnostics and therapy may allow better prevention and management of radiation-related thyroid injury [1].

4.2 Etiology

The thyroid gland is extremely susceptible to radiation and can be compromised in a wide radiation dose range. Radiation, both internal and external, has been linked to thyroiditis, especially in higher doses. In general, radiation-induced thyroiditis is rare, and the incidence is about 1%.

M. Sakr, *Thyroiditis*, https://doi.org/10.1007/978-3-032-19513-5_4

Radiation treatment of neck cancer such as tonsillar carcinoma and lymphoma can cause thyroiditis, followed by destruction of thyroid cells and consequently hypothyroidism. Patients who receive radioactive iodine (RAI) (internal radiation therapy) for ablation of Graves' disease or toxic multinodular goiter (MNG) occasionally develop severe thyroid pain 7–10 days after therapy due to the development of acute thyroiditis. Radiation-induced thyroiditis can occur with external or internal irradiation therapies (^{131}I) and at varying doses [1, 3]. Historically, hypothyroidism after external beam radiotherapy (EBRT) of the thyroid gland in adulthood was considered not to develop below a dose threshold of 10–20 Gy [4, 5]. More recent data from patients receiving EBRT suggest a dose threshold for an increased risk of hypothyroidism of 10 Gy [6]. Data from patients with Graves' disease after radioactive iodine (RAI-^{131}I) therapy (internal radiotherapy) indicate that hypothyroidism rarely occurs below thyroid doses of 50 Gy [7].

Irradiation to the thyroid during therapy for breast cancer can also induce hypothyroidism. Recently, Digkas et al. (2024) [8] reported that during the follow-up (median 7.9 years), 5.7% (1212/21,268) patients with early breast cancer developed hypothyroidism. No association of the systemic oncological treatment in terms of either chemotherapy or endocrine therapy and hypothyroidism development could be identified. However, a higher risk of hypothyroidism was identified among patients treated with RT of the regional lymph nodes and not among those treated only with RT to the breast/chest wall. The risk of hypothyroidism in the cohort treated with RT of the regional lymph nodes was present irrespective of the use of adjuvant chemotherapy treatment. They concluded that the implementation of hypothyroidism surveillance among the breast cancer survivors treated with RT of the regional lymph nodes can be considered as reasonable in the follow-up program.

4.3 Pathogenesis

Radiation can destroy thyroid tissue with consequent hypothyroidism, and, besides this mechanism, radiation may lead to hypothyroidism indirectly, by induction of autoimmune thyroiditis. The primary damage caused by the thyroid gland's irradiation is thyroiditis [9]. Apart from that, autoimmune reactions including thyroid atrophy, hypothyroidism, and even thyroid cancer may be induced via radiation exposure [1, 3, 10]. The probability and severity of such complications depend on a variety of factors, such as the dose of radiation delivered, duration, and which sites of the head and neck obtained radiation such as Hodgkin Lymphoma (HL), rhabdomyosarcoma (RMS), and naso-pharyngeal carcinoma [11]. Other variables such as age, gender, and thyroid volume all play a role in the probability of these dysfunctions occurring [12]. Furthermore, it is believed that concomitant chemotherapy causes hypothyroidism by increasing the sensitivity of the thyroid gland to radiation [13].

4.3.1 Autoimmune Thyroiditis

In addition to the deterministic effects such as necrosis and apoptosis, radiation exposure can cause autoimmune processes in which autoantibodies are produced against cellular components of thyrocytes. Binding of these auto-antibodies to their target antibody-dependent cell-mediated cytotoxicity may lead to thyroiditis with subsequent hypothyroidism. This process is not fully understood [14], but its nature may be stochastic, not limited to threshold radiation doses [3]. On the other hand, relatively high radiation doses may induce autoimmune hyperthyroidism as well; this complication is well-known, but rather rare (approximately 1%) in the radioiodine treatment of autonomous hyper-functioning thyroid nodules [15]. In these cases, TSH receptor-stimulating antibodies become prevalent, instead of antibodies that induce destruction of thyrocyte components [16].

4.3.2 Thyroid Atrophy

Regarding radiation-induced thyroid atrophy, deterministic radiation effects (tissue reactions) usually appear shortly after exposure and are characterized by a dose threshold and a clear dose–effect association. Above the threshold, cells and tissues tend to be more frequently and severely damaged, and to more often lose their function as the radiation dose increases. In a recent comprehensive review about the effects of radioactive iodine (RAI-^{131}I) treatment of the diseased thyroid gland, Riley et al. (2019) [14] reported that ^{131}I induces cell death by both direct and indirect damage to thyrocyte DNA, largely through apoptosis. Some studies, however, have described detailed findings of cell death by necrosis following ^{131}I. In this sense, thyroid atrophy with subsequent hypothyroidism is a typical deterministic radiation effect.

4.4 Incidence

4.4.1 Radioactive Iodine (RAI) Therapy

Bonnema and Hegedüs (2012) [17] systematically reviewed the literature on the effects, side effects, and factors affecting therapeutic outcome of radioiodine therapy in benign thyroid diseases. Regarding hypothyroidism in patients treated with RAI for Graves' disease, the effect/time curve was exponential, with a steep increase after the first year post-^{131}I (24%). Approximately; 59% of patients become hypothyroid after 10 years, and 85% after 25 years of exposure [18]. This curve is less steep and more linear in patients with non-immunogenic hyperthyroidism (toxic nodules or goiter), with the percentage of a 4% hypothyroid patients after 1 year, 15% after 10 years, and 32% after 25 years [18].

4.4.2 External Beam Radiotherapy (EBRT)

If external beam radiation therapy (EBRT) of the cervical region is used to treat head and neck cancers, lymphomas, or malignancies of the central nervous system (CNS), exposure of non-target tissues, such as the thyroid gland, cannot be prevented. Hypothyroidism can, therefore, develop months to years after EBRT [19]. In a prospective study from Denmark involving 203 patients with head and neck cancer, the estimated 5-year incidence of EBRT-induced hypothyroidism was 26%. The median thyroid dose amounted to 40 Gy (minimum–maximum: 1.2–68.0 Gy).

Lin et al. (2018) [20] recently published a prospective observational study of 68 patients with naso-pharyngeal cancer for 48 months post-EBRT. In their study, the mean TSH levels increased shortly after RT, peaked at 18–24 months, and then decreased, albeit remaining elevated above an upper level of normal of 4.0 U/L.

Vogelius et al. (2011) [6] reviewed risk factors for hypothyroidism in a meta-analysis involving patients with a variety of malignant diseases needing EBRT of the neck region. They reported that hypothyroidism rarely occurs at doses < 10 Gy; however, there was marked heterogeneity among studies, the most likely cause being differences in follow-up time and intensity. More recently, Inskip et al. (2018) [21] published a report about the incidence of both overt and subclinical hypothyroidism in a large cohort of childhood cancer survivors (n = 12,015) who had been treated with EBRT of the neck, the base of the skull, or both. The cumulative proportion affected with hypothyroidism was highest in patients irradiated for Hodgkin's disease (32.3%) and cancers of the central nervous system (17.7%). The incidence was significantly associated with the radiation dose to the thyroid and the pituitary. Risks of EBRT-induced hypothyroidism were inversely associated with age at exposure and remained elevated for more than 25 years after exposure.

There are several reasons why lower thyroid doses of EBRT induce hypothyroidism with comparable frequency as do four- to fivefold higher doses of "internal radiotherapy" with ^{131}I. There is evidence from studies in children that in patients treated with EBRT, hypothyroidism may be induced directly by irradiation of the thyroid and indirectly too, if the pituitary, which controls the thyroid, is in the radiation field (e.g., in tumors of the skull base). Another reason may be that ß-particles of ^{131}I taken up by thyroid cells have a short range of only 0.4 mm in tissue, so that blood vessels supplying the thyroid are out of range, which is not the case in EBRT, where structures adjacent to the thyroid also are irradiated [21].

4.4.3 Diagnostic Radiation Exposure

Relative to planar radiography, computed tomography (CT) scans of the head and neck region may expose the thyroid gland to comparably high doses of up to 10–20 mGy in adults, as noted earlier by Sinnott et al. (2010) [22] and Su et al. [23]. Doses in children are higher, up to 30–50 mGy [24], and in both pediatric and adult patients, the use of iodinated contrast media may increase doses by up to 35% [25]. Nevertheless, these doses are much lower—by three to four orders of magnitude—compared to those associated with EBRT or RAI. No publications report an increased incidence of thyroiditis or hypothyroidism after diagnostic radiation exposure of the thyroid by CT scan [10].

4.4.4 Atomic Bombing Survivors (Hiroshima and Nagasaki)

Imaizumi et al. (2017) [26] summarized the current knowledge about thyroid dysfunction and autoimmune thyroiditis among atomic bomb survivors from Hiroshima and Nagasaki. The mean age at the examination of these survivors was 68.2 ± 2.7 years. Thyroid radiation doses ranged from 0 to 4.0 Gy, with a mean of 0.182 Gy. Hypothyroidism (subclinical or overt) was detected in 4.8% (129/2668) of the exposed people. Of the patients with overt hypothyroidism, 44% (57/129; 2.1% of the overall cohort) were thyroid autoantibody-positive and 56% (72/129; 2.7% of the overall cohort) thyroid autoantibody-negative. Additionally, 21.5% (573/2668) of the subgroup were antibody-positive without thyroid dysfunction. Most importantly, no significant association of TSH concentration or antibody detectability with thyroid radiation dose was found.

4.4.5 Nuclear Reactor Accidents (Chernobyl Accident, 1986)

After the Chernobyl accident of 1986, hypothyroidism was detected in 4/83 (4.8%) of the emergency workers with the highest radiation exposure among those treated for acute radiation syndrome at Burnasyan Federal Medical Biophysical Center of the Federal Medical Biological Agency in Moscow. Hypothyroidism developed during the first 5 years in three of the four cases, developing later in one case. The highest thyroid dose reported in these four patients amounted to 11 Gy; however, thyroid doses for the whole cohort of 83 ARS patients were not available [27].

Oustroumova et al. investigated subjects from the Ukraine (n = 11,853) [28] or Belarus (n = 10,827) [29] who were children and adolescents <18 years old at the time of the Chernobyl accident. They reported significant associations between the presence of subclinical hypothyroidism (TSH >4 mU/L) and thyroid hormone levels within the reference range, and cumulative thyroid radiation doses in both cohorts. In the Ukrainian cohort [28], 6.1% (719/11,853) had subclinical hypothyroidism, and 0.1% (14/11,853) had overt hypothyroidism with decreased levels (<10 pmol/L) of serum-free thyroxin. In the Belarus cohort [29], 2.8% (301/10,827) had subclinical hypothyroidism and 0.2% (18/10,827) had overt hypothyroidism. The risk for hypothyroidism decreased with increasing age at exposure or examination and was similar for males and females. TPO-Abs were found in 5.7% of the subjects investigated, with no positive association of the antibodies' presence with the radiation dose.

4.5 Clinical Picture

4.5.1 History-Taking/Symptoms

There are three phases in most thyroiditis types. They include thyrotoxic, hypothyroid, and euthyroid. Radiation-induced thyroiditis and Hashimoto's thyroiditis usually stay in the hypo-thyroid phase. The euthyroid phase may follow the thyrotoxic phase before hypothyroidism or after inflammation stabilizes and the thyroid gland recovers.

History of recent radiation to the neck or radioactive iodine (RAI) treatment could indicate radiation-induced thyroiditis, and symptoms will depend on its phase. The common symptoms of the "thyrotoxicosis phase" include palpitation, enhanced appetite, weight loss, anxiety, irritability, sleep disturbances (e.g., insomnia), sweating, heat sensitivity, and fine tremors. The common symptoms of the "hypothyroid phase" include fatigue, weight gain, constipation, depression, dry skin, cold sensitivity, muscle weakness, and focus issues [30]. Neck pain and tenderness usually develop 5–10 days following radiation treatment. Symptoms are usually mild and subside spontaneously in a week.

4.5.2 Physical Examination

On local physical examination of the thyroid gland, the majority of patients with radiation-induced thyroiditis have a tender and inflamed gland.

4.6 Evaluation/Work-Up

4.6.1 Thyroid Panel

The thyroid panel thoroughly investigates the different thyroid hormones (TSH, T3, T4, free T3, and free T4) as well as antibodies that may be associated with thyroiditis. Since there are different phases of thyroiditis, this functional laboratory test should be considered one of the main laboratory tests for radiation-induced thyroiditis.

4.6.2 Inflammatory Markers

Inflammatory markers should also be assessed when investigating acute thyroiditis. Two markers are commonly used: C-reactive protein (CRP) and erythrocyte sedimentation rate (ESR).

Typically, CRP levels may be elevated during the acute phase of thyroiditis, when the condition first occurs, and ESR may be elevated after the acute phase.

4.6.3 Micro-nutrient Panel

Nutrients such as vitamin D, zinc, and others are needed for optimal thyroid function. Although nutrient deficiencies are not the underlying cause of radiation-induced thyroiditis, this test should be included as a comprehensive approach to addressing this condition. This micro-nutrient panel will analyze various nutrients associated with thyroid function and overall health.

4.6.4 Imaging Studies

Imaging of the thyroid by a thyroid ultrasound is necessary to assess the health of the thyroid gland itself.

4.7 Treatment

4.7.1 Conventional Treatment of Radiation-Induced Thyroiditis

Generally, therapy should be directed toward the primary disease rather than the thyroid, but administration of thyroid hormone may be necessary if destruction of thyroid tissue is sufficient to produce hypothyroidism. The conventional treatment of radiation-induced thyroiditis commonly involves medications and is based on the phase of thyroiditis and its symptoms.

Treatment of radiation-induced thyroiditis is mainly symptomatic with non-steroidal anti-inflammatory drugs (NSAIDs) or prednisone in severe cases. Beta-blockers are often used during the thyrotoxic phase to decrease the associated symptoms such as palpitation and tremors. Medications such as levothyroxine may be prescribed during the hypothyroid phase to increase T4 levels, which are usually low during this phase [30].

In any case, follow-up of thyroid function after EBRT or RAI is mandatory so that patients with hypothyroidism needing thyroid hormone replacement will not be overlooked. In populations exposed to accidental radiation, a conservative threshold dose of 3–5 Gy for the most vulnerable group of children and adolescents is proposed, which should be implemented in emergency management plans including long-term follow-up of this group [10].

4.7.2 Functional Medicine Treatment of Radiation-Induced Thyroiditis

Functional medicine approaches for radiation-induced thyroiditis include personalized nutrition, targeted supplements to support the thyroid, and other integrative approaches such as exercise.

4.7.2.1 Nutrition Considerations

As thyroiditis involves inflammation, the right nutritional plan can help reduce it. The "Mediterranean diet" is an excellent choice. It includes fresh fruits, vegetables, herbs, and healthy fats like olive oil, nuts, fatty fish, whole grains, beans, and legumes. This type of diet has anti-inflammatory effects, which can be helpful in radiation-induced thyroiditis.

If there is an autoimmune component, a gluten-free diet might help, as cutting out gluten can lessen the autoimmune process and inflammation. Also, adding iodine-rich foods like seaweed can improve thyroid function. Ideally, iodine should be incorporated into a treatment protocol as part of the nutritional plan for these patients.

4.7.2.2 Supplements

The following supplements are helpful for patients with radiation-induced thyroiditis:

- *Zinc*: Zinc has been shown to have anti-inflammatory effects and reduce CRP levels, which can be helpful in radiation-induced thyroiditis. This nutrient also plays a role in thyroid regulation. The recommended dose to reduce inflammation is up to 40–50 mg/day [31].
- *L-Carnitine*: This form of amino acid has been shown to help manage thyroiditis, especially in its thyrotoxicosis phase, and can reduce the symptoms associated with this phase. The recommended dose is 2–4 g daily [32].
- *Vitamin D*: Insufficient vitamin D levels have been linked with thyroid dysfunction and should be considered as part of a treatment therapy for thyroiditis. Sufficient vitamin D levels can be beneficial during the hypo-thyroid phase. A vitamin D dose of 50,000 IU is helpful with hypothyroid patients [33].
- *Omega 3*: This supplement has been shown to reduce pro-inflammatory cytokines and may help reduce inflammatory responses in thyroiditis. This essential fatty acid can also reduce CRP markers related to inflammation. The general daily recommended dose is 1000 mg.

References

1. Jereczek-Fossa BA, Alterio D, Jassem J, Gibelli B, Tradati N, Orecchia R. Radiotherapy-induced thyroid disorders. Cancer Treat Rev. 2004;30(4):369–84.
2. Nakhla SF, Fadel SH, Al-adawi MH, Morsi MI. Evaluation of radiation-induced thyroid disorders in non-thyroid head and neck cancers in childhood. Int J Cancer Biomed Res. 2022;6(3):11–8.
3. Nagayama Y. Radiation-related thyroid autoimmunity and dysfunction. J Radiat Res. 2018;59(2):98–107.
4. Clifton KH. Thyroid and mammary radiobiology: radiogenic damage to glandular tissue. Br J Cancer Suppl. 1986;7:237–50.

5. Ron E, Brenner A. Non-malignant thyroid diseases after a wide range of radiation exposures. Radiat Res. 2010;174:877–88.
6. Vogelius IR, Bentzen SM, Maraldo MV, Petersen PM. Specht L risk factors for radiation-induced hypothyroidism: a literature-based meta-analysis. Cancer. 2011;117:5250–60.
7. Peters H, Fischer C, Bogner U, Reiners C, Schleusener H. Treatment of Graves' hyperthyroidism with radioiodine: results of a prospective randomized study. Thyroid. 1997;7:247–51.
8. Digkas E, Smith DR, Wennstig AK, Matikas A, Tegnelius E, Valachis A. Incidence and risk factors of hypothyroidism after treatment for early breast cancer: a population-based cohort study. Breast Cancer Res Treat. 2024;204:79–87.
9. Bakhshandeh M, Hashemi B, Mahdavi SR, Nikoofar A, Edraki HR, Kazemnejad A. Evaluation of thyroid disorders during head-and-neck radiotherapy by using functional analysis and ultrasonography. Int J Radiat Oncol Biol Phys. 2012;83(1):198–203.
10. Reiners C, Drozd V, Yamashita S. Hypothyroidism after radiation exposure: brief narrative review. J Neural Transm (Vienna). 2020;127(11):1455–66.
11. Stubblefield MD. Clinical evaluation and management of radiation fibrosis syndrome. Phys Med Rehabil Clin N Am. 2017;28(1):89–100.
12. Miller MC, Agrawal A. Hypothyroidism in postradiation head and neck cancer patients: incidence, complications, and management. Curr Opin Otolaryngol Head Neck Surg. 2009;17(2):111–5.
13. Alterio D, Jereczek-Fossa BA, Franchi B, D'Onofrio A, Piazzi V, Rondi E, et al. Thyroid disorders in patients treated with radiotherapy for head-and-neck cancer: a retrospective analysis of seventy-three patients. Int J Radiat Oncol Biol Phys. 2007;67(1):144–50.
14. Riley AS, McKenzie GAG, Green V, Schettino G, England RJA, Greenman J. The effect of radioiodine treatment on the diseased thyroid gland. Int J Radiat Biol. 2019;95:1718–27.
15. Dunkelmann S, Wolf R, Koch A, Kittner C, Groth P, Schuemichen C. Incidence of radiation-induced Graves' disease in patients treated with radioiodine for thyroid autonomy before and after introduction of a high-sensitivity TSH receptor antibody assay. Eur J Nucl Med Mol Imaging. 2004;31:1428–34.
16. Nagayama Y. Thyroid autoimmunity and thyroid cancer—the pathogenic connection: a 2018 update. Horm Metab Res. 2018;50:922–31.
17. Bonnema SJ, Heged L. Radioiodine therapy in benign thyroid diseases: effects, side effects, and factors affecting therapeutic outcome. Endocr Rev. 2012;33(6):80–92.
18. Metso S, Jaatinen P, Huhtala H, Luukkaala T, Oksala H, Salmi J. Long-term follow-up study of radioiodine treatment of hyperthyroidism. Clin Endocrinol. 2004;61:641–8.
19. Rønjom MF, Brink C, Bentzen SM, Hegedüs L, Overgaard J, Petersen JB, et al. External validation of a normal tissue complication probability model for radiation-induced hypothyroidism in an independent cohort. Acta Oncol. 2015;5:1301–9.
20. Lin Z, Yang Z, He B, Wang D, Gao X, Tam SY, et al. Pattern of radiation-induced thyroid gland changes in nasopharyngeal carcinoma patients in 48 months after radiotherapy. PLoS One. 2018;13:e0200310.
21. Inskip PD, Veiga LHS, Brenner AV, Sigurdson AJ, Ostroumova E, Chow EJ, et al. Hypothyroidism after radiation therapy for childhood cancer: a report from the childhood cancer survivor study. Radiat Res. 2018;190:117–32.
22. Sinnott B, Ron E, Schneider AB. Exposing the thyroid to radiation: a review of its current extent, risks, and implications. Endocr Rev. 2010;31:756–73.
23. Su YP, Niu HW, Chen JB, Fu YH, Xiao GB, Sun QF. Radiation dose in the thyroid and the thyroid cancer risk attributable to CT scans for pediatric patients in one general hospital of China. Int J Environ Res Public Health. 2014;11:2793–803.
24. Spampinato MV, Tipnis S, Tavernier J, Huda W. Thyroid doses and risk to paediatric patients undergoing neck CT examinations. Eur Radiol. 2015;25:1883–90.
25. Dawson P, Punwani S. The thyroid dose burden in medical imaging: a re-examination. Eur J Radiol. 2009;69:74–9.

26. Imaizumi M, Ohishi W, Nakashima E, Sera N, Neriishi K, Yamada M, et al. Thyroid dysfunction and autoimmune thyroid diseases among atomic bomb survivors exposed in childhood. J Clin Endocrinol Metab. 2017;102:2516–24.
27. United Nations Scientific Committee on the Effects of Atomic Radiation. Sources and effects of ionizing radiation. UNSCEAR 2008 report to the general assembly with scientific annexes. Volume II Scientific annexes C, D and E. New York: United Nations; 2011.
28. Ostroumova E, Brenner A, Oliynyk V, McConnell R, Robbins J, Terekhova G, et al. Subclinical hypothyroidism after radioiodine exposure: Ukrainian-American cohort study of thyroid cancer and other thyroid diseases after the Chornobyl accident (1998–2000). Environ Health Perspect. 2009;117:745–50.
29. Ostroumova E, Rozhko A, Hatch M, Furukawa K, Polyanskaya O, McConnell RJ, et al. Measures of thyroid function among Belarusian children and adolescents exposed to iodine-131 from the accident at the Chernobyl nuclear plant. Environ Health Perspect. 2013;121:865–71.
30. Ma C, Xie J, Wang H, Li J, Chen S. Radioiodine therapy versus antithyroid medications for Graves' disease. Cochrane Database Syst Rev. 2016;2(2):CD010094.
31. Mousavi SM, Djafarian K, Mojtahed A, Varkaneh HK, Shab-Bidar S. The effect of zinc supplementation on plasma C-reactive protein concentrations: a systematic review and meta-analysis of randomized controlled trials. Eur J Pharmacol. 2018;834:10–6.
32. Benvenga S, Amato A, Calvani M, Trimarchi F. Effects of carnitine on thyroid hormone action. Ann N Y Acad Sci. 2004;1033:158–67.
33. Talaei A, Ghorbani F, Asemi Z. The effects of vitamin D supplementation on thyroid function in hypothyroid patients: a randomized, double-blind, placebo-controlled trial. Indian J Endocrinol Metab. 2018;22(5):584–8.

Subacute (de Quervain's) Thyroiditis

5

5.1 Introduction

The term "subacute thyroiditis" (SAT) is used for several different causes of thyroiditis: de Quervain's (granulomatous) thyroiditis, silent thyroiditis, post-partum thyroiditis, and palpation thyroiditis [1]. "De Quervain's thyroiditis" is commonly known as (painful) "subacute thyroiditis" (SAT), but also termed "subacute non-suppurative thyroiditis," "granulomatous thyroiditis," "pseudo-tuberculous thyroiditis," "pseudo-giant cell thyroiditis," "giant cell thyroiditis," "migratory thyroiditis," "creeping thyroiditis," and "struma granulomatosa."

de Quervain's thyroiditis is a spontaneously remitting inflammatory condition of the thyroid gland that may last for a week to several months and is characterized by a triphasic course of transient thyrotoxicosis, followed by hypothyroidism and by a return to euthyroidism [2–4]. It is the most common cause of "painful" thyroiditis and a common cause of thyroid dysfunction, mainly thyrotoxicosis. It is most likely of post-viral origin and characteristically has the tendency to recur. The gland is typically involved as a whole, and thyroidal radioactive iodine uptake (RAIU) is much depressed. Transient hyper-thyroxinemia, elevation of the serum thyroglobulin (Tg) concentration and the erythrocyte sedimentation rate (ESR), and sometimes the white cell count (WBC) during the early acute phase are characteristic if not pathognomonic. The incidence rate of SAT has maintained an upward trend in recent years. Recurrence and prolonged treatment time have become severe problems for the treatment of SAT [5, 6].

5.2 Epidemiology

Subacute thyroiditis (SAT) is encountered in up to 5% of patients with thyroid disease [7]. Woolner et al. (1957) [8] collected 162 cases diagnosed on clinical grounds at the Mayo Clinic over a 5-year period; during the same time, 1250 patients with Graves' disease were seen. Thus, SAT had approximately one-eighth the incidence

M. Sakr, *Thyroiditis*, https://doi.org/10.1007/978-3-032-19513-5_5

of Graves' disease in this clinical population. Between 1970 and 1997, in the Epidemiology Project in Olmsted County (Minnesota), 94 patients with SAT were identified [9]. They reported an incidence of 12.1 cases/100,000/year with a 3–6 times higher incidence in women than in men (19.1 and 4.1 per 100,000/year, respectively). It is most common in young adulthood (24/100,000/year) and middle age (35/100,000/year), with a peak incidence between the second and fifth decade of life, and it decreases in frequency with increasing age. Although the disease has been described by many authors at all ages, it is rare in children [4, 10]. Several authors reported that female patients have outnumbered male patients in a ratio of 1.9–6:1, with a preponderance of cases in the third to fifth decades of life [3, 8, 11–13].

During an evaluation of the different causes of hypothyroidism over a 4-year period in Denmark, Carle et al. reported, in 2006, an incidence of SAT of 1.8% in a cohort of 685 patients with hypothyroidism [14]. Moreover, SAT has been reported by some researchers as a rare cause of hyperthyroidism in pregnancy [15, 16].

Some investigators have reported a higher rate of SAT during the summer months, reflecting the peak incidence of coxsackie virus A and B and echovirus infections [17]. In the Italian series by Martino et al. (1987) [18], the reported onset of SAT was predominant between June and September, with almost 50% of the cases between July and August, thus confirming the overlapping seasonal distribution of SAT and enterovirus infections. Similarly, Japanese data from 1061 SAT patients by Iitaka et al. (1996) [19] indicated a higher frequency of SAT cases in summer than in winter. However, other authors found no significant differences in distribution throughout the year. Although seasonal differences may be observed in a mild climate contrast like Italy's, no statistically significant seasonal variation was found in studies from Minnesota [12] and Finland [20] where the periodic climatic contrast is much more severe [21].

5.3 Etiology/Pathophysiology

5.3.1 Overview

A post-viral cytokine-mediated inflammation of the thyroid is suspected as the cause of SAT because of the seasonal frequency and association with upper respiratory tract infection or sore throats, though definite evidence is lacking [22]. In 50% of patients, antibodies against mumps, measles, influenza, adenovirus, Coxsackie virus, or echovirus are found. Earlier suggestions that the disease may represent a bacterial infection have been disproven. A strong association with genetic predisposition with the haplotype HLA-Bw35 has also been reported [23]. An autoimmune reaction is also unlikely. The development during the illness of cell-mediated immunity against various thyroid cell particulate fractions or crude antigens appears to be related to the release of these materials during tissue destruction [24, 25].

5.3.2 Viral Cause

5.3.2.1 Mumps and Other Viruses

Although the search for a viral cause has usually been unrewarding, a few cases have been associated with the virus that causes mumps [3, 26]. The disease has occurred in an epidemic form. High titers of mumps antibodies have been found in some patients with SAT, and occasionally parotitis or orchitis are associated with the thyroiditis. The mumps virus has been cultured directly from thyroid tissue involved in SAT. Although the mumps virus may be one discrete etiologic factor, the disease has also been reported in association with other viral conditions, including measles, influenza, H1N1 influenza [27], adenovirus infection, infectious mononucleosis (IMN) [28], myocarditis, human immuno-deficiency virus (HIV) [29], cat scratch fever, and coxsackie virus [30]. In addition, SAT has been reported following hand-foot-mouth disease due to coxsackie B4 [31], cytomegalovirus (CMV) [32], hepatitis E virus [33, 34], and scrub typhus infection [35]. Case reports suggesting SAT as a rare facet of Dengue expanded syndrome have also been published [36–38].

Recently (2020), SAT has been associated with SARS-COV-2/COVID 19 infection [39]. Two previous (1998) comprehensive studies [40, 41] did not find evidence of enteroviruses in 27 patients and Epstein-Barr virus (EBV) or CMV in 10 patients, respectively, but a single case report by Espino Montoro et al. (2000) has implicated EBV in a case of SAT with typical clinical features [42], and CMV has been reported in 2008 by Al Maawali et al. in an infant [43].

Numerous attempts to culture viruses from cases not associated with mumps have failed. Virus-like particles have been demonstrated in the follicular epithelium of a single patient suffering from SAT [30]. However, viral antibody titers to common respiratory tract viruses are often elevated in these patients. Since the titers fall promptly, and multiple viral antibodies may appear in the same patient, the titer elevation may represent an anamnestic response to the inflammatory condition. It is likely that the thyroid gland could respond with thyroiditis after invasion by a variety of different viruses, but no single agent is likely to be causative [44].

5.3.2.2 SARS-COV-2 Infection and Subacute Thyroiditis

Severe acute respiratory syndrome coronavirus 2 (SARSCoV-2) has infected more than 190 million people worldwide, and the pandemic is still spreading. The first case of SAT after a SARS-CoV-2 infection was published from Italy in 2020 [39]. Although additional cases were soon reported, this entity is likely under-recognized [45–47].

A case series of four patients with SAT after SARS-COV-2 infection was published by Brancatella et al. (2020) [39]. In this case series, all four patients were female (age, 29–46 years). SAT developed 16–36 days after the resolution of coronavirus disease 2019 (COVID-19). Neck pain radiated to the jaw, and palpitations were the main presenting symptoms and were associated with fever and asthenia. One patient was hospitalized because of atrial fibrillation. Laboratory exams during the acute phase of SAT, available for three patients, were typical of destructive thyroiditis: thyroid hormones, and particularly free thyroxin, were increased, TSH was low to undetectable, serum thyroglobulin was high, and TSH receptor antibodies were undetectable.

At neck ultrasound (performed in all patients), the thyroid was enlarged, with diffuse and bilateral hypoechoic areas. At color Doppler ultrasonography (performed in three patients), thyroid vascularization was absent. One patient had a thyroid scintiscan with 99mtechnetium (^{99m}Tc), which showed absent uptake, as typical of the destructive phase of SAT. Symptoms subsided in all patients a few days after starting treatment (prednisone 25 mg/day in three patients and non-steroidal anti-inflammatory drug [NASID] in one patient). Six weeks after the onset of SAT symptoms, inflammatory markers had returned to normal range in all patients. Two patients were euthyroid and two were diagnosed with subclinical hypothyroidism. No patient experienced a relapse of COVID-19.

Expression of the mRNA encoding for the ACE-2 receptor has been documented in thyroid follicular cells, making them a potential target for SARS-COV-2 entry [48]. The expression of ACE-2 mRNA in follicular cells was confirmed by analyzing primary cultures of thyroid cells, which expressed the ACE-2 mRNA at levels similar to those in thyroid tissues. It is important to note that, as recently demonstrated in 2020, SARS-CoV-2 infection requires the ACE-2 receptor to coexist with type II serine protease trans-membranes (TMPRSS2) [49].

More recently (2021), three cases of SAT were reported from Turkey after inactivated SARS-CoV-2 vaccination (CoronaVac®) was administered. Three female healthcare workers presented with anterior neck pain and fatigue 4–7 days after SARS-CoV-2 vaccination and were diagnosed with SAT, as a part of an autoimmune/inflammatory syndrome induced by adjuvants (ASIA syndrome). This can be seen as a post-vaccination phenomenon that occurs after exposure to adjuvants in vaccines that increase the immune responses. However, two of these patients were in the post-partum period, which may have facilitated the development of ASIA syndrome after the SARS-CoV-2 vaccination [50]

5.3.3 Genetic Predisposition

The association of SAT with specific genetic backgrounds has been postulated since 1975, when predisposition to SAT was found to be related to human leukocyte antigen (HLA) genes [51]. HLA alleles were demonstrated not only to increase the risk of SAT, but also to correlate with SAT clinical course and its risk of recurrence [51]. Histocompatibility studies show that 72% of patients with subacute thyroiditis manifest HLA-BW35 [52]. There are two main hypotheses: (i) the HLA-B35-restricted viral antigen presentation hypothesis suggests that viral antigens may cross-react with host antigens, resulting in tissue destruction; (ii) viral infection may cause direct damage to thyroidal tissue, releasing high quantities of self-antigens, that may be recognized as foreign by HLA-B35, leading to the development of an autoimmune process and further tissue damage [53]. Familial occurrence of SAT associated with HLA-B35 has been reported by several investigators [53–56].

The correlation between SAT occurrence and the presence of HLA-B*18:01 and DRB1*01, as well as HLA-C*04:01 has been demonstrated, with the latter one being in linkage disequilibrium with a well-known SAT risk haplotype HLA-B*35 [5]. These new three antigens, together with the known HLA-B*35, allow confirmation of a genetic predisposition in almost all patients with SAT. The haplotypes HLA-B*18:01, -DRB1*01, and HLA-B*35 are all independent SAT risk factors. Recent studies demonstrated for the first time that the risk of SAT recurrence is indeed HLA-dependent, and the high-risk group includes patients with co-occurrence of HLA-B*18:01 and -B*35 [5]. It seems that the presence of HLA B18:01 significantly changes the course of SAT. The risk of recurrence was significantly influenced by the presence of HLA-B*18:01, but only with the concurrent presence of HLA-B*35. However, the demonstration that the co-occurrence of HLA-B*18:01 and -B*35 carries the risk of SAT recurrence should be confirmed in further studies.

A susceptibility to SAT seems to be genetically influenced, and it has been suggested that SAT might occur by transmission of viral infection in genetically predisposed individuals [43]. A reported association between SAT and acute febrile neutrophilic dermatosis (Sweet's syndrome) [57, 58] may imply a common role for cytokines in both these conditions.

Several authors have also reported other possible associations between SAT and haplotypes such as HLA-Dw1, HLA-DRw8, HLA-B67, and HLA-Cw3. However, these studies applied mostly serological methods, and only some associations were confirmed when high-resolution methods were used [59].

5.3.4 Immune Alteration

New treatments, particularly those in which there is manipulation of the immune system, have led to the development of a SAT-like clinical course [60]. Infusion of interleukin-2 (IL-2) caused hyper-thyroxinemia with a low radioiodine uptake in six patients who received this in combination with tumor necrosis factor-alpha (TNF-α) or gamma (γ) interferon [61]. The patients proceeded through the pattern of hyperthyroidism followed by transient hypothyroidism, with a re-establishment of normal thyroid function typical of patients with autoimmune painless thyroiditis. However, none of the patients had detectable anti-thyroid antibodies. This condition is thus intermediate between subacute lymphocytic (painless) thyroiditis and subacute thyroiditis, which is typically painful.

The advent of immunotherapy has revolutionized cancer therapy. Immune checkpoint inhibitors (ICI) are a group of monoclonal antibodies that target the receptors cytotoxic T-lymphocyte antigen 4 (CTLA-4) and programmed cell death protein 1 (PD-1) or its associated ligand (PD-L-1). The thyroid gland is the endocrine gland most frequently affected in association with immune checkpoint inhibitors (ICIs). With the increase in use of immunotherapy for various malignancies, thyroid immune-related adverse events (irAE) have been reported to be on the rise [62]. Thyroid dysfunction has been more frequently associated with PD-1 inhibitors rather than CTLA-4 inhibitors [63]. About 20% of the patients receiving PD-1 inhibitors present with thyroid dysfunction, occurring early in the course of treatment (median onset 6 weeks after first infusion) [64, 65]. The exact underlying patho-physiological mechanisms for the development of thyroid irAEs are still unclear. It has been suggested to be secondary to destructive, immune-mediated thyroiditis and may include T-cell, NK-cell, and/or monocyte-mediated pathways [66]. However, the onset and clinical manifestations are highly variable and not all patients develop the classic thyroiditis-like presentation [67]. Based on the limited data available, the PD-1 inhibitor- induced thyroiditis may histologically present as a granulomatous inflammation with active destruction of thyroid follicles [68].

In a study by de Filette et al. (2016), thyroid function was prospectively monitored in patients with melanoma receiving PD-1 inhibitor therapy. The authors reported that most patients presenting with thyrotoxicosis developed hypothyroidism within 1–3 months [64]. A recent study by Muir et al. (2021) looked at thyroid dysfunction in patients with melanoma undergoing CTLA-4 or PD-1-based treatment and reported many distinct phenotypes [69]. Of the 1246 patients studied, 42% developed thyroid irAEs. The most common presentation was subclinical hyperthyroidism followed by overt hyperthyroidism, subclinical hypothyroidism, and overt hypothyroidism.

The most common thyroid dysfunction in SAT is thyrotoxicosis followed by hypothyroidism. Incidences of hypothyroidism were lower with the anti-CTLA-4 antibody (2.5–5.2%) than with anti-PD-1/anti-PD-L1 (3.9–8.5%), while combination therapy was associated with the highest estimated incidence (10.2–16.4%). Similarly, for thyrotoxicosis, differences according to the class of ICIs had been reported, with ipilimumab having low frequencies (0.2–1.7%), anti-PD-1/anti-PD-L1 drugs having higher frequencies (0.6–3.7%), and combination therapy having the highest frequency (8.0–11.1%) [70]. Moreover, the risk of thyrotoxicosis was significantly greater with anti-PD-1 antibodies than with anti-PD-L1 antibodies, and differences among anti-PD-1 drugs were also observed, with nivolumab having a lower risk for hyperthyroidism than pembrolizumab [70].

In the majority of the patients who develop thyroid dysfunction, ICI therapy can be continued, unless they experience symptoms of severe thyrotoxicosis or there is concern for thyroid storm [71]. Current guidelines recommend initiation of beta-blockers for symptomatic relief, and if there is persistence of hypothyroidism, levothyroxine should be initiated after ruling out adrenal insufficiency, which can also occur with ICI therapy.

Patients have developed SAT after influenza vaccination, suggesting immune alteration as a contributory factor. The exact mechanism is not known, but the presumed pathogenesis of SAT after vaccinations may involve the autoimmune/inflammatory syndrome induced by adjuvants (ASIA) [72], an immune reaction triggered by a class of excipients named adjuvants, primarily used in vaccines, which could cause dysregulation of both the innate and adaptive immune systems [73]. A second hypothesis involves molecular mimicry; a recent in vitro study [74] found that antibodies directed against SARS-CoV-2 antigens could cross-react with self-tissue antigens, including thyroid peroxidase (TPO). This mechanism represents a potential pathogenic trigger for immune-mediated adverse events both after SARS-CoV-2 infections [75] and SARS-CoV-2 vaccination. A possible association between HLA genotypes and vaccine-induced SAT has been described [76, 77].

In patients with chronic hepatitis C, studies following interferon therapy (IFN) have shown that a minority (15%) developed a destructive thyroiditis while others had a mild elevation of thyroid-stimulating hormone (TSH) [61–71, 78–81]. Interferon (IFN) can exacerbate previous thyroid autoimmunity and cause destructive thyroidal changes de novo. Subacute thyroiditis has also been noted in patients treated with combination therapy of IFN plus ribavirin for this disease [82, 83] as well as during treatment of hepatitis B with interferon-α [84]. Peginterferon alpha-2a has been reported to cause SAT [85], and the condition has been seen in Takayasu's arteritis suggesting an immune abnormality [86]. On the other hand, SAT has also been reported in patients receiving long-term immunosuppressive therapy suggesting a minimal role for activating autoimmunity in the condition [87, 88]. A phase 2 trial conducted with alemtuzumab, a monoclonal anti-CD52 antibody for relapsing and remitting type of multiple sclerosis found that 34% of the subjects developed thyroid dysfunction and 4% had SAT [89]. The use of TNF inhibitor therapy has been reported to be associated with thyroid dysfunction that closely resembles SAT [90, 91]. A recent report of SAT associated with the use of the kinase inhibitor, dasatinib, has been published by Vazquez Friol et al. in 2020 [92]. Other reports of the occurrence of a SAT-like picture with renal cell carcinoma [93], following the administration of cardiac catheterization dye [94] after gastric bypass [95] or after ginger ingestion [96] do not clearly contribute to an enhanced understanding of its etiology.

It is worth mentioning that vitamin D has been proposed as a protective factor. Calapkulu et al. (2020) [97] recently reported that 25(OH) vitamin D levels in SAT patients are significantly lower compared to the healthy control group, though with no effect on disease prognosis, development of permanent hypothyroidism, development or recurrence rate. This could be a consequence of the protective effect of vitamin D on respiratory tract infections [98].

5.4 Pathology

5.4.1 Gross Appearance

The thyroid gland may be adherent to its capsule or to the strap muscles, but it can usually be dissected free, a feature distinguishing subacute thyroiditis (SAT) from Riedel's thyroiditis. The involved tissue appears yellowish or white in color and is firmer in consistency than normal. The thyroid gland is enlarged, usually bilaterally and uniform, but may be asymmetrical, with predominant involvement of one lobe. Although the lesion may extend to the capsular surface, it can also be confined to the thyroid parenchyma or merely be palpable as a suspiciously hard area.

Macroscopically, yellow-white, solidified foci of different sizes are visible, which occur focally, asymmetrically, or less often, bilaterally. The macroscopic pathological picture of SAT frequently bears a striking resemblance to a thyroid malignancy. The lesion is firm-to-hard in consistency, pale white in color, and has poorly defined margins that encroach irregularly on the adjacent normal thyroid.

5.4.2 Histological Appearance

Histologically, there is a characteristic picture of a granulomatous inflammatory reaction in SAT with focal destruction of the follicular epithelial cells. Due to the destruction of the follicles in the early stages of the disease, colloid emerges; neutrophils dominate, which can form granulomas with central micro-abscesses [99]. In the florid phase, lymphocytes, histiocytes, and plasma cells predominate in the inflammatory infiltrate. The typical granulomas of this phase consist of cell necrosis, macrophages, multi-nucleated colloid phagocytic giant cells, and lymphocytes [100]. The regeneration phase is characterized by focal fibrosis of the affected thyroid area with regenerative cell and nuclear changes in the immediately adjacent unaffected thyroid tissue. The characteristic juxta-position of the different histological stages of inflammation indicates that the disease is evolving in parallel zones [99].

Microscopically, a mixture of subacute, chronic, and granulomatous inflammatory changes associated with zones of parenchymal destruction and scar tissue may be seen. Early infiltration with polymorphonuclear leukocytes (PNLs) is replaced by lymphocytes and macrophages. The normal follicles may be largely replaced by an inflammatory reaction, but a few small follicles containing colloid remain (Fig. 5.1). The most distinctive microscopic feature is the granuloma, consisting of giant cells clustered about foci of degenerating thyroid follicles (Fig. 5.1). Mast cells play an important part in the repair process of thyroid tissue affected by the disease via production of growth factors and biomolecules which modulate thyroid folliculogenesis and angiogenesis [101]. The early literature contains reports of tuberculous thyroiditis, a diagnosis largely based on the granulomatous tissue reaction, from which the term "pseudo-tuberculous thyroiditis" arose [8].

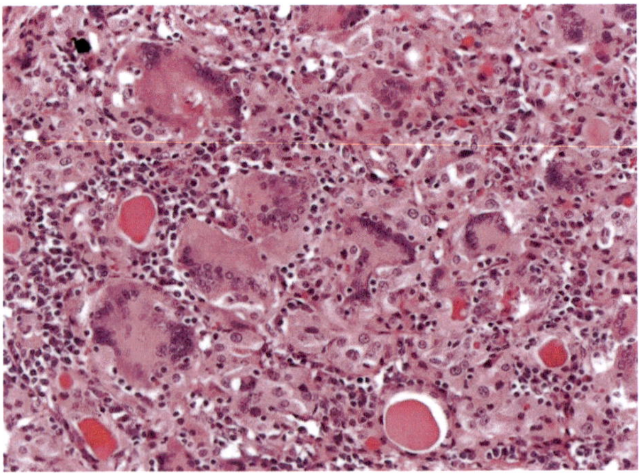

Fig. 5.1 Subacute thyroiditis. Microscopic findings show numerous foreign body giant cells and chronic inflammatory infiltrate consisting of lymphocytes and plasma cells. A few residual thyroid follicles with colloid can be seen. H&E stain

5.4.3 Electron Microscopy

Three-dimensional cytomorphological analysis of fine needle aspiration biopsy (FNAB) samples from patients with SAT examined with scanning and transmission electron microscopy has shown a loss of a uniform, honeycomb cellular arrangement and variation in size and a decrease or shortening of micro-villi in follicular cells together with the appearance of round or ovoid giant cells [102].

5.5 Pathogenesis

Data on the mechanism of inflammation and the pathogenesis of SAT at the cellular level are sparse. However, a study of apoptosis and expression of Bcl 1–2 family proteins in 11 patients with SAT suggests that apoptotic mechanisms may be involved in the development of SAT [103]. Growth factor-rich monocytes/macrophages (containing vascular endothelial growth factor [VEGF], beta-fibroblast growth factor [β-FGF], platelet-derived growth factor [PDGF], and transforming growth factor-beta 1 [TGF- β1]) are involved in the granulomatous stage [104]. Epidermal growth factor [EGF] is important in the regenerative stage as it has mitogenic effects on the thyrocyte. VEGF and beta FGF contribute to angiogenesis at both these stages of the disease.

Factors influencing the severity of the acute phase response during the course of SAT include serum interleukin-1 (IL-1) receptor antagonist, which may have a significant anti-inflammatory role [105]; also, a decrease in tumor necrosis factor-alpha (TNF-α) results in earlier resolution of experimentally induced granulomatous thyroiditis [106]. TNF-related apoptosis-inducing ligand (TRAIL) has also been shown to promote resolution of granulomatous autoimmune thyroiditis in animal models [107].

5.6 Clinical Presentation

5.6.1 Phases of Subacute Thyroiditis (Natural History)

Subacute thyroiditis (SAT) is a self-limited inflammatory thyroid disease that usually has a three-phase course. The first phase of the acute inflammatory process destroys the thyroid follicles and releases thyroid hormones into the circulatory system, resulting in thyrotoxicosis. Then, the thyroid is depleted of stored thyroid hormone, and a phase of hypothyroidism typically occurs. Finally, thyroid hormones and thyroid-stimulating hormone (TSH) levels return to normal as the disease subsides, usually within 12 months [7, 108]. However, some patients may experience recurrence or permanent hypothyroidism during follow-up [109].

5.6.2 Symptoms

Characteristically, the patient with SAT has severe *pain* and extreme tenderness in the thyroid region. At times, the pain begins in one pole and then spreads rapidly to involve the rest of the gland ("creeping thyroiditis"). Pain may radiate to the jaw or the ears. Malaise, fatigue, myalgia and arthralgia are common. A minority of patients have been noted to present with painless or minimally painful SAT following viral symptomatology [110]. These may be regarded as "atypical" SAT patients, but the natural history of their disease is not known. Subacute thyroiditis has been reported to occur during the first trimester of pregnancy [15]. When the symptom is difficulty in swallowing, the disorder may be initially mistaken for pharyngitis. Transient vocal cord paresis may occur [111]. A mild to moderate fever is expected, and at times is high, swinging fever with temperatures above 40.0 °C.

The disease may reach its peak within 3–4 days, subside, and disappear within a week, but more typically, a gradual onset extends over 1–2 weeks and continues with fluctuating intensity for 3–6 weeks. Several recurrences of diminishing intensity extending over many months have also been reported.

5.6.3 Physical Examination

The thyroid gland is typically enlarged two or three times the normal size or larger and is tender to palpation, sometimes exquisitely so. It is typically smooth and firm, but thyroid adherence to surrounding structures, a common feature of Riedel's thyroiditis, is usually minimal or absent. Occasionally, the condition may be confined to one lobe [112, 113]. Approximately, 50% of the patients present during the first weeks of the illness, with symptoms of thyrotoxicosis, including nervousness, heat intolerance, palpitations—(including ventricular tachycardia) [114], tremors, and increased sweating. These symptoms are caused by excessive release of preformed thyroid hormone from the thyroid gland during the acute phase of the inflammatory process. At least three cases of thyroid storm due to SAT have been described in the literature [115, 116], and adverse cardiac outcomes have been reported even in individuals without pre-existing cardiac history or lesions [117].

As the disease process subsides, transient hypothyroidism occurs in approximately 25% of the patients. Ultimately thyroid function returns to normal, and permanent hypothyroidism occurs in less than 10% of cases [2, 11], and recurrence may be noted in approximately 4% [12]. Occasionally, atypical SAT may present as fever of unknown origin [118–120] even in the absence of anterior neck pain or thyrotoxicosis, or associated with other findings and mimicking conditions such as temporal arteritis [121].

In trained athletes, adrenergic manifestations of thyrotoxicosis could be masked by the frequently observed resting bradycardia; less typical signs and symptoms such as undesired weight loss, fatigue, and performance level decrease can be present [122]. In addition, it should be noted that long-term immunosuppressive therapy may lead to a milder clinical presentation of SAT with low pyrexia and minimal neck pain, regardless of the severity of thyrotoxicosis [87].

5.7 Investigations/Diagnosis

5.7.1 Laboratory Studies

5.7.1.1 Inflammatory Markers

Laboratory examination usually discloses a striking elevation of the erythrocyte sedimentation rate (ESR), at times above 100 mm/h, or an elevated level of serum C-reactive protein (CRP), which [123] are useful diagnostic clues. The identification of CRP in salivary samples can also provide a convenient source for documenting the presence of abnormal levels in patients with SAT [124].

5.7.1.2 Hematological Parameters

White blood count (WBC) could also be elevated, with about half of the patients presenting neutrophilia and a positive correlation with granulocyte colony–stimulating factor (G-CSF), at least in the active phase of SAT before treatment [125]. Hematological parameters, such as higher platelet-to-lymphocyte ratio and neutrophil-to-lymphocyte ratio values, are typical in SAT patients compared to healthy control subjects, as well as a lower mean platelet volume value [126, 127], correlating with ESR and CRP parameters [128]. Interleukin-6 (IL-6), a mediator of acute phase response, is also increased in SAT, though no correlation was found between serum concentration of IL-6 and serum-free thyroid hormone values [129].

5.7.1.3 Thyroid Function Tests

In absence of a tissue diagnosis, the characteristic combination of elevated ESR, high serum T4, T3 (T3:T4 <20), and thyroglobulin (Tg) concentrations in the presence of low thyroidal radioactive iodine uptake (RAIU), TSH, and an absent or low titer of circulating thyroid peroxidase (TPO) and Tg antibodies are the most helpful parameters. As compared to Graves' disease, SAT often displays a lower T3/T4 ratio, typically <20 [130, 131]. Peak levels of laboratory abnormalities are reached within 1 week after disease onset, according to a study by Nishihara et al. (2008) [132] analyzing 852 cases of SAT. While the estimation of thyrotropin receptor antibodies (TRAb) in a thyrotoxic patient may be clinically useful in identifying Graves' disease, there have been reports of positive TRAb in patients with SAT although the frequency of this finding is low [133–137].

5.7.1.4 Thyroid Antibodies

Some patients show a positive thyroid antibody pattern. Recently, Stasiak et al. (2019) [138] reported 15.5% anti-thyroid peroxidase antibodies (TPOAb) and 33.3% anti-thyroglobulin antibodies (TgAb) positivity in SAT patients. A Turkish study by Erden et al. (2007) [139] on the local population reported about 4% positivity for TPOAb and about 20% positivity for TgAb. In another more recent study by Nishihara et al. (2019) [140], patients' samples were moderately positive for TgAb in a first phase, with titers decreasing or disappearing afterwards.

In most cases, this transient antibody positivity might be a consequence of thyroid antigen release following thyroid follicle damage, rather than a veritable autoimmune disease [141]. To note, antibody titers were significantly lower than those observed in Hashimoto's thyroiditis [140]. In the same study by Stasiak et al. (2019) [138], TSH receptor antibody (TRAb) levels were increased in 6% of patients with SAT.

5.7.1.5 Other Laboratory Findings

Mild anemia and hyper-globulinemia may be present in patients with SAT. Liver function test abnormalities are found in approximately 50% of patients and return to normal in a few months [142].

5.7.2 Imaging Studies

Nuclear medicine imaging and US are the main diagnostic tools for SAT, and provide clinical guidance for diagnosis and treatment of this disease, with the latter being easier to operate, more economical, better tolerated, and with wider applications [143].

5.7.2.1 Ultrasonography

In patients with SAT, Doppler flow assessment ultrasonography (US) has shown an absence of vascular flow in the acute phase (Fig. 5.2), and the utility of this finding in the differential diagnosis of unclear cases has been emphasized [144, 145].

Standard ultrasonographic images are characterized by a hypoechoic appearance of the affected tissue (Fig. 5.3), the volume of which correlates with the severity of clinical discomfort [146, 147]. The pressure exerted during US may cause

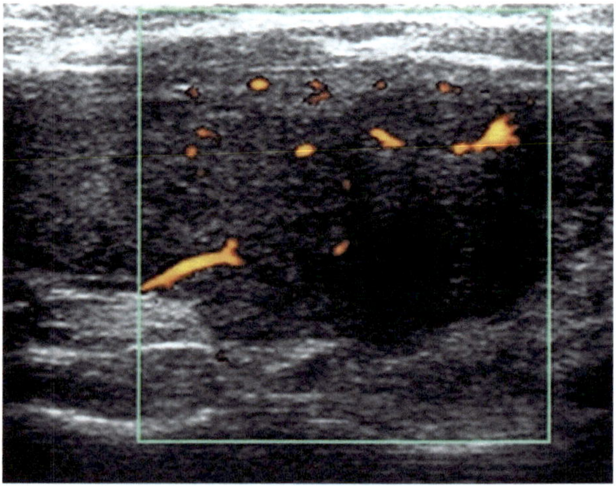

Fig. 5.2 Typical Doppler sonographic pattern of subacute thyroiditis showing hypoechoic blurred areas with decreased or absent vascularization

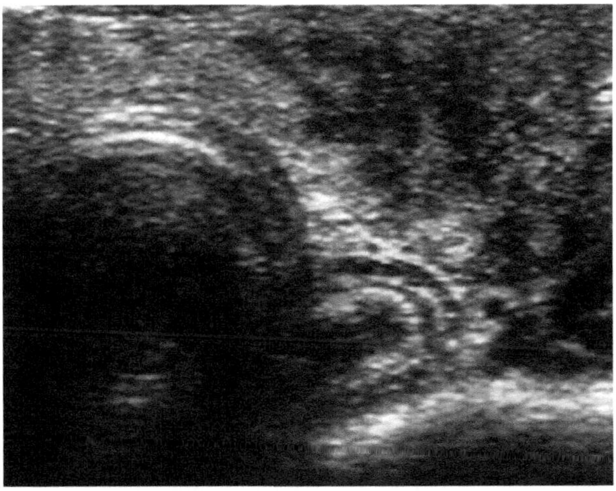

Fig. 5.3 Typical sonographic patterns of subacute thyroiditis showing hypoechoic, strongly heterogeneous, areas with poorly defined margins

tenderness and pain exacerbation, which is a specific sign [143]. On the contrary, enhanced vascular signal may be appreciated during disease recovery. According to Omori et al. (2008) [146], hypoechoic area extensions reflect the degree of inflammation and correlate with the intensity of pain experienced by the patient and with the increase in FT4 levels. The presence of multiple ill-defined hypoechoic areas allows clinicians to distinguish SAT from Hashimoto's thyroiditis and Graves' disease, which typically show a diffuse, homogeneous, hypoechoic texture instead [148]. These features are typical of SAT; thus, even in cases with no clinical symptoms, SAT should be considered as a differential diagnosis for every lesion presenting these characteristics [149].

In some patients with SAT, a nodular space-occupying lesion can be observed, and some of these lesions may mimic thyroid malignancy, given also their hypoechogenicity at US and firmness on palpation [150]. On the other hand, it is worth mentioning that the presence of supposed inflammatory nodules on US during SAT does *not* exclude the concomitant presence of suspicious neoplastic nodules, as US changes in SAT might even hide a co-existing papillary thyroid carcinoma (PTC) or less commonly a thyroid lymphoma [151–153].

The evaluation of cervical lymphadenopathy can also be challenging because inflammatory lymphadenopathies in SAT are extremely common. However, specific patterns of malignancy, e.g., cystic appearance, hyper-echoic punctuations, loss of hilum, and peripheral vascularization of lymph nodes, should raise concerns about the possibility of a co-existing thyroid cancer [154, 155].

Ultrasonographic follow-up is recommended after symptom resolution and laboratory value normalization to identify an underlying nodular disease [152]. Despite the variety of sonographic interval changes in the lesions, most lesions show progressive regression [156] as well as a reduction in size and number of hypoechoic areas [149]. In some cases, however, hypoechoic areas continue to increase or do not disappear, thus suggesting the need for further medical treatment or possibly identifying early disease recurrence [157].

5.7.2.2 Sono-elastography

The application of newer technologies such as sono-elastography has the capacity to demonstrate markedly decreased elasticity (enhanced stiffness) in SAT lesions [158]. However, a study conducted by Xie et al. (2011) [159] demonstrated that even US elastography cannot provide conclusive information about the differential diagnoses of SAT and thyroid cancer. In fact, especially in the early phase of SAT, because of the intra-follicular cellular infiltration with partial or complete loss of colloid, thyroid tissue shows increased stiffness, which is also a typical finding in thyroid cancer. In SAT, however, a subsequent restoration to normal values is generally observed [158].

5.7.2.3 Scintigraphy

Thyroid scintigraphy is another valuable option and, especially in the early stages of SAT, it represents the most useful diagnostic tool. Thyroid tissue can absorb and concentrate Iodine-131 (^{131}I), and is able to uptake ^{99m}Tc-pertechnetate [143]. The value of a ^{99m}Tc-pertechnetate scintigraphy as a marker of disease activity and severity has been described [160]. Pertechnetate scanning (Fig. 5.4), which is inexpensive and convenient, typically reveals little to no uptake, and thus no thyroid tissue visualization during the first phase of SAT process [160, 161], a finding consistently reported in the literature [27, 31, 117, 162–164]. This pattern is common to other forms of destructive thyroiditis such as type-2 amiodarone-induced thyroid dysfunction.

The very low radioactive iodine uptake reflects the inability of the damaged thyroid follicles to concentrate iodine [165]. According to the stage of the disease, the tracer uptake loss can be seen in the whole or in part of the gland. It is also possible that even when SAT affects only a certain part of the gland, e.g., one lobe of the

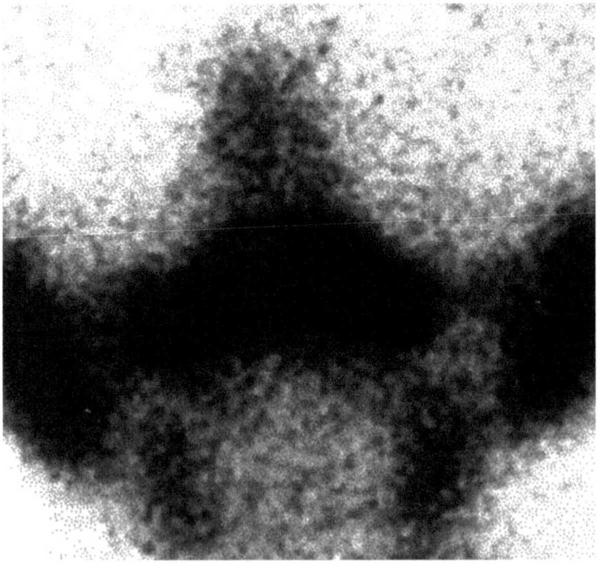

Fig. 5.4 Iodine-131 (^{131}I) radionuclide scan of the thyroid gland in a patient with subacute thyroiditis showing virtually no uptake of radioactive iodine by the gland

thyroid, the scan shows a complete lack of uptake in the whole gland due to the suppression of TSH levels and the consequent lack of stimulation of thyroid cells [166]. On the contrary, cases of increased thyroid function, such as in Graves' disease, are typically associated with normal or high thyroid tracer uptake [167].

As opposed to ^{131}I and ^{99m}Tc-pertechnetate, which show reduced or absent uptake during the acute stage of SAT, further imaging studies have shown diffuse increased uptake of ^{99m}Tc- Sestamibi [161] and ^{99m}Tc-tetrofosmin [160] in the thyroid region of patients in the acute phase (thyrotoxic) of SAT suggesting an ability of both agents to detect the inflammatory process associated with the disease [160, 161].

5.7.2.4 Computed Tomography (CT) Scan

On CT scans, the normal thyroid gland has a high attenuation (80–100 HU) because the normal thyroid gland concentrates iodine almost 100 times more than does the serum. In SAT, CT scan shows diffusely swollen thyroid glands with a low attenuation corresponding to 45 HU (Fig. 5.5). This can be explained on the basis of follicular cell destruction and loss of iodine concentration within the thyroid gland. After the administration of contrast material, the normal thyroid gland has marked enhancement, and this is attributed to its rich vascularity. Moderate enhancement of the thyroid gland on the contrast-enhanced scans suggests the diffuse inflammatory nature of the disease process.

5.7.2.5 Magnetic Resonance Imaging (MRI)/Positron Emission Tomography (PET) Scan

Subacute thyroiditis with thyrotoxicosis may also be distinguished from Graves' hyperthyroidism by using T1- and T2-diffusion weighted magnetic resonance imaging (MRI) and as an intense area of uptake on F-FDG PET/CT [164, 168], although these investigations are usually *not* necessary. Altered F-18 FDG uptake in skeletal muscle and reduced hepatic uptake have been observed during the hyperthyroid phase [169, 170].

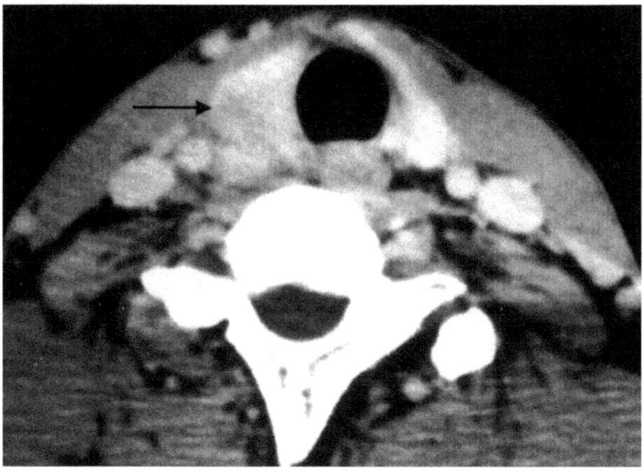

Fig. 5.5 Contrast-enhanced computed tomography (CT) scan showings enlarged right thyroid lobe with decreased attenuation (arrow) in a 32-year-old lady with subacute thyroiditis

Rarely, a sensor-navigated 124-iodine positron emission tomography/ultrasound (I-124-PET/US) fusion has been implemented to establish this diagnosis [171].

5.7.3 Cyto-histopathology

Clinical and laboratory data are usually adequate for SAT diagnosis and fine needle aspiration (FNA) is rarely indicated [172]. Fine-needle aspiration biopsy (FNAB) is often diagnostic although patients are often alarmed at the prospect of this test due to the pain in the thyroid. However, FNA may be helpful in ruling out malignancy [173].

Cytological features alone are often non-specific [174] and can vary as the disease stage evolves [175, 176], so the interpretation may be challenging, especially because SAT findings can resemble other benign or malignant thyroid lesions [174]. In everyday practice, cytopathology may be useful in selected cases to differentiate SAT from other conditions, such as painful Hashimoto's or Riedel's thyroiditis [177], acute suppurative thyroiditis (AST) [178], or malignancies [179]. Correct communication between the endocrinologist and the pathologist is critical so that US and cellular specimen findings can be interpreted in the specific clinical context.

The typical, yet not pathognomonic, histological findings during a full-blown SAT include intra-vacuolar follicular cell granules, epithelioid granulomas (Fig. 5.6), and multi-nucleated giant cells (Fig. 5.7) in an inflammatory background [180]. Degenerated follicular cells with atypia and scant colloid can also be observed (Fig. 5.8) [175]. Conversely, fire-flare cells, hypertrophic follicular cells, oncocytic cells, and transformed lymphocytes are usually absent [180]. As inflammation decreases, a variable range of fibrosis with epithelioid granulomas can be observed,

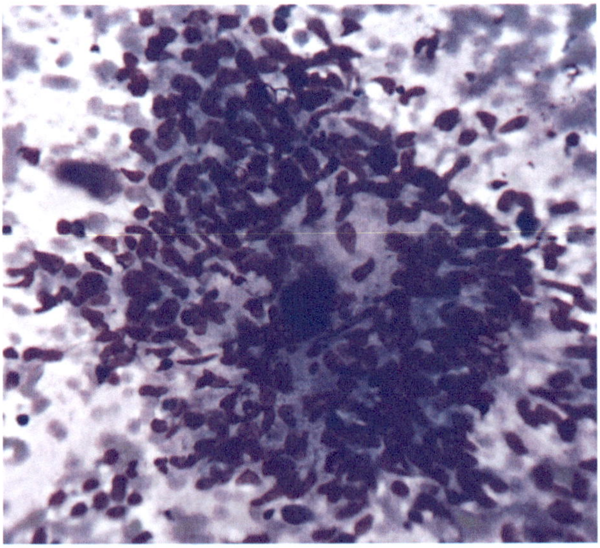

Fig. 5.6 Microscopy of subacute (granulomatous) thyroiditis showing a granuloma with scant colloid. May-Grünwald Giemsa (MGG) stain, 40X

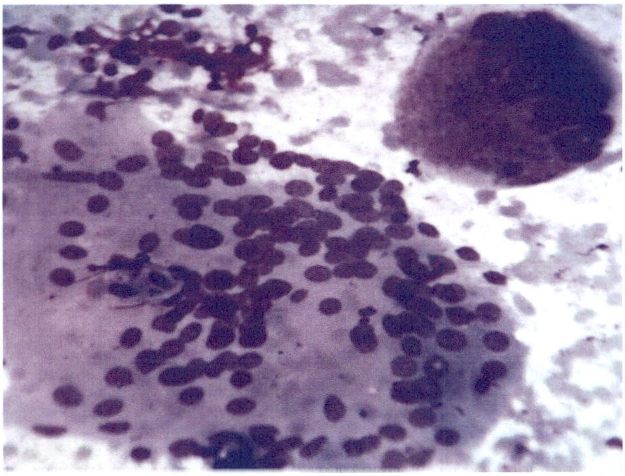

Fig. 5.7 Cytology of subacute thyroiditis showing a large multi-nucleated giant cell with abundant cytoplasm. May-Grünwald Giemsa (MGG) stain, 40X

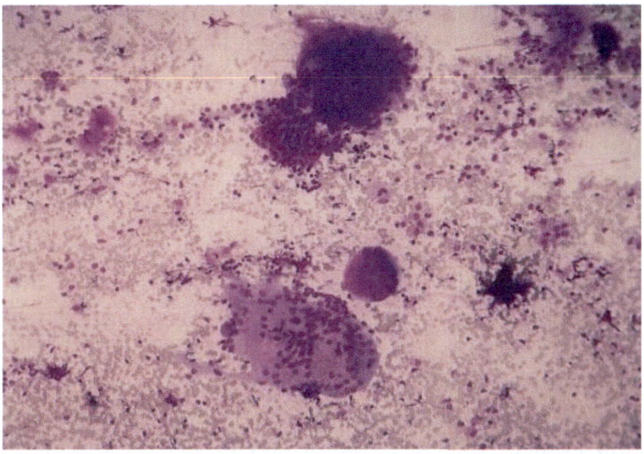

Fig. 5.8 Cytology of subacute thyroiditis (low power view) showing multi-nucleated giant cells, degenerated follicular epithelial cells, and scant colloid May-Grünwald Giemsa (MGG) stain, 10X

while growth factors promote follicular cell regeneration and thyroid tissue repair [101]. In the late phase of SAT, typical cytological features are fibrous tissue fragments, fibroblasts, regenerative epithelial cells, multi-nucleated giant cells, and lymphocytes [174].

Multi-nucleated giant cells and non-caseating granulomas are *not* entirely specific to SAT and can be observed in other benign and malignant thyroid conditions, such as Hashimoto's thyroiditis, multinodular goiter (MNG) with degenerative changes, papillary thyroid carcinoma (PTC), and even anaplastic thyroid carcinoma (ATC) [149, 181]. Well-formed granulomas or caseous necrosis are *not* seen in granulomatous thyroiditis (Fig. 5.9). As SAT and PTC can co-exist in about 0.5% of patients [153, 182]. PTC cytological features (papillary structure, swirl pattern, powdery chromatin, and intra-nuclear cytoplasmic pseudo-inclusions) should be excluded prior to diagnosing SAT [174]. It should be noted that early reactive cellular atypia and late regenerative micro-follicles observed in SAT may lead to a false cytological diagnosis [174, 176].

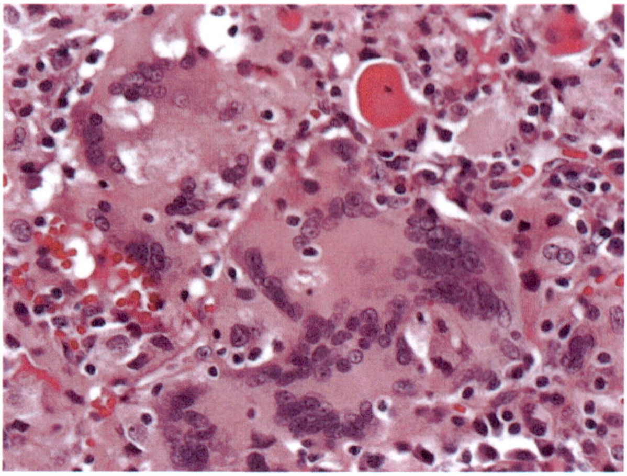

Fig. 5.9 Microscopy of subacute thyroiditis (high magnification). Note that well-formed granulomas or caseous necrosis are not seen in granulomatous (subacute) thyroiditis. H&E stain

As previously described in 1997 by Lu et al. [182], ultrasonographic improvement of the thyroid echo-structure usually occurs earlier than cytological healing. Nishihara et al. (2008) [153] analyzed sequential ultrasonographic and histopathological findings in five SAT cases complicated by PTC. The authors concluded that ultrasonographic precocious hypoechoic lesions observed in SAT could reflect the early inflammatory change such as neutrophilic infiltration. Histological evidence of granulomas and fibrosis was still seen about 3 months after SAT onset; residual fibrosis persisted for several additional months, interestingly with no ultrasonographic evidence of hypoechoic lesions. Further, the authors suggested that the inflammatory and regenerative processes of SAT in thyroid cells did *not* affect papillary thyroid carcinomas [153]. For this reason, if US had been performed during the active SAT phase and suspicious hypoechoic areas had been identified after clinical and biochemical SAT resolution, US re-examination and fine-needle aspiration biopsy (FNAb) of persistent hypoechoic areas of at least 10 mm would be recommended.

5.8 Differential Diagnosis

5.8.1 Diagnostic Criteria

The patient presenting with painful neck symptoms is frequently empirically treated with antibiotics with minimal evaluation in general practice only later to be found to have thyroid-related disease [163]. With an acutely enlarged, tender thyroid, RAIU near zero, and elevated serum T4, T3 (T3:T4 <20), Tg concentrations, and ESR, the diagnosis of SAT is almost certain. Stasiak et al. (2021) [51] recently proposed updated SAT diagnostic criteria. Two main criteria (elevation of ESR or CRP and hypoechoic areas with blurred margin and decreased vascularization at US) should be met, together with at least one additional criterion (hard thyroid swelling, pain and tenderness of the thyroid gland or lobe, elevation of serum FT4 and suppression of TSH, decreased radioiodine uptake, FNAb result typical for SAT).

It is noteworthy that SAT diagnosis should be considered in patients during or after SARS-CoV-2 infection with unexpected symptoms or laboratory markers of thyrotoxicosis. Besides, SAT can occasionally present without neck pain [12], remarkably so in SAT cases caused by SARS-CoV-2 [183]. Thus, the presence of pain should not be treated as a SAT essential diagnostic criterion. Furthermore, as SAT may be the only manifestation of COVID-19, testing for SARS-CoV-2 infection could be considered in patients with SAT diagnosed during an epidemic flare [51].

Circulating thyroid auto-antibodies are absent, or the titer is low. Rarely, a fever of unknown origin may suggest "temporal arteritis" but is actually due to SAT [121]. Additionally, because of the radiation of painful thyroid into the jaw area, the presence of "dental pain" may be confused with SAT [184].

5.8.2 Delay in Diagnosis of SAT

Despite the availability of efficient diagnostic tools, differential diagnosis could be challenging, especially for a non-endocrinologist, and thus could delay proper diagnosis and adequate treatment [185]. Lack of awareness or recognition of this disorder, e.g., by primary care physicians, may cause misdiagnoses, with the most common error being pharyngitis diagnoses and subsequent antibiotic overuse [185, 186]. Indeed, neck pain and laboratory results, especially in SAT cases with no thyrotoxic symptoms, can be easily confused with common infective processes. Two recent studies by Stasiak et al. (2019) [187] and Bostan et al. (2021) [185] reported a delay in SAT diagnosis of over 2 weeks in 73–82% of cases and unnecessary antibiotic prescriptions in about 47–59% of patients. Furthermore, a lack of improvement in patients' symptoms can lead to repeated visits to different specialists, thus increasing healthcare costs [188].

5.8.3 Diagnostic Alternatives

Among the diagnostic alternatives, the following disorders must be considered and their possibility excluded:

5.8.3.1 Hashimoto's Thyroiditis

The thyroid in Hashimoto's thyroiditis may be slightly tender and painful, but this event is rare, and the typical disturbances in iodine metabolism and ESR are rarely found. Markers of inflammation such as CRP, as measured in the saliva, are normal in Hashimoto's thyroiditis when compared to controls, but are grossly elevated in the patient with SAT [124]. Standard thyroid US may appear similar with hypoechoic tissue in both Hashimoto's thyroiditis and SAT. Doppler measured blood flow is usually robust in Hashimoto's thyroiditis (and Graves' disease) but minimal in SAT while assessment by sono-elastography reveals that the SAT gland is profoundly stiffer than Hashimoto's thyroiditis tissue, which is itself somewhat stiffer than normal controls [85]. The radio nuclide thyroid uptake and scanning in Hashimoto's thyroiditis is variable with elevated, depressed, or normal results reported. On the other hand, ^{18}F-FDG-PET in Hashimoto's is similar to that seen in SAT with usually very positive uptake reported [189, 190]. Likewise, MRI does *not* differentiate between Hashimoto's thyroiditis and SAT [191] and is therefore, like $^{131/123}$I and PET scanning, of little value in separating the patient with painful Hashimoto's thyroiditis from the SAT patient.

5.8.3.2 Hemorrhage in a Cyst/Nodule

Hemorrhage into a cyst in a nodular thyroid gland may be acutely painful and therefore confused with SAT although the condition may be associated with an initially autonomously functioning nodule [192]. The clinical presentation of a nodule hemorrhage is usually sudden and transient. A fluctuant mass may be found in the involved region, which may be confirmed as fluid-filled and avascular by US, and further differentiated as the ESR is normal.

5.8.3.3 Hyperthyroidism

Occasionally, SAT mimics endogenous hyperthyroidism (Graves' or toxic nodular goiter) in a patient whose RAIU is suppressed by the administration of exogenous iodine [193, 194]. This event occurs particularly in thyrotoxicosis induced by iodine (Jod-Basedow phenomenon) [195]. The sudden onset of SAT, the presence of toxic symptoms without the typical signs of long-term hyperthyroidism, the tender gland, the constitutional symptoms, and the high ESR are helpful in making the differentiation. In some instances, measurement of antibodies and thyroid-stimulating immunoglobulins, and observation of the course of the illness, may be required to confirm the diagnosis.

5.8.3.4 Variant of Autoimmune Thyroiditis

The single disease entity that is probably most difficult to differentiate from SAT is a variant of lymphocytic thyroiditis [196]. This condition is unrelated to iodine ingestion and most likely is a variant of autoimmune thyroiditis. The patient presents with goiter, thyrotoxicosis, and a low RAIU. The biochemical course of the disease is indistinguishable from that of SAT and proceeds from a thyrotoxic phase through a hypothyroid phase to spontaneous remission with normalization of thyroid function. The goiter is, however, typically painless, and there are no associated systemic symptoms. This condition has been formerly confused with subacute (de Quervain's) thyroiditis, which likely has led to the descriptive terms of silent, painless, or atypical SAT to refer to this entity. The most helpful distinguishing features, short of histological evidence of biopsy material, are the absence of pain, the positivity of anti-thyroid antibodies, and a normal ESR.

5.8.3.5 Acute Suppurative Thyroiditis

It is also important to exclude acute suppurative thyroiditis [197] since this could be worsened by corticosteroid treatment and require antibiotics and/or surgical drain of the abscess. Localized SAT, with induration, mild tenderness, and depressed iodine uptake visualized on scan, can clearly be very suggestive of acute suppurative thyroiditis or even thyroid cancer. One series indicated a surprisingly high frequency of focal involvement observed among those with SAT [150]. Indeed, this differential is quite difficult when incidentally discovered lesions are evaluated. Typical US images in early acute suppurative thyroiditis show unifocal lesions collection of small amounts of fluid around the affected thyroid lobe with a unifocal hypoechoic lesion [198].

A comparison between the clinical and work-up (laboratory, imaging, and cytology) findings of patients with subacute thyroiditis (SAT) and acute suppurative thyroiditis (AST) is provided in Table 5.1 [2, 195, 196, 199–202].

5.8.3.6 Focal Thyroid Lesions

Focal thyroid lesions incidentally identified by 18F-FDG-PET/CT are said to have malignant potential in up to 14–63% of cases [203, 204]. Among the other diagnostic findings reported to account for such FDG-PET incidentalomas is focal SAT [168]. Usually, the degree of pain and tenderness, elevated ESR, leukocytosis, and remission or spread to other parts of the gland make clinical differentiation possible. Traditional US may reveal localized hypoechoic area in the thyroid, and gray-scale and Doppler sonography may be helpful in this situation [144, 186]. Sonoelastography of these nodular lesions yields abnormally inelastic results in both SAT as well as thyroid cancer [159]. Occasionally, magnetic resonance imaging [191], where the image of SAT is characterized by low intensity, may assist the clinician in the differential diagnosis of these nodular lesions. The hypoechoic area on US can reflect the degree of inflammation and thyroid hormone levels [146]. However, FNA may be necessary for a definitive differentiation between these two processes, as well as the other entities noted above [205].

5.8.3.7 Thyroid Cancer

It is also important to rule out primary or secondary lymphoma involvement [206] or malignancy [207, 208] before the diagnosis of SAT. Improper diagnosis of SAT in patients with thyroid malignancies of poor prognosis, in particular anaplastic thyroid carcinoma (ATC), non-thyroid cancer infiltrating the gland or metastasizing to the thyroid, is rare, but may constitute a life-threatening problem. In addition, these conditions, because of their typical rapid growth, can stretch the capsule and infiltrate surrounding tissue, causing the same neck pain characteristic of SAT [209]. Thus, differentiating these conditions may not be so straightforward. Since SAT can involve the entire thyroid gland but can also present in an asymmetric manner, the disease should be differentiated from a carcinoma, as such asymmetry is also typical of malignancies [186]. Moreover, there is considerable imaging overlap in the two conditions at both US and technetium scans. Thyroid malignancies, such as differentiated thyroid cancer (DTC), or rarer conditions such as medullary

Table 5.1 Features differentiating acute suppurative thyroiditis and subacute thyroiditis

Criteria	Characteristics	Acute thyroiditis	Subacute thyroiditis
History	Preceding URTI	88%	17%
	Fever	100%	54%
	Sore throat	90%	36%
	Hyperthyroidism symptoms	Uncommon	47%
Thyroid gland examination	Painful thyroid swelling	100%	77%
	Left side involvement	85 + %	Not specific
	Migrating thyroid tenderness	Possible	27%
	Erythema of overlying skin	83%	Not usually
Laboratory tests	Leukocytosis	57%	25–50%
	ESR (>30 mm/h)	100%	85%
	Abnormal thyroid hormone levels	5–10%	60%
	Alkaline phosphatase, transaminases increased	Rare	Common
Imaging studies	^{123}I uptake low	Common	~100%
	Abnormal thyroid scan	92%	Non-visualized
	Thyroid US helpful in diagnosis	75%	Non-specific
	Gallium scan positive	~100%	~100%
	^{18}F-FDG-PET	Positive	Positive
	Barium swallow showing fistula	Common	0
	CT scan useful	Varies	Not indicated
Needle aspiration	Purulent, bacteria or fungi present	~100%	0
	Lymphocytes, macrophages, some polys, giant cells	0	~100%
Clinical course	Response to glucocorticoids	Transient	100%
	I&D required	85%	No
	Recurrence following I&D	16%	No
	Pyriform sinus fistula discovered	96%	No

URTI upper respiratory tract infection, *ESR* erythrocyte sedimentation rate, *US* ultrasound, *18F-FDG-PET* [18F] fluorodeoxyglucose positron emission tomography, *CT* computed tomography, *I&D* incision and drainage

thyroid carcinoma (MTC) or ATC, have been reported in few cases and thus should be considered for differential diagnosis [165]. A case of leukemic thyroiditis in recurrent acute lymphocytic leukemia (ALL) mimicking SAT has also been described earlier by Byrd et al. (1997) [210]. The correct diagnosis can be provided by FNAB, evaluated by an experienced cytopathologist, and an adequate US quality examination, thus minimizing unnecessary surgery and subsequent morbidity risk [211].

5.8.3.8 Other Pathologies

On FNA, the differential diagnosis of SAT further includes thyroid amyloidosis [212], palpation thyroiditis, iodine-induced thyroiditis, radiation-induced thyroiditis, or exogenous thyrotoxicosis (factitious or iatrogenic) [167], in addition to other granulomatous diseases such as sarcoidosis, tuberculosis (TB) [213], and rheumatoid diseases.

Urine iodine levels could be helpful in differential diagnosis, with levels lower than 500 mcg/L in SAT and higher in iodide-induced thyroiditis (e.g., amiodarone or other drugs or products containing iodide, iodide contrast agent, etc.) [17].

5.9 Management

The goals of SAT management are pain relief and symptom control. Treatment guidelines are mostly based on observational data and expert opinion with limited trials being available.

5.9.1 Medical Treatment

5.9.1.1 First-Line Treatment: Analgesic Therapy

Subacute thyroiditis (SAT) is usually self-limiting and, in some patients, no treatment is required [212]. However, for many, some form of analgesic therapy is warranted to treat the symptoms of the disease until it resolves. At times, this relief of symptoms can be achieved with non-steroidal anti-inflammatory drugs (NSAIDs) such as salicylic acid (600 mg orally every 6 h) or ibuprofen (400–800 mg orally every 8 h), for patients with mild to moderate symptoms [214]. Beta-blockers can be used in severe cases of hyperthyroidism to control thyrotoxic symptoms [214]. Using NSAIDs alone, a complete resolution of pain is expected within 5 weeks, with a reported range of 1–20 weeks [12].

5.9.1.2 Second-Line Treatment: Corticosteroids

In the case of lack of response to anti-inflammatory therapy and/or in patients with more severe symptoms, and after acute suppurative thyroiditis (AST) has been definitively ruled out, the second-line treatment by corticosteroid (prednisone) administration should be employed [3, 10]. Large doses promptly relieve the symptoms through non-specific anti-inflammatory effects. Treatment is generally begun with a single daily dose of 40 mg prednisone for 1–2 weeks, and then gradually tapered over a period of 2–4 weeks. The relief of the tenderness in the neck is so dramatic as to be virtually diagnostic of SAT. A dose as low as 15 mg with tapering by 5 mg every 2 weeks [214, 215] of prednisolone has been shown to be as effective [216], and further studies should be conducted to determine the lowest effective doses.

The regimen of about 6 weeks of prednisone has been recommended by international guidelines for SAT treatment [214], but this scheme has been debated in recent years. In a recent randomized controlled trial by Duan and colleagues (2020) [217], conducted on patients with moderate-to-severe symptoms of SAT, fewer side-effects of glucocorticoids and similar efficacy and recurrence rates were observed with short-term prednisone (30 mg/day prednisone for 1 week, followed by 1 week of NSAIDs) when compared to the 6-week treatment. Other studies proposed the use of prednisolone, with different initial dosages, such as 30 mg/day [218], 20 mg/day [219], and 15 mg/day [216], resulting in comparable effectiveness and fewer potential side effects. However, 20% of patients that were treated with 15 mg/day as an initial dose required a longer time before discontinuing the glucocorticoid treatment [216]. In another study by Hepsen et al. (2020) [220], patients were enrolled in either the 16 or 48 mg methylprednisolone groups, and it was observed that low-dose steroid therapy could as well achieve complete symptom resolution and even better outcomes in SAT. Moreover, the high-dose steroid treatment was associated with a higher rate of recurrence, whereas no difference was observed in permanent hypothyroidism rates between the two groups [220]. Therapeutic algorithm for the management of subacute thyroiditis is shown in Fig. 5.10.

Few investigators have also proposed intra-thyroidal steroid injection as an alternative therapeutic approach for SAT, suggesting it could provide a faster, safer, and generally better tolerated approach [221], with most of the patients requiring only one injection to achieve complete cure [221, 222].

Compared to the use of NSAIDs, the use of steroids has been shown to reduce time to resolution of symptoms [223], but if glucocorticoid treatment is tapered too

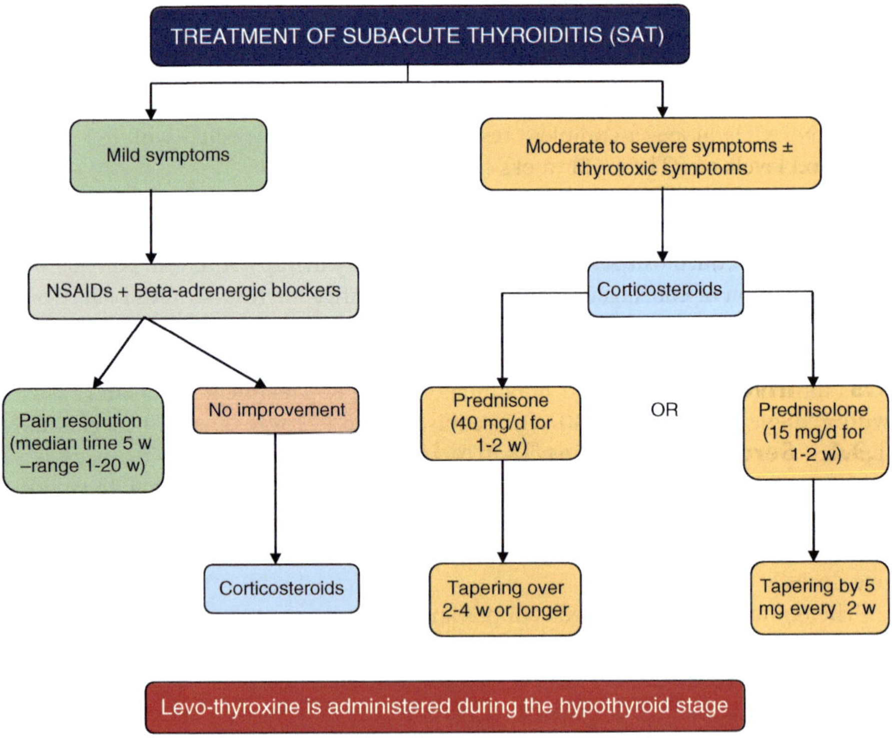

Fig. 5.10 Therapeutic algorithm for the management of subacute thyroiditis (SAT)

fast or interrupted, a recurrence of pain is often observed [224], requiring resumption of therapy and the need to increase the dose again, which results in prolongation of treatment duration [12].

Several studies have focused on the recurrence rates of SAT among different treatment groups. A recent systematic review and cohort study meta-analysis by Zhang et al. (2021) [225] reported a pooled SAT recurrence rate of 12.0%, with a higher risk of recurrence in the glucocorticoids group (approximately 20%) compared to the NSAIDs group. A recent study by Sencar et al. (2019) evaluated the results of the steroid and NSAID treatments in SAT in relation to persistent hypothyroidism and recurrence, and concluded that NSAIDs fail to provide clinical remission in more than half of SAT patients, and symptomatic response to NSAIDs is lower in patients with higher ESR and CRP levels. Despite the high recurrence rate observed in steroid-treated SAT patients, steroid treatment appears to be protective against permanent hypothyroidism. Steroid therapy should therefore be considered, especially in anti-TPO-positive SAT patients and those with high level ESR and CRP [226].

The results of another study by Arao et al. (2016) showed that SAT recurrence rate during prednisolone therapy correlated with the number of days required for tapering the dose of prednisolone to 5 mg/day, but not with the starting dose of prednisolone, suggesting a relatively longer period of steroid tapering could prevent the recurrence of SAT [227].

5.9.1.3 New Therapeutic Approaches

A newer therapeutic approach with local injection of lidocaine and dexamethasone through an insulin syringe has been reported to alleviate symptoms earlier than standard treatment with systemically administered prednisone and needs further evaluation in larger studies [228].

Colchicine 1 mg/day, due to the inhibition it can exert on tumor necrosis factor-alpha (TNF-α) and pro-inflammatory cytokines signaling, has been proposed as a therapeutic adjunctive tool in patients with steroid-refractory recurrent SAT [218].

Eventually, iopanoic acid, ipodate sodium, and *Prunella vulgaris* have also been proposed as adjunctive tools in selected cases [194, 229].

5.9.1.4 Levothyroxine

Levothyroxine could be prescribed in the hypothyroid phase of SAT but should be withdrawn during the follow-up, generally in 3–6 months. Long-term therapy should be applied only if hypothyroidism endures. Permanent hypothyroidism rate is *not* affected by the use of NSAIDs or corticosteroid treatment, but overall, patients that require corticosteroid therapy show more often the need for replacement therapy, probably because of the severity of SAT in such cases [230].

5.9.2 Surgical Treatment

Surgical intervention is *not* the primary treatment of SAT, but rarely this has been performed due to the presence of "indeterminate" cytology on FNA [211, 231, 232] or due to the presence of severe pain [233]. In 2015, Mazza et al. [233] reported an unusual case of SAT resistance to high-dose steroids that was treated with total thyroidectomy. Surgery could thus represent a rare alternative option for a few selected patients with SAT resistant to steroid treatment and with persistent pain [231]. Experience from the Mayo Clinic [231] has shown that if surgery is performed for a clinically indeterminate thyroid nodule, resection is safe and with low morbidity. Because of the possibility of associated papillary thyroid carcinoma (PTC), further cytological examination should be performed in patients presenting with a persistent hypoechoic area larger than 1 cm by US [153].

5.9.3 Radioactive Iodine (RAI)

In the single report in the literature, Dumitriu et al. (1990) [234] described very few cases of "recurrent" SAT treated with radioactive iodine (RAI). After 2–3 recurrences, occurring despite glucocorticoid treatment, RAI was administered to these patients with no reports of any further relapse.

5.10 Follow-Up/Prognosis

5.10.1 Recovery/Transient Hypothyroidism

In the majority of patients with SAT, there is a complete and spontaneous recovery and a return to normal thyroid function. However, the thyroid glands of patients with SAT may exhibit irregular scarring between islands of residual functioning parenchyma, although the patient has no symptoms. In terms of thyroid dysfunction following SAT, hypothyroidism is the main event, but in most cases, it is "temporary." A recent study by Zhao et al. (2020) that followed 61 patients for 2 years following diagnosis of SAT explored the early indicators of hypothyroidism and the final changes in thyroid volume in SAT patients [235]. They reported that the thyroid gland volumes of SAT patients, especially those with hypothyroidism, were smaller than those of healthy controls after the acute stage of the disease. They also suggested that the higher early maximum TSH value within 3 months after SAT onset may be a risk factor for the incidence of hypothyroidism 2 years later.

Görges et al. (2019) [236] investigated the long-term follow-up of patients with SAT for up to 30 years, concluding that 25% of patients develop hypothyroidism in the long term. Recently (2021), a Chinese study by Tang et al. [237] reported that patients with higher CRP and lower TSH levels were at a higher risk of developing hypothyroidism. A possible role of TRAb in the development of prolonged hypothyroidism was previously hypothesized by Tamai et al. (1991) [24], in particular regarding TSH-blocking antibodies (TSH-BAb). According to this study, increased TSH-blocking antibody activity was correlated with a prolonged period of hypothyroidism, whereas hypothyroidism without TSH-BAb was more transient [24]. The extent of hypo-echogenic areas in the thyroid may represent another possible marker for developing thyroid dysfunction after SAT. A small study conducted by Teixeira et al. (1985) [238] demonstrated a low thyroid reserve detectable even after 5 years of follow-up after the spontaneous course of SAT. These findings could be related to the progression toward thyroid fibrosis even in apparently healed patients [238].

5.10.2 Recurrence Rate

Recurrence is usually defined as the "relapse of episodes of pain with elevated inflammatory laboratory parameters (ESR or CRP) and US findings" [226]. Many studies have reported recurrence rates, but depending on the studied population, discrepancies in the SAT recurrence rate vary significantly between studied groups, ranging from 0% to over 30%, usually occurring within 1 year after diagnosis [239, 240]. Recurrence of SAT can seriously affect the lives of patients and create psychological troubles for them. Thus, the determination of the risk groups for recurrent SAT can guide clinicians in preventing recurrence and providing early diagnosis and proper treatment.

Zhang et al. (2021) [225] conducted a systematic review and meta-analysis of cohort studies to estimate SAT recurrence rates and summarize the risk factors for SAT recurrence. A total of 18 studies reported the recurrence rate of SAT. The recurrence rates varied from 0% [239] to 34.8% [240]. The pooled recurrence rate was 12.0% with significant heterogeneity ($p < 0.01$). Moreover, the risk of recurrence in patients treated with glucocorticoids is higher than that of patients treated with NSAIDs [238, 241]. Treatment-related factors, HLA haplotype (HLA-B*18:01, HLA-B*35, and HLA-A*26) [5, 242, 243], the sialic acid level [244], or the TSH level [245], at the termination of treatment, further extension of the hypoechoic area, and increase in thyroid volume [240] were all potential predictors for recurrence of SAT. In such high-risk patients, it is suggested that the steroid treatment regimen should be intensified with a slower dose reduction [243]. There was no significant difference in age [227, 241, 245–247] or gender [5, 227, 241, 244, 245, 247, 248] between the recurrence group and the non-recurrence group, although recurrence rate was less in males than in females. Further randomized controlled trials, prospective cohort studies, and studies on the molecular and cellular mechanisms are needed to explore the association between these factors and SAT recurrence. This recent meta-analysis study (2021) [225] shed light on the choice of therapeutic optimization for clinicians to reduce recurrence and has important implications for improving the quality of life of SAT patients in the future.

5.10.3 Permanent Hypothyroidism

Some studies have described the development of "permanent" hypothyroidism in approximately 10% (range 5–15%) of patients with SAT requiring permanent replacement with Levo-thyroxine [12, 249]. Since this can also occur several years after diagnosis, long-term follow-up, i.e., annual monitoring of thyroid function tests, in these patients is important as late-onset hypothyroidism may occur [249].

The choice of treatment, use of steroids, NSAID, or both, may *not* predict the development of permanent hypothyroidism [230]. In an interesting work carried out retrospectively on 252 patients, Nishihara and colleagues (2009) [250] reported that permanent hypothyroidism occurred in 5.9%. All of these had bilateral hypoechoic areas on thyroid US at initial presentation, suggesting that this may be a useful prognostic marker for the potential development of thyroid dysfunction after SAT [250]. They added that the rates of thyroid dysfunction after SAT were significantly lower in patients receiving prednisone. In this study, steroid-treated SAT patients had a higher recurrence rate, but developed permanent hypothyroidism less frequently. Therefore, the authors concluded that steroid therapy should be considered, especially in most severe cases, such as anti-TPO-positive SAT patients and patients with high levels of ESR and CRP.

Permanent hypothyroidism was reported by Bogazzi et al. (2009) to be significantly less common in SAT compared to the outcome noted in amiodarone-induced thyrotoxicosis type 2 (destructive thyroiditis) [251]. It is of interest that elevated levels of serum Tg may persist well over a year after the initial diagnosis, indicating that disordered follicular architecture and/or low-grade inflammation can persist for a relatively long period [252].

5.10.4 Autoimmune Thyroid Dysfunction (Graves' Disease—Hashimoto's Thyroiditis)

The study of a contemporary and relatively large series of patients with SAT by Benbassat et al. (2007) [253] defined that the degree of biochemical thyrotoxicosis is associated with a prolonged disease duration and a more profound hypothyroid phase.

A minority (<1%) of patients presenting with clinical SAT in Japan have been reported to return ($n = 7$) with findings consistent with Graves' disease after a mean of 4.7 months [254]. Review of the other 26 cases summarized in the report of Nakano et al. (2011) indicates a similar interval between the diagnosis of SAT and subsequent Graves' disease presentation, a clearly elevated RAIU in the Graves' disease phase of all the reports where an uptake is reported (14/26 [54%]) and a change in thyroid antibody positivity in 50% of those evaluated in both (6/26 [23%]) the SAT and Graves' disease presentation [254]. Combining the case series by Nakano et al. with their review of the literature, 21/31 [68%] of cases labeled as SAT were diagnosed clinically without a RAIU assessment, and a further 4/12 [33%] of those diagnosed as SAT with a RAIU available had an uptake greater than

10% at the time of diagnosis [254]. This brings into question the true incidence of this reported transition from presumably non-autoimmune SAT to clearly immune-mediated Graves' disease.

It should also be noted that cases of autoimmune thyroid dysfunction development after SAT have been described [255], including Hashimoto's thyroiditis [256] and Graves' disease [257, 258], and also arising several years after SAT onset [259]. Possibly, destructive thyroiditis, inducing the release of self-antigens, may trigger thyroid autoimmunity.

5.11 Summary and Conclusions

Subacute thyroiditis (SAT) is a destructive inflammatory disorder of the thyroid gland, characterized by neck pain and symptoms caused by thyroid hormone excess (transient thyrotoxicosis). It is usually self-limiting and displays a characteristic triphasic clinical course: an initial thyrotoxic phase, a transient hypothyroidism phase, and, in 85–95% of patients, the subsequent restoration to baseline thyroid function within a mean of 12 months.

Viruses are considered the main trigger of SAT, especially considering its frequent association with recent viral infections of the upper respiratory tract. Genetic susceptibility also seems to have a central role in pathogenesis, as SAT is often associated with some HLA haplotypes, peculiarly HLA-B35.

Soon after the onset of the recent pandemic, many cases of SAT induced by SARS-CoV-2 have also been published. SAT diagnosis should be considered in patients during or after SARS-CoV-2 infection with typical symptoms or laboratory markers of thyrotoxicosis, even without thyroid pain, which is not always present. As SARS-CoV-2 may trigger different types of thyroid damage, thyroid function tests should be performed in most patients hospitalized due to COVID-19, especially in those referred to ICUs. Since SAT may be the only manifestation of COVID-19, testing for SARS-CoV-2 infection could be considered in patients with SAT diagnosed during the pandemic. SAT has also been reported after several vaccinations, including some cases following SARS-CoV-2 vaccination, whether for mRNA, the viral vector, or the inactivated virus vaccine. Potential explanations for post-vaccination SAT have been proposed, yet distinct mechanisms remain unclear, with ASIA syndrome (autoimmune/inflammatory syndrome induced by adjuvants) and molecular mimicry currently being the two main pathogenetic hypotheses. The SARS-CoV-2 vaccine-associated SAT is a recent discovery: this condition shares epidemiological and clinical characteristics with the classic post-viral SAT but is triggered by peculiar mechanisms associated with immunization. Though SAT in such cases should not raise concern regarding vaccination, this condition needs to be recognized in order to avoid incongruous treatment, monitor long-term thyroid function, and notify these cases for pharmacovigilance.

There is a wide span of possible differential diagnoses of SAT. Notably, false positive diagnoses of SAT in patients with malignancies of poor prognosis may constitute a life-threatening problem. Considerable similarities exist between US characteristics of SAT and malignant thyroid nodules including thyroid lymphoma, such as undefined lesion margins or hypo-echogenicity. Therefore, it is recommended that patients with SAT nodular ultrasonographic pattern undergo US not only for the initial evaluation but also after recovery, since the resolution of US findings alongside the resolution of symptoms is the definitive proof of benignity. In selected patients with focal masses, FNAb should be considered to rule out a malignancy and should be performed in all doubtful cases and in patients who show no improvement in the short-term. In such cases, the patient's history is of paramount importance and may suggest important clues aiding the differential diagnosis.

The first-line treatment of SAT is by NSAIDs, which can be used in patients with mild or moderate forms of the disorder, while symptomatic treatment in the acute phase could benefit from β-blockers for thyrotoxic symptoms. Methimazole, acting on thyroid hormone production, but not on fT4/fT3 peripheral effect, is *not* useful to reduce the systemic thyroid hormone excess. The use of glucocorticoids is recommended in moderate to severe cases, with adequate tapering, and for refractory or severe pain and thyrotoxic symptoms.

The optimal treatment protocol and regimen have been a matter of debate in recent years. Steroids offer faster pain relief and tend to shorten disease duration, but their use has been correlated with higher recurrence rates in different series. Studies have often shown opposing results concerning the correlation of the treatment modalities with permanent hypothyroidism. Since no sure predictive factors have been noticed so far, it is worth remembering that permanent hypothyroidism usually develops within 1 year after SAT, but given the fact that later onset has also been described, long-term follow-up with annual monitoring of thyroid function tests in these patients is recommended.

References

1. Intenzo C, dePapp A, Jabbour S, Miller J, Kim S, Capuzzi D. Scintigraphic manifestations of thyrotoxicosis. Radiographic. 2003;23(4):857–69.
2. Szabo SM, Allen DB. Thyroiditis. Differentiation of acute suppurative and subacute. Case report and review of the literature. Clin Pediatr Phila. 1989;28(4):171–4.
3. Volpe R. The management of subacute (De Quervain's) thyroiditis. Thyroid. 1993;3(3):253–5.
4. Ogawa E, Katsushima Y, Fujiwara I, Iinuma K. Subacute thyroiditis in children: patient report and review of the literature. J Pediatr Endocrinol Metab. 2003;16(6):897–900.
5. Stasiak M, Tymoniuk B, Stasiak B, Lewinski A. The risk of recurrence of subacute thyroiditis is HLA-dependent. Int J Mol Sci. 2019;20:1089.
6. Saklamaz A. Is there a drug effect on the development of permanent hypothyroidism in subacute thyroiditis? Acta Endocrinol (Buchar). 2017;13:119–23.
7. Greene JN. Subacute thyroiditis. Am J Med. 1971;51(1):97–108.
8. Woolner LB, Mc CW, Beahrs OH. Granulomatous thyroiditis (De Quervain's thyroiditis). J Clin Endocrinol Metab. 1957;17(10):1202–21.
9. Golden SH, Robinson KA, Saldanha I, Anton B, Ladenson PW. Clinical review: prevalence and incidence of endocrine and metabolic disorders in the United States: a comprehensive review. J Clin Endocrinol Metab. 2009;94(6):1853–78.

10. Wasniewska M, Vigone MC, Cappa M, Cassio A, Scognamillo R, Aversa T, Rubino M, De Luca F. Acute suppurative thyroiditis in childhood: spontaneous closure of sinus pyriform fistula may occur even very early. J Pediatr Endocrinol Metab. 2007;20(1):75–7.
11. Singer PA. Thyroiditis. Acute, subacute, and chronic. Med Clin North Am. 1991;75(1):61–77.
12. Fatourechi V, Aniszewski JP, Fatourechi GZ, Atkinson EJ, Jacobsen SJ. Clinical features and outcome of subacute thyroiditis in an incidence cohort: Olmsted County, Minnesota, study. J Clin Endocrinol Metab. 2003;88(5):2100–5.
13. Qari FA, Maimani AA. Subacute thyroiditis in Western Saudi Arabia. Saudi Med J. 2005;26(4):630–3.
14. Carle A, Laurberg P, Pedersen IB, Knudsen N, Perrild H, Ovesen L, Rasmussen LB, Jorgensen T. Epidemiology of subtypes of hypothyroidism in Denmark. Eur J Endocrinol. 2006;154(1):21–8.
15. Anastasilakis AD, Karanicola V, Kourtis A, Makras P, Kampas L, Gerou S, Giomisi A. A case report of subacute thyroiditis during pregnancy: difficulties in differential diagnosis and changes in cytokine levels. Gynecol Endocrinol. 2011;27(6):384–90.
16. Hiraiwa T, Kubota S, Imagawa A, Sasaki I, Ito M, Miyauchi A, Hanafusa T. Two cases of subacute thyroiditis presenting in pregnancy. J Endocrinol Investig. 2006;29(10):924–7.
17. Tabassom A, Chippa V, Edens MA. De Quervain thyroiditis. In: StatPearls [Internet]. Treasure Island: StatPearls Publishing; 2022. https://www.ncbi.nlm.nih.gov/books/NBK526066/.
18. Martino E, Buratti L, Bartalena L, Mariotti S, Cupini C, Aghini-Lombardi F, et al. High prevalence of subacute thyroiditis during summer season in Italy. J Endocrinol Investig. 1987;10:321–3.
19. Iitaka M, Momotani N, Ishii J, Ito K. Incidence of subacute thyroiditis recurrences after a prolonged latency: 24-year survey. J Clin Endocrinol Metab. 1996;81:466–9.
20. Oksa H, Järvenpää P, Metsähonkala L, Pasternack A, Leinikki P. No seasonal distribution in subacute de Quervain's thyroiditis in Finland. J Endocrinol Investig. 1989;12:495.
21. Greer MA. Subacute thyroiditis. West J Med. 1991;155:83.
22. Volpé R, Row VV, Ezrin C. Circulating viral and thyroid antibodies in subacute thyroiditis. J Clin Endocrinol Metab. 1967;27(9):1275–84.
23. Ohsako N, Tamai H, Sudo T, Mukuta T, Tanaka H, Kuma K, et al. Clinical characteristics of subacute thyroiditis classified according to human leukocyte antigen typing. J Clin Endocrinol Metab. 1995;80(12):3653–6.
24. Tamai H, Nozaki T, Mukuta T, Morita T, Matsubayashi S, Kuma K, et al. The incidence of thyroid stimulating blocking antibodies during the hypothyroid phase in patients with subacute thyroiditis. J Clin Endocrinol Metab. 1991;73(2):245–50.
25. Galluzzo A, Giordano C, Andronico F, Filardo C, Andronico G, Bompiani G. Leukocyte migration test in subacute thyroiditis: hypothetical role of cell-mediated immunity. J Clin Endocrinol Metab. 1980;50(6):1038–41.
26. Parmar RC, Bavdekar SB, Sahu DR, Warke S, Kamat JR. Thyroiditis as a presenting feature of mumps. Pediatr Infect Dis J. 2001;20(6):637–8.
27. Dimos G, Pappas G, Akritidis N. Subacute thyroiditis in the course of novel H1N1 influenza infection. Endocrine. 2010;37(3):440–1.
28. Volta C, Carano N, Street ME, Bernasconi S. Atypical subacute thyroiditis caused by Epstein-Barr virus infection in a three-year-old girl. Thyroid. 2005;15(10):1189–91.
29. Bouillet B, Petit JM, Piroth L, Duong M, Bourg JB. A case of subacute thyroiditis associated with primary HIV infection. Am J Med. 2009;122(4):e5–6.
30. Satoh M. Virus-like particles in the follicular epithelium of the thyroid from a patient with subacute thyroiditis (de Quervain's). Acta Pathol Jpn. 1975;25:499–501.
31. Engkakul P, Mahachoklertwattana P, Poomthavorn P. de Quervain thyroiditis in a young boy following hand-foot-mouth disease. Eur J Pediatr. 2011;170(4):527–9.
32. Andre R, Opris A, Costantino F, Hayem G, Breban M. Cytomegalovirus subacute thyroiditis in a patient treated by infliximab for psoriatic arthritis. Joint Bone Spine. 2016;83(1):109–10.
33. Martinez-Artola Y, Poncino D, Garcia ML, Munne MS, Gonzalez J, Garcia DS. Acute hepatitis E virus infection and association with a subacute thyroiditis. Ann Hepatol. 2015;14(1):141–2.

34. Mo ZM, Dong YX, Chen XL, Yao HY, Zhang B. Acute transverse myelitis and subacute thyroiditis associated with dengue viral infection: a case report and literature review. Exp Ther Med. 2016;12(4):2331–5.
35. Kim S, Park TS, Baek HS, Jin HY. Subacute painful thyroiditis accompanied by scrub typhus infection. Endocrine. 2013;44(2):546–8.
36. Mangaraj S. Subacute thyroiditis complicating dengue fever – case report and brief review of literature. Trop Dr. 2021;51(2):254–6.
37. Sheraz F, Tahir H, Saqi J, Daruwalla V. Dengue fever presenting atypically with viral conjunctivitis and subacute thyroiditis. J Coll Physicians Surg Pak. 2016;26(6):S33–4.
38. Assir MZ, Jawa A, Ahmed HI. Expanded dengue syndrome: subacute thyroiditis and intracerebral hemorrhage. BMC Infect Dis. 2012;12:240.
39. Brancatella A, Ricci D, Viola N, Sgro D, Santini F, Latrofa F. Subacute thyroiditis after SARS-COV-2 infection. J Clin Endocrinol Metab. 2020;105(7):276.
40. Luotola K, Hyoty H, Salmi J, Miettinen A, Helin H, Pasternack A. Evaluation of infectious etiology in subacute thyroiditis--lack of association with coxsackievirus infection. APMIS. 1998;106(4):500–4.
41. Mori K, Yoshida K, Funato T, Ishii T, Nomura T, Fukuzawa H, et al. Failure in detection of Epstein-Barr virus and cytomegalovirus in specimen obtained by fine needle aspiration biopsy of thyroid in patients with subacute thyroiditis. Tohoku J Exp Med. 1998;186(1):13–7.
42. Espino Montoro A, Medina Perez M, Gonzalez Martin MC, Asencio Marchante R, Lopez Chozas JM. Subacute thyroiditis associated with positive antibodies to the Epstein-Barr virus. An Med Interna. 2000;17(10):546–8.
43. Al Maawali A, Al Yaarubi S, Al Futaisi A. An infant with cytomegalovirus-induced subacute thyroiditis. J Pediatr Endocrinol Metab. 2008;21(2):191–3.
44. Desailloud R, Hober D. Viruses and thyroiditis: an update. Virol J. 2009;6:5.
45. Ippolito S, Dentali F, Tanda ML. SARS-CoV-2: a potential trigger for subacute thyroiditis? Insights from a case report. J Endocrinol Investig. 2020;43(8):1171–2.
46. Asfuroglu Kalkan E, Ates I. A case of subacute thyroiditis associated with Covid-19 infection. J Endocrinol Investig. 2020;43(8):1173–4.
47. Ruggeri RM, Campenni A, Siracusa M, Frazzetto G, Gullo D. Subacute thyroiditis in a patient infected with SARS-COV-2: an endocrine complication linked to the COVID-19 pandemic. Hormones (Athens). 2021;20(1):219–21.
48. Rotondi M, Coperchini F, Ricci G, Denegri M, Croce L, Ngnitejeu ST, Villani L, Magri F, Latrofa F, Chiovato L. Detection of SARS-COV-2 receptor ACE-2 mRNA in thyroid cells: a clue for COVID-19-related subacute thyroiditis. J Endocrinol Investig. 2021;44(5):1085–90.
49. Ma D, Chen CB, Jhanji V, Xu C, Yuan XL, Liang JJ, Huang Y, Cen LP, Ng TK. Expression of SARS-CoV-2 receptor ACE2 and TMPRSS2 in human primary conjunctival and pterygium cell lines and in mouse cornea. Eye (Lond). 2020;34(7):1212–9.
50. Iremli BG, Sendur SN, Unluturk U. Three cases of subacute thyroiditis following SARS-CoV-2 vaccine: postvaccination ASIA syndrome. J Clin Endocrinol Metab. 2021;106(9):2600–5.
51. Stasiak M, Lewiński A. New aspects in the pathogenesis and management of subacute thyroiditis. Rev Endocr Metab Disord. 2021;22:1027–39.
52. Buc M, Nyulassy S, Hnilica P, Stefanovic J. HLA-BW35 and subacute de Quervain's thyroiditis. Diabete Metab. 1976;2(3):163.
53. Kramer AB, Roozendaal C, Dullaart RP. Familial occurrence of subacute thyroiditis associated with human leukocyte antigen-B35. Thyroid. 2004;14:544–7.
54. Hamaguchi E, Nishimura Y, Kaneko S, Takamura T. Subacute thyroiditis developed in identical twins two years apart. Endocr J. 2005;52(5):559–62.
55. Kabalak T, Ozgen AG. Familial occurrence of subacute thyroiditis. Endocr J. 2002;49(2):207–9.
56. Zein EF, Karaa SE, Megarbane A. Familial occurrence of painful subacute thyroiditis associated with human leukocyte antigen-B35. Presse Med. 2007;36(5 Pt 1):808–9.
57. Kalmus Y, Kovatz S, Shilo L, Ganem G, Shenkman L. Sweet's syndrome and subacute thyroiditis. Postgrad Med J. 2000;76(894):229–30.

58. Richard J, Lazarte S, Calame A, Lingvay I. Sweet's syndrome and subacute thyroiditis: an unrecognized association? Thyroid. 2010;20(12):1425–6.
59. Stasiak M, Tymoniuk B, Michalak R, Stasiak B, Kowalski ML, Lewiński A. Subacute thyroiditis is associated with HLA-B*18:01, -DRB1*01 and -C*04:01—the significance of the new molecular background. J Clin Med. 2020;9:534.
60. Vassilopoulou-Sellin R, Sella A, Dexeus FH, Theriault RL, Pololoff DA. Acute thyroid dysfunction (thyroiditis) after therapy with interleukin-2. Horm Metab Res. 1992;24(9):434–8.
61. Amenomori M, Mori T, Fukuda Y, Sugawa H, Nishida N, Furukawa M, Kita R, Sando T, Komeda T, Nakao K. Incidence and characteristics of thyroid dysfunction following interferon therapy in patients with chronic hepatitis C. Intern Med. 1998;37(3):246–52.
62. Martins F, Sofiya L, Sykiotis GP, Lamine F, Maillard M, Fraga M, et al. Adverse effects of immune-checkpoint inhibitors: epidemiology, management and surveillance. Nat Rev Clin Oncol. 2019;16(9):563–80.
63. Gonzalez-Rodriguez E, Rodriguez-Abreu D. Spanish Group for Cancer I-B. Immune checkpoint inhibitors: review and management of endocrine adverse events. Oncologist. 2016;21(7):804–16.
64. de Filette J, Jansen Y, Schreuer M, Everaert H, Velkeniers B, Neyns B, Bravenboer B. Incidence of thyroid-related adverse events in melanoma patients treated with pembrolizumab. J Clin Endocrinol Metab. 2016;101(11):4431–9.
65. Lee H, Hodi FS, Giobbie-Hurder A, Ott PA, Buchbinder EI, Haq R, Tolaney S, et al. Characterization of thyroid disorders in patients receiving immune checkpoint inhibition therapy. Cancer Immunol Res. 2017;5(12):1133–40.
66. Delivanis DA, Gustafson MP, Bornschlegl S, Merten MM, Kottschade L, Withers S, et al. Pembrolizumab-induced thyroiditis: comprehensive clinical review and insights into underlying involved mechanisms. J Clin Endocrinol Metab. 2017;102(8):2770–80.
67. Muir CA, Menzies AM, Clifton-Bligh R, Tsang VHM. Thyroid toxicity following immune checkpoint inhibitor treatment in advanced cancer. Thyroid. 2020;30(10):1458–69.
68. Neppl C, Kaderli RM, Trepp R, Schmitt AM, Berger MD, Wehrli M, et al. Histology of nivolumab-induced thyroiditis. Thyroid. 2018;28(12):1727–8.
69. Muir CA, Clifton-Bligh RJ, Long GV, Scolyer RA, Lo SN, Carlino MS, et al. Thyroid immune-related adverse events following immune checkpoint inhibitor treatment. J Clin Endocrinol Metab. 2021;106(9):e3704–13.
70. Stelmachowska-Banas M, Czajka I. Management of endocrine immune-related adverse events of immune checkpoint inhibitors: an updated review. Endocr Connect. 2020;9(10):R207–28.
71. Deligiorgi MV, Panayiotidis MI, Trafalis DT. Endocrine adverse events related with immune checkpoint inhibitors: an update for clinicians. Immunotherapy. 2020;12(7):481–510.
72. Das L, Bhadada SK, Sood A. Post-COVID-vaccine autoimmune/inflammatory syndrome in response to adjuvants (ASIA syndrome) manifesting as subacute thyroiditis. J Endocrinol Investig. 2021;45:465–7.
73. Shoenfeld Y, Agmon-Levin N. 'ASIA'—autoimmune/inflammatory syndrome induced by adjuvants. J Autoimmun. 2011;36:4–8.
74. Vojdani A, Kharrazian D. Potential antigenic cross-reactivity between SARS-CoV-2 and human tissue with a possible link to an increase in autoimmune diseases. Clin Immunol. 2020;217:108480.
75. Dotan A, Muller S, Kanduc D, David P, Halpert G, Shoenfeld Y. The SARS-CoV-2 as an instrumental trigger of autoimmunity. Autoimmun Rev. 2021;20:102792.
76. Şendur SN, Özmen F, Oğuz SH, Iremli BG, Malkan Y, Gürlek A, et al. Association of human leukocyte antigen genotypes with severe acute respiratory syndrome coronavirus 2 vaccine-induced subacute thyroiditis. Thyroid. 2022;32:640–7.
77. Stasiak M, Zawadzka-Starczewska K, Lewiński A. Clinical manifestation of subacute thyroiditis triggered by SARS-CoV-2 infection can be HLA-dependent. Viruses. 2021;13:2447.
78. Hernan Martinez J, Corder E, Uzcategui M, Garcia M, Sostre S, Garcia A. Subacute thyroiditis and dyserythropoesis after influenza vaccination suggesting immune dysregulation. Bol Asoc Med P R. 2011;103(2):48–52.

79. Hsiao JY, Hsin SC, Hsieh MC, Hsia PJ, Shin SJ. Subacute thyroiditis following influenza vaccine (Vaxigrip) in a young female. Kaohsiung J Med Sci. 2006;22(6):297–300.
80. Momani MS, Zayed AA, Bakri FG. Subacute thyroiditis following influenza vaccine: a case report and literature review. Ital J Med. 2015;9(4):384–6.
81. Shen L, Bui C, Mansberg R, Nguyen D, Alam-Fotias S. Thyroid dysfunction during interferon alpha therapy for chronic hepatitis C. Clin Nucl Med. 2005;30(8):546–7.
82. Kryczka W, Brojer E, Kowalska A, Zarebska-Michaluk D. Thyroid gland dysfunctions during antiviral therapy of chronic hepatitis C. Med Sci Monit. 2001;7(Suppl 1):221–5.
83. Parana R, Cruz M, Lyra L, Cruz T. Subacute thyroiditis during treatment with combination therapy (interferon plus ribavirin) for hepatitis C virus. J Viral Hepat. 2000;7(5):393–5.
84. Omur O, Daglyoz G, Akarca U, Ozcan Z. Subacute thyroiditis during interferon therapy for chronic hepatitis B infection. Clin Nucl Med. 2003;28(10):864–5.
85. Moser C, Furrer J, Ruggieri F. Neck pain and fever after peginterferon alpha-2a. Praxis (Bern 1994). 2007;96(6):205–7.
86. Ohta Y, Ohya Y, Fujii K, Tsuchihashi T, Sato K, Abe I, Iida M. Inflammatory diseases associated with Takayasu's arteritis. Angiology. 2003;54(3):339–44.
87. Obuobie K, Al-Sabah A, Lazarus JH. Subacute thyroiditis in an immunosuppressed patient. J Endocrinol Investig. 2002;25(2):169–71.
88. Ozdogu H, Boga C, Bolat F, Ertorer ME. Wegener's granulomatosis with a possible thyroidal involvement. J Natl Med Assoc. 2006;98(6):956–8.
89. Daniels GH, Vladic A, Brinar V, Zavalishin I, Valente W, Oyuela P, Palmer J, Margolin DH, Hollenstein J. Alemtuzumab-related thyroid dysfunction in a phase 2 trial of patients with relapsing-remitting multiple sclerosis. J Clin Endocrinol Metab. 2014;99(1):80–9.
90. Kawashima J, Naoe H, Sasaki Y, Araki E. A rare case showing subacute thyroiditis-like symptoms with amyloid goiter after anti-tumor necrosis factor therapy. Endocrinol Diabetes Metab Case Rep. 2015;2015:140117.
91. Senlis M, Ottaviani S, Gardette A, Palazzo E, Coustet B, Dieude P. Subacute thyroiditis in psoriatic arthritis treated by adalimumab. Joint Bone Spine. 2017;84(6):745–6.
92. Vazquez Friol MDC, Bravo Blazquez I, Tejera Perez C. Subacute thyroiditis by dasatinib. Med Clin (Barc). 2020;155(6):270–1.
93. Algun E, Alici S, Topal C, Ugras S, Erkoc R, Sakarya ME, et al. Coexistence of subacute thyroiditis and renal cell carcinoma: a paraneoplastic syndrome. CMAJ. 2003;168(8):985–6.
94. Calvi L, Daniels GH. Acute thyrotoxicosis secondary to destructive thyroiditis associated with cardiac catheterization contrast dye. Thyroid. 2011;21(4):443–9.
95. Carneiro JR, Macedo RG, Da Silveira VG. Thyrotoxicosis after gastric bypass. Obes Surg. 2004;14(5):699–701.
96. Sanavi S, Afshar R. Subacute thyroiditis following ginger (Zingiber officinale) consumption. Int J Ayurveda Res. 2010;1(1):47–8.
97. Calapkulu M, Sencar ME, Sakiz D, Unsal IO, Ozbek M, Cakal E. The importance of vitamin D level in subacute thyroiditis disease and the effect of vitamin D on disease prognosis. Endocr Pract. 2020;26:1062–9.
98. Ginde AA, Mansbach JM, Camargo CA Jr. Association between serum 25-hydroxyvitamin D level and upper respiratory tract infection in the Third National Health and Nutrition Examination Survey. Arch Intern Med. 2009;169:384–90.
99. Synoracki S, Ting S, Schmid KW. Inflammatory diseases of the thyroid gland. Pathologe. 2016;37(3):15–223.
100. Harach HR, Williams ED. The pathology of granulomatous diseases of the thyroid gland. Sarcoidosis. 1990;7(1):19–27.
101. Toda S, Tokuda Y, Koike N, Yonemitsu N, Watanabe K, Koike K, et al. Growth factor-expressing mast cells accumulate at the thyroid tissue-regenerative site of subacute thyroiditis. Thyroid. 2000;10(5):381–6.
102. Chang TC, Lai SM, Wen CY, Hsiao YL. Three-dimensional cytomorphology in fine needle aspiration biopsy of subacute thyroiditis. Acta Cytol. 2004;48(2):155–60.

103. Koga M, Hiromatsu Y, Jimi A, Toda S, Koike N, Nonaka K. Immunohistochemical analysis of Bcl-2, Bax, and Bak expression in thyroid glands from patients with subacute thyroiditis. J Clin Endocrinol Metab. 1999;84(6):2221–5.
104. Toda S, Nishimura T, Yamada S, Koike N, Yonemitsu N, Watanabe K, et al. Immunohistochemical expression of growth factors in subacute thyroiditis and their effects on thyroid folliculogenesis and angiogenesis in collagen gel matrix culture. J Pathol. 1999;188(4):415–22.
105. Luotola K, Mantula P, Salmi J, Haapala AM, Laippala P, Hurme M. Allele 2 of interleukin-1 receptor antagonist gene increases the risk of thyroid peroxidase antibodies in subacute thyroiditis. APMIS. 2001;109(6):454–60.
106. Chen K, Wei Y, Sharp GC, Braley-Mullen H. Decreasing TNF-alpha results in less fibrosis and earlier resolution of granulomatous experimental autoimmune thyroiditis. J Leukoc Biol. 2007;81(1):306–14.
107. Fang Y, Sharp GC, Yagita H, Braley-Mullen H. A critical role for TRAIL in resolution of granulomatous experimental autoimmune thyroiditis. J Pathol. 2008;216(4):505–13.
108. Gorges J, Ulrich J, Keck C, Muller-Wieland D, Diederich S, Janssen O. Long-term outcome of subacute thyroiditis. Exp Clin Endocrinol Diabetes. 2019;128:703–8.
109. Lio S, Pontecorvi A, Caruso M, Monaco F, D'Armiento M. Transitory subclinical and permanent hypothyroidism in the course of subacute thyroiditis (De Quervain). Acta Endocrinol. 1984;106:67–70.
110. Daniels GH. Atypical subacute thyroiditis: preliminary observations. Thyroid. 2001;11(7):691–5.
111. Dedivitis RA, Coelho LS. Vocal fold paralysis in subacute thyroiditis. Braz J Otorhinolaryngol. 2007;73(1):138.
112. Nakamura S, Saio Y, Ishimori M. Recurrent hemithyroiditis: a case report. Endocr J. 1998;45(4):595–600.
113. Sari O, Erbas B, Erbas T. Subacute thyroiditis in a single lobe. Clin Nucl Med. 2001;26(5):400–1.
114. Alper AT, Hasdemir H, Akyol A, Cakmak N. Incessant ventricular tachycardia due to subacute thyroiditis. Int J Cardiol. 2007;116(1):e22–4.
115. Sherman SI, Simonson L, Ladenson PW. Clinical and socioeconomic predispositions to complicated thyrotoxicosis: a predictable and preventable syndrome? Am J Med. 1996;101(2):192–8.
116. Swinburne JL, Kreisman SH. A rare case of subacute thyroiditis causing thyroid storm. Thyroid. 2007;17(1):73–6.
117. Kim HJ, Jung TS, Hahm JR, Hwang SJ, Lee SM, Jung JH, et al. Thyrotoxicosis-induced acute myocardial infarction due to painless thyroiditis. Thyroid. 2011;21(10):1149–51.
118. Mizokami T, Okamura K, Sato K, Hirata T, Yamasaki K, Fujishima M. Localized painful giant-cell thyroiditis without inflammatory signs in a euthyroid patient followed by serial sonography. J Clin Ultrasound. 1998;26(6):329–32.
119. Muqtadir F, Ahmed A, Gufran K, Bin Hamza MO. Case of subacute thyroiditis presenting as the cause of pyrexia of unknown origin. J Evol Med Dent Sci. 2015;4(88):15373–5.
120. Popovska-Jovicic B, Canovic P, Gajovic O, Rakovic I, Mijailovic Z. Fever of unknown origin: most frequent causes in adults patients. Vojnosanit Pregl. 2016;73(1):21–5.
121. Cunha BA, Chak A, Strollo S. Fever of unknown origin (FUO): de Quervain's subacute thyroiditis with highly elevated ferritin levels mimicking temporal arteritis (TA). Heart Lung. 2010;39(1):73–7.
122. Duhig TJ, McKeag D. Thyroid disorders in athletes. Curr Sports Med Rep. 2009;8:16–9.
123. Pearce EN, Bogazzi F, Martino E, Brogioni S, Pardini E, Pellegrini G, et al. The prevalence of elevated serum C-reactive protein levels in inflammatory and noninflammatory thyroid disease. Thyroid. 2003;13(7):643–8.
124. Rao NL, Shetty S, Upadhyaya K, Prasad RM, Lobo EC, Kedilaya HP, et al. Salivary C-reactive protein in Hashimoto's thyroiditis and subacute thyroiditis. Int J Inflam. 2010;2010:514659.

125. Sakane S, Murakami Y, Sasaki M, Yamano Y, Takamatsu J, Kuma K, et al. Serum concentrations of granulocyte colony-stimulating factor (G-CSF) determined by a highly-sensitive chemiluminescent immunoassay during the clinical course of subacute thyroiditis. Endocr J. 1995;42:391–6.
126. Calapkulu M, Sencar ME, Sakiz D, Duger H, Unsal IO, Ozbek M, et al. The prognostic and diagnostic use of hematological parameters in subacute thyroiditis patients. Endocrine. 2019;68:138–43.
127. Taşkaldiran I, Omma T, Önder E, Firat SN, Koç G, Kiliç MK, et al. Neutrophil to lymphocyte ratio, monocyte to lymphocyte ratio, platelet to lymphocyte ratio in different etiological causes of thyrotoxicosis. Turk J Med Sci. 2019;49:1687–92.
128. Cengiz H, Varım C, Demirci T, Cetin S. Hemogram parameters in the patients with subacute thyroiditis. Pak J Med Sci. 2019;36:240–5.
129. Bartalena L, Brogioni S, Grasso L, Martino E. Increased serum interleukin-6 concentration in patients with subacute thyroiditis: relationship with concomitant changes in serum T4-binding globulin concentration. J Endocrinol Investig. 1993;16:213–8.
130. Amino N, Yabu Y, Miki T, Morimoto S, Kumahara Y, Mori H, et al. Serum ratio of triiodothyronine to thyroxine, and thyroxine-binding globulin and calcitonin concentrations in graves' disease and destruction-induced thyrotoxicosis. J Clin Endocrinol Metab. 1981;53:113–6.
131. Hennessey J. Subacute thyroiditis, acute and subacute, and Riedel's thyroiditis. South Dartmouth: MDText.com, Inc.; 2018.
132. Nishihara E, Ohye H, Amino N, Takata K, Arishima T, Kudo T, et al. Clinical characteristics of 852 patients with subacute thyroiditis before treatment. Intern Med. 2008;47:725–9.
133. Fujii S, Miwa U, Seta T, Ohoka T, Mizukami Y. Subacute thyroiditis with highly positive thyrotropin receptor antibodies and high thyroidal radioactive iodine uptake. Intern Med. 2003;42(8):704–9.
134. Iitaka M, Momotani N, Hisaoka T, Noh JY, Ishikawa N, Ishii J, et al. TSH receptor antibody-associated thyroid dysfunction following subacute thyroiditis. Clin Endocrinol. 1998;48(4):445–53.
135. Kamijo K. TSH-receptor antibody measurement in patients with various thyrotoxicosis and Hashimoto's thyroiditis: a comparison of two two-step assays, coated plate ELISA using porcine TSH-receptor and coated tube radioassay using human recombinant TSH-receptor. Endocr J. 2003;50(1):113–6.
136. Takasu N, Kamijo K, Sato Y, Yoshimura H, Nagata A, Ochi Y. Sensitive thyroid-stimulating antibody assay with high concentrations of polyethylene glycol for the diagnosis of Graves' disease. Clin Exp Pharmacol Physiol. 2004;31(5–6):314–9.
137. Fang F, Yan S, Zhao L, Jin YB, Wang YF. Concurrent onset of subacute thyroiditis and Graves' disease. Am J Med Sci. 2016;352(2):224–6.
138. Stasiak M, Michalak R, Stasiak B, Lewinsk A. Clinical characteristics of subacute thyroiditis is different than it used to be-current state based on 15 years own material. Neuro Endocrinol Lett. 2019;39:489–95.
139. Erdem N, Erdogan M, Ozbek M, Karadeniz M, Cetinkalp S, Ozgen AG, et al. Demographic and clinical features of patients with subacute thyroiditis: results of 169 patients from a single University Center in Turkey. J Endocrinol Investig. 2007;30:546–50.
140. Nishihara E, Amino N, Kudo T, Kohsaka K, Ito M, Fukata S, et al. Moderate frequency of anti-thyroglobulin antibodies in the early phase of subacute thyroiditis. Eur Thyroid J. 2019;8:268–72.
141. Prajapati S, Hernandez-Prera JC. Putting all the pieces together: clinical, macroscopic and microscopic characteristics of subacute thyroiditis. Head Neck Pathol. 2018;13:231–4.
142. Matsumoto Y, Amino N, Kubota S, Ikeda N, Morita S, Nishihara E, Ohye H, Kudo T, Ito M, Fukata S, Miyauchi A. Serial changes in liver function tests in patients with subacute thyroiditis. Thyroid. 2008;18(7):815–6.
143. Zhuo L, Nie Y, Ma L, Shen L, Zhou X, Li F. Diagnostic value of nuclear medicine imaging and ultrasonography in subacute thyroiditis. Am J Transl Res. 2021;13:5629–34.

144. Kunz A, Blank W, Braun B. De Quervain's subacute thyroiditis -- colour Doppler sonography findings. Ultraschall Med. 2005;26(2):102–6.
145. Park SY, Kim EK, Kim MJ, Kim BM, Oh KK, Hong SW, Park CS. Ultrasonographic characteristics of subacute granulomatous thyroiditis. Korean J Radiol. 2006;7(4):229–34.
146. Omori N, Omori K, Takano K. Association of the ultrasonographic findings of subacute thyroiditis with thyroid pain and laboratory findings. Endocr J. 2008;55(3):583–8.
147. Cappelli C, Pirola I, Gandossi E, Formenti AM, Agosti B, Castellano M. Ultrasound findings of subacute thyroiditis: a single institution retrospective review. Acta Radiol. 2014;55(4):429–33.
148. Li JH, Daniels GH, Barbesino G. Painful subacute thyroiditis is commonly misdiagnosed as suspicious thyroid nodular disease. Mayo Clin Proc Innov Qual Outcomes. 2021;5:330–7.
149. Park SY, Kim E-K, Kim MJ, Kim BM, Oh KK, Hong SW, et al. Ultrasonographic characteristics of subacute granulomatous thyroiditis. Korean J Radiol. 2006;7:229–34.
150. Park HK, Kim DW, Lee YJ, Ha TK, Kim DH, Bae SK, et al. Suspicious sonographic and cytological findings in patients with subacute thyroiditis: two case reports. Diagn Cytopathol. 2014;43:399–402.
151. Ucan B, Delibasi T, Cakal E, Arslan MS, Bozkurt NC, Demirci T, et al. Papillary thyroid cancer case masked by subacute thyroiditis. Arq Bras Endocrinol Metabol. 2014;58:851–4.
152. Valentini RB, De Macedo BM, Izquierdo RF, Meyer ELS. Painless thyroiditis associated to thyroid carcinoma: role of initial ultrasonography evaluation. Arch Endocrinol Metab. 2016;60:178–82.
153. Nishihara E, Hirokawa M, Ohye H, Ito M, Kubota S, Fukata S, et al. Papillary carcinoma obscured by complication with subacute thyroiditis: sequential ultrasonographic and histopathological findings in five cases. Thyroid. 2008;18(11):1221–5.
154. Ohta T, Nishioka M, Nakata N, Fukuda K, Shirakawa T. Significance of perithyroidal lymph nodes in benign thyroid diseases. J Med Ultrason. 2018;45(1):81–7.
155. Leboulleux S, Girard E, Rose M, Travagli JP, Sabbah N, Caillou B, et al. Ultrasound criteria of malignancy for cervical lymph nodes in patients followed up for differentiated thyroid cancer. J Clin Endocrinol Metab. 2007;92:3590–4.
156. Lee YJ, Kim DW. Sonographic characteristics and interval changes of subacute thyroiditis. J Ultrasound Med. 2016;35:1653–9.
157. Solbiati L, Osti V, Cova L, Tonolini M. Ultrasound of thyroid, parathyroid glands and neck lymph nodes. Eur Radiol. 2001;11:2411–24.
158. Ruchala M, Szczepanek-Parulska E, Zybek A, Moczko J, Czarnywojtek A, Kaminski G, et al. The role of sonoelastography in acute, subacute and chronic thyroiditis – a novel application of the method. Eur J Endocrinol. 2012;166(3):425–32.
159. Xie P, Xiao Y, Liu F. Real-time ultrasound elastography in the diagnosis and differential diagnosis of subacute thyroiditis. J Clin Ultrasound. 2011;39:435–40.
160. Hiromatsu Y, Ishibashi M, Miyake I, Nonaka K. Technetium-99m tetrofosmin imaging in patients with subacute thyroiditis. Eur J Nucl Med. 1998;25(10):1448–52.
161. Hiromatsu Y, Ishibashi M, Nishida H, Kawamura S, Kaku H, Baba K, Kaida H, Miyake I. Technetium-99m sestamibi imaging in patients with subacute thyroiditis. Endocr J. 2003;50(3):239–44.
162. Alonso O, Mut F, Lago G, Aznarez A, Nunez M, Canepa J, Touya E. 99Tc(m)-MIBI scanning of the thyroid gland in patients with markedly decreased pertechnetate uptake. Nucl Med Commun. 1998;19(3):257–61.
163. Janssen OE. Atypical presentation of subacute thyroiditis. Dtsch Med Wochenschr. 2011;136(11):519–22.
164. Song YS, Jang SJ, Chung JK, Lee DS. F-18 fluorodeoxyglucose (FDG) positron emission tomography (PET) and Tc-99m pertechnate scan findings of a patient with unilateral subacute thyroiditis. Clin Nucl Med. 2009;34(7):456–8.
165. Peter SA. Painful subacute thyroiditis (de Quervain's thyroiditis). J Natl Med Assoc. 1992;84:877.

166. Mariani G, Tonacchera M, Grosso M, Fiore E, Falcetta P, Montanelli L, et al. The role of nuclear medicine in the clinical management of benign thyroid disorders. Part 2. Nodular goiter, hypothyroidism, and subacute thyroiditis. J Nucl Med. 2021;62:886–95.
167. De Leo S, Lee SY, Braverman LE. Hyperthyroidism. Lancet. 2016;388:906–18.
168. Yeo SH, Lee SK, Hwang I, Ahn EJ. Subacute thyroiditis presenting as a focal lesion on [18F] fluorodeoxyglucose whole-body positron-emission tomography/CT. AJNR Am J Neuroradiol. 2011;32(4):E58–60.
169. Kim MH, Kim DW, Park SA, Kim CG. Transiently altered distribution of F-18 FDG in a patient with subacute thyroiditis. Nucl Med Mol Imaging. 2018;52(1):82–4.
170. Yoshida K, Yokoh H, Toriihara A, Fujii H, Harata N, Isogai J, et al. F-18-FDG PET/CT imaging of atypical subacute thyroiditis in thyrotoxicosis. A case report. Medicine (Baltimore). 2017;96(30):e7535.
171. Freesmeyer M, Opfermann T. Diagnosis of de Quervain's subacute thyroiditis via sensor-navigated (124)iodine PET/ultrasound (I-124-PET/US) fusion. Endocrine. 2015;49(1):293–5.
172. Yeo S, Lee S, Hwang I, Ahn E. Subacute thyroiditis presenting as a focal lesion on [18F] fluorodeoxyglucose whole-body positron-emission tomography/CT. Am J Neuroradiol. 2010;32:E58–60.
173. Shabb NS, Salti I. Subacute thyroiditis: fine-needle aspiration cytology of 14 cases presenting with thyroid nodules. Diagn Cytopathol. 2006;34(1):18–23.
174. Sahin D, Akpolat I. Diagnostic cytological features and differential diagnosis of subacute granulomatous (De Quervain's) thyroiditis. Diagn Cytopathol. 2019;47:1251–8.
175. Vural C, Paksoy N, Gök ND, Yazal K. Subacute granulomatous (De Quervain's) thyroiditis: fine-needle aspiration cytology and ultrasonographic characteristics of 21 cases. Cytojournal. 2015;12:9.
176. Öfner C, Hittmair A, Kröll I, Bangerl I, Zechmann W, Totsch M, et al. Fine needle aspiration cytodiagnosis of subacute (De Quervain's) thyroiditis in an endemic goitre area. Cytopathology. 1994;5:33–40.
177. Zimmerman RS, Brennan MD, McConahey WM, Goellner JR, Gharib H. Hashimoto's thyroiditis: an uncommon cause of painful thyroid unresponsive to corticosteroid therap. Ann Intern Med. 1986;104:355–7.
178. Houghton DJ, Gray HW, MacKenzie K. The tender neck: thyroiditis or thyroid abscess? Clin Endocrinol. 1998;48:521–4.
179. Jin M, Kim TY. Anaplastic thyroid carcinoma with initial ultrasonography features mimicking subacute thyroiditis. Endocrinol Metab. 2021;36:201–2.
180. García Solano J, Giménez Bascuñana A, Sola Pérez J, Campos Fernández J, Martínez Parra D, Sánchez Sánchez C, et al. Fine-needle aspiration of subacute granulomatous thyroiditis (De Quervain's thyroiditis): a clinico-cytologic review of 36 cases. Diagn Cytopathol. 1997;16:214–20.
181. Shabb NS, Salti I. Subacute thyroiditis: fine-needle aspiration cytology of 14 cases presenting with thyroid nodules. Diagn Cytopathol. 2005;34:18–23.
182. Lu C-P, Chang T-C, Wang C-Y, Hsiao Y-L. Serial changes in ultrasound-guided fine needle aspiration cytology in subacute thyroiditis. Acta Cytol. 1997;41:238–43.
183. Christensen J, O'Callaghan K, Sinclair H, Hawke K, Love A, Hajkowicz K, et al. Risk factors, treatment and outcomes of subacute thyroiditis secondary to COVID-19: a systematic review. Intern Med J. 2021;52:522–9.
184. Tesfaye H, Cimermanova R, Cholt M, Sykorova P, Pechova M, Prusa R. Subacute thyroiditis confused with dental problem. Cas Lek Cesk. 2009;148(9):438–41.
185. Bostan H, Sencar ME, Calapkulu M, Hepsen S, Duger H, Unsal IO, et al. Two important issues in subacute thyroiditis management: delayed diagnosis and inappropriate use of antibiotics. Eur Thyroid J. 2021;10:323–9.
186. Zacharia TT, Perumpallichira JJ, Sindhwani V, Chavhan G. Gray-scale and color Doppler sonographic findings in a case of subacute granulomatous thyroiditis mimicking thyroid carcinoma. J Clin Ultrasound. 2002;30:442–4.

187. Stasiak M, Michalak R, Stasiak B, Lewiński A. Time-lag between symptom onset and diagnosis of subacute thyroiditis–how to avoid the delay of diagnosis and unnecessary overuse of antibiotics. Horm Metab Res. 2019;52:32–8.
188. Spitzer M, Alexanian S, Farwell AP. Thyrotoxicosis with post-treatment hypothyroidism in a patient with acute suppurative thyroiditis due to porphyromonas. Thyroid. 2012;22(1):97–100.
189. Meller J, Sahlmann CO, Scheel AK. 18F-FDG PET and PET/CT in fever of unknown origin. J Nucl Med. 2007;48(1):35–45.
190. Yasuda S, Shohtsu A, Ide M, Takagi S, Takahashi W, Suzuki Y, Horiuchi M. Chronic thyroiditis: diffuse uptake of FDG at PET. Radiology. 1998;207(3):775–8.
191. Tezuka M, Murata Y, Ishida R, Ohashi I, Hirata Y, Shibuya H. MR imaging of the thyroid: correlation between apparent diffusion coefficient and thyroid gland scintigraphy. J Magn Reson Imaging. 2003;17(2):163–9.
192. Liel Y. The survivor: association of an autonomously functioning thyroid nodule and subacute thyroiditis. Thyroid. 2007;17(2):183–4.
193. Pereira O, Prasad DS, Bal AM, McAteer D, Abraham P. Fatal descending necrotizing mediastinitis secondary to acute suppurative thyroiditis developing in an apparently healthy woman. Thyroid. 2010;20(5):571–2.
194. Yung BC, Loke TK, Fan WC, Chan JC. Acute suppurative thyroiditis due to foreign body-induced retropharyngeal abscess presented as thyrotoxicosis. Clin Nucl Med. 2000;25(4):249–52.
195. Savoie JC, Massin JP, Thomopoulos P, Leger F. Iodine-induced thyrotoxicosis in apparently normal thyroid glands. J Clin Endocrinol Metab. 1975;41(4):685–91.
196. Woolf PD. Transient painless thyroiditis with hyperthyroidism: a variant of lymphocytic thyroiditis? Endocr Rev. 1980;1(4):411–20.
197. Szabo SM, Allen DB. Thyroiditis. Differentiation of acute suppurative and subacute. Case report and review of the literature. Clin Pediatr. 1989;28:171–4.
198. Masuoka H, Miyauchi A, Tomoda C, Inoue H, Takamura Y, Ito Y, et al. Imaging studies in sixty patients with acute suppurative thyroiditis. Thyroid. 2011;21:1075–80.
199. Fragu P, Rougier P, Schlumberger M, Tubiana M. Evolution of thyroid 127I stores measured by X-ray fluorescence in subacute thyroiditis. J Clin Endocrinol Metab. 1982;54(1):162–6.
200. Gordin A, Lamberg BA. Serum thyrotrophin response to thyrotrophin releasing hormone and the concentration of free thyroxine in subacute thyroiditis. Acta Endocrinol. 1973;74(1):111–21.
201. Intenzo CM, Park CH, Kim SM, Capuzzi DM, Cohen SN, Green P. Clinical, laboratory, and scintigraphic manifestations of subacute and chronic thyroiditis. Clin Nucl Med. 1993;18(4):302–6.
202. Rapoport B, Block MB, Hoffer PB, DeGroot LJ. Depletion of thyroid iodine during subacute thyroiditis. J Clin Endocrinol Metab. 1973;36(3):610–1.
203. King DL, Stack BC Jr, Spring PM, Walker R, Bodenner DL. Incidence of thyroid carcinoma in fluorodeoxyglucose positron emission tomography-positive thyroid incidentalomas. Otolaryngol Head Neck Surg. 2007;137(3):400–4.
204. Van den Bruel A, Maes A, De Potter T, Mortelmans L, Drijkoningen M, Van Damme B, Delaere P, Bouillon R. Clinical relevance of thyroid fluorodeoxyglucose-whole body positron emission tomography incidentaloma. J Clin Endocrinol Metab. 2002;87(4):1517–20.
205. Mordes DA, Brachtel EF. Cytopathology of subacute thyroiditis. Diagn Cytopathol. 2012;40(5):433–4.
206. Guarda MLA, Baskin MHJ. Inflammatory and lymphoid lesions of the thyroid gland: cytopathology by fine-needle aspiration. Am J Clin Pathol. 1987;87:14–22.
207. Kasagi K. Painful Hashimoto's thyroiditis. Intern Med. 2006;45:351–2.
208. Meier DA, Nagle CE. Differential diagnosis of a tender goiter. J Nucl Med. 1996;37:1745.
209. Stasiak M, Michalak R, Lewinski A. Thyroid primary and metastatic malignant tumours of poor prognosis may mimic subacute thyroiditis-time to change the diagnostic criteria: case reports and a review of the literature. BMC Endocr Disord. 2019;19:86.

210. Byrd JC, Dow NS, Gaertner E, Hargis JB, Raber TR, Burrell L, et al. Leukemic thyroiditis as the initial relapsing sign in a patient with acute lymphocytic leukemia and blast expression of the neural cell adhesion molecule. Am J Hematol. 1997;55:212–5.
211. Ranganath R, Shaha MA, Xu B, Migliacci J, Ghossein R, Shaha AR. de Quervain's thyroiditis: a review of experience with surgery. Am J Otolaryngol. 2016;37:534–7.
212. Samuels MH. Subacute, silent, and postpartum thyroiditis. Med Clin North Am. 2012;96:223–33.
213. Gupta N, Sharma K, Barwad A, Sharma M, Rajwanshi A, Dutta P, et al. Thyroid tuberculosis-role of PCR in diagnosis of a rare entity. Cytopathology. 2010;22:392–6.
214. Ross DS, Burch HB, Cooper DS, Greenlee MC, Laurberg P, Maia AL, et al. 2016 American Thyroid Association guidelines for diagnosis and management of hyperthyroidism and other causes of thyrotoxicosis. Thyroid. 2016;26:1343–421.
215. Volpé R. The management of subacute (DeQuervain's) thyroiditis. Thyroid. 1993;3:253–5.
216. Kubota S, Nishihara E, Kudo T, Ito M, Amino N, Miyauchi A. Initial treatment with 15 mg of prednisolone daily is sufficient for most patients with subacute thyroiditis in Japan. Thyroid. 2013;23(3):269–72.
217. Duan L, Feng X, Zhang R, Tan X, Xiang X, Shen R, et al. Short-term versus 6-week prednisone in the treatment of subacute thyroiditis: a randomized controlled trial. Endocr Prac. 2020;26:900–8.
218. Tian Z, Su Y, Zhang M, Zhang X, Guan Q. Successful management of recurrent subacute thyroiditis by adding colchicine to glucocorticoid treatment: a case series study. Horm Metab Res. 2020;52:712–7.
219. Koirala KP. Treatment of acute painful thyroiditis with low dose prednisolone: a study on patients from Western Nepal. J Clin Diagn Res. 2015;9:MC01.
220. Hepsen S, Akhanli P, Sencar ME, Duger H, Sakiz D, Kizilgul M, et al. The evaluation of low- and high-dose steroid treatments in subacute thyroiditis: a retrospective observational study. Endocr Pract. 2020;27:594–600.
221. Li J, Zhang J, Jiang L, Li Z, Li F, Chen H, et al. Efficacy and safety of ultrasound-guided intrathyroidal injection of glucocorticoids versus routine oral administration of glucocorticoids for subacute thyroiditis: protocol of systematic review and meta-analysis. Medicine (Baltimore). 2019;98:e18564.
222. Forkert IO, Melekhovets OK, Kalynychenko DO, Melekhovets YV, Kovalenko EL. Painful subacute thyroiditis treatment approach. Wiad Lek. 2021;74:1921–4.
223. Sato J, Uchida T, Komiya K, Goto H, Takeno K, Suzuki R, et al. Comparison of the therapeutic effects of prednisolone and nonsteroidal anti-inflammatory drugs in patients with subacute thyroiditis. Endocrine. 2017;55(1):218–23.
224. Topuzovic N, Smoje J, Karner I. The therapeutic approach in subacute (de Quervain's) thyroiditis. J Nucl Med. 1997;38:1665.
225. Zhang J, Ding G, Li J, Li X, Ding L, Li X, et al. Risk factors for subacute thyroiditis recurrence: a systematic review and meta-analysis of cohort studies. Front Endocrinol. 2021;12:783439.
226. Sencar ME, Calapkulu M, Sakiz D, Hepsen S, Kus A, Akhanli P, et al. An evaluation of the results of the steroid and non-steroidal anti-inflammatory drug treatments in subacute thyroiditis in relation to persistent hypothyroidism and recurrence. Sci Rep. 2019;9(1):16899.
227. Arao T, Okada Y, Torimoto K, Kurozumi A, Narisawa M, Yamamoto S, et al. Prednisolone dosing regimen for treatment of subacute thyroiditis. J UOEH. 2015;37:103–10.
228. Ma SG, Bai F, Cheng L. A novel treatment for subacute thyroiditis: administration of a mixture of lidocaine and dexamethasone using an insulin pen. Mayo Clin Proc. 2014;89(6):861–2.
229. Shen X, Yang R, An J, Zhong X. Analysis of the molecular mechanisms of the effects of Prunella vulgaris against subacute thyroiditis based on network pharmacology. Evid Based Complement Altern Med. 2020;2020:9810709.
230. Saklamaz A. Is there a drug effect on the development of permanent hypothyroidism in subacute thyroiditis? Acta Endocrinol. 2017;13:119–23.
231. Duininck TM, van Heerden JA, Fatourechi V, Curlee KJ, Farley DR, Thompson GB, et al. de Quervain's thyroiditis: surgical experience. Endocr Pract. 2002;8(4):255–8.

232. Park HK, Kim DW, Lee YJ, Ha TK, Kim DH, Bae SK, et al. Suspicious sonographic and cytological findings in patients with subacute thyroiditis two case reports. Diagn Cytopathol. 2015;43(5):399–402.
233. Mazza E, Quaglino F, Suriani A, Palestini N, Gottero C, Leli R, Taraglio S. Thyroidectomy for painful thyroiditis resistant to steroid treatment: three new cases with review of the literature. Case Rep Endocrinol. 2015;2015:138327.
234. Dumitriu L, Gudovan E, Ursu H. Radioiodine treatment in recurrences of subacute thyroiditis. Endocrinologie. 1990;28:21–3.
235. Zhao N, Wang S, Cui XJ, Huang MS, Wang SW, Li YG, Zhao L, Wan WN, Li YS, Shan ZY, Teng WP. Two-years prospective follow-up study of subacute thyroiditis. Front Endocrinol (Lausanne). 2020;11:47.
236. Görges J, Ulrich J, Keck C, Müller-Wieland D, Diederich S, Janssen OE. Long-term outcome of subacute thyroiditis. Exp Clin Endocrinol Diabetes. 2019;128:703–8.
237. Tang C, Dong Y, Lu L, Zhang N. C-reactive protein and thyroid-stimulating hormone levels as risk factors for hypothyroidism in patients with subacute thyroiditis. Endocr Connect. 2021;10:965–72.
238. Teixeira VL, Romaldini J, Rodrigues HF, Tanaka LM, Farah CS. Thyroid function during the spontaneous course of subacute thyroiditis. J Nucl Med. 1985;26:457–60.
239. Qari FA, Maimani AA. Subacute thyroiditis in Western Saudi Arabia. Saudi Med J. 2005;26:630–3.
240. Bennedbaek FN, Hegedüs L. The value of ultrasonography in the diagnosis and follow-up of subacute thyroiditis. Thyroid. 1997;7:45–50.
241. Erdem N, Erdogan M, Ozbek M, Karadeniz M, Cetinkalp S, Gokhan Ozgen A, et al. Demographic and clinical features of patients with subacute thyroiditis: results of 169 patients from a single University Center in Turkey. J Endocrinol Investig. 2007;30:546–50.
242. Yamamoto M, Saito S, Sakurada T, Tamura M, Kudo Y, Yoshida K, et al. Recurrence of subacute thyroiditis over 10 years after the first attack in three cases. Endocrinol Jpn. 1988;35:833–9.
243. Stasiak M, Tymoniuk B, Stasiak B, Lewiński A. The risk of recurrence of subacute thyroiditis is HLA-dependent. Int J Mol Sci. 2019;20:1089.
244. Tajiri J, Noguchi S, Morita M, Tamaru M, Murakami T, Murakami N. Serum sialic acid levels in the diagnosis and follow-up of subacute granulomatous thyroiditis. Endocr J. 1993;40:83–7.
245. Hepsen S, Akhanli P, Sencar ME, Duger H, Sakiz D, Kizilgul M, et al. The evaluation of low- and high-dose steroid treatments in subacute thyroiditis: a retrospective observational study. Endocr Pract. 2021;27:594–600.
246. Iitaka M, Momotani N, Ishii JKI. Incidence of subacute thyroiditis recurrences after a prolonged latency: 24-year survey. J Clin Endocrinol Metab. 1996;81:466–9.
247. Sencar ME, Calapkulu M, Sakiz D, Akhanli P, Hepsen S, Duger H, et al. The contribution of ultrasonographic findings to the prognosis of subacute thyroiditis. Arch Endocrinol Metab. 2020;64:306–11.
248. Mizukoshi T, Noguchi S, Murakami T, Futata T, Yamashita H. Evaluation of recurrence in 36 subacute thyroiditis patients managed with prednisolone. Intern Med. 2001;40:292–5.
249. Engkakul P, Mahachoklertwattana P, Poomthavorn P. Eponym. Eur J Pediatr. 2010;170:427–31.
250. Nishihara E, Amino N, Ohye H, Ota H, Ito M, Kubota S, et al. Extent of hypoechogenic area in the thyroid is related with thyroid dysfunction after subacute thyroiditis. J Endocrinol Investig. 2009;32:33–6.
251. Bogazzi F, Dell'Unto E, Tanda ML, Tomisti L, Cosci C, Aghini-Lombardi F, et al. Long-term outcome of thyroid function after amiodarone-induced thyrotoxicosis, as compared to subacute thyroiditis. J Endocrinol Investig. 2006;29(8):694–9.
252. Izumi M, Larsen PR. Correlation of sequential changes in serum thyroglobulin, triiodothyronine, and thyroxine in patients with Graves' disease and subacute thyroiditis. Metabolism. 1978;27(4):449–60.

253. Benbassat CA, Olchovsky D, Tsvetov G, Shimon I. Subacute thyroiditis: clinical characteristics and treatment outcome in fifty-six consecutive patients diagnosed between 1999 and 2005. J Endocrinol Investig. 2007;30:631–5.
254. Nakano Y, Kurihara H, Sasaki J. Graves' disease following subacute thyroiditis. Tohoku J Exp Med. 2011;225(4):301–9.
255. Mathew AA, Papaly R, Maliakal A, Chandra L, Antony MA. Elevated Graves' disease-specific thyroid-stimulating immunoglobulin and thyroid stimulating hormone receptor antibody in a patient with subacute thyroiditis. Cureus. 2021;13:e19448.
256. Minciullo PL, Ruggeri RM, Vita G, Benvenga S, Gangemi S. Development of Hashimoto's thyroiditis after subacute thyroiditis: an unusual patient. Thyroid. 2009;19:73–4.
257. Iitaka M, Kakinuma S, Yamanaka K, Fujimaki S, Oosuga I, Wada S, et al. Induction of autoimmune hypothyroidism and subsequent hyperthyroidism by TSH receptor antibodies following subacute thyroiditis: a case report. Endocr J. 2001;48:139–42.
258. Hallengren B, Planck T, Åsman P, Lantz M. Presence of thyroid-stimulating hormone receptor antibodies in a patient with subacute thyroiditis followed by hypothyroidism and later Graves' disease with ophthalmopathy: a case report. Eur Thyroid J. 2015;4:197–200.
259. Fukata S, Matsuzuka F, Kobayashi A, Hirai K, Kuma K, Sugawara M. Development of Graves' disease after subacute thyroiditis: two unusual cases. Eur J Endocrinol. 1992;126:495–6.

6 Subacute Lymphocytic (Silent/Painless) Thyroiditis

6.1 Pathogenesis

Silent (painless) lymphocytic thyroiditis is a well-known cause of subacute thyroiditis that affects mostly women in the post-partum period. The majority of patients pass through a tri-phasic course starting with a transient hyperthyroid phase, followed by a longer hypothyroid phase; most, but not all, recover spontaneously to the euthyroid state. The disorder is self-limited and often goes undiagnosed. Suspicion of the diagnosis generally depends on clinical findings, typically once hypothyroidism has occurred [1–3].

Management of painless thyroiditis depends on patient presentation and disease phase. In general, treatment is *not* necessary for asymptomatic or mildly symptomatic patients. Because silent lymphocytic thyroiditis lasts only a few months, treatment is conservative. Anti-thyroid medications are not used as they are ineffective. Surgery and radioactive iodine (RAI) therapy are contraindicated [1, 2]. A beta-blocker is often needed in the hyperthyroid phase, and thyroid hormone replacement is typically needed in the hypothyroid phase. This disorder usually recurs after subsequent pregnancies. Recurrent disease is treated in the same manner as the initial occurrence, though patients with "multiple" recurrences may opt for surgery or RAI ablation of the thyroid (after recovering from the thyrotoxic phase) [1, 2].

6.2 Classification

Silent (painless) thyroiditis is classified into (1) sporadic type, which includes thyroiditis unrelated to pregnancy, (2) post-partum thyroiditis and gestational painless thyroiditis [4]; (3) exogenous (drug-induced) painless thyroiditis [5]; and (4) "others" including that induced by neck radiation, trauma and post-^{131}I therapy for Graves' disease [6]. Table 6.1 summarizes the novel classification of silent thyroiditis introduced by Kamijo in 2019.

M. Sakr, *Thyroiditis*, https://doi.org/10.1007/978-3-032-19513-5_6

Table 6.1 Novel classification of painless thyroiditis

Sporadic painless thyroiditis
1. Unrelated to pregnancy
(a) Autoimmune (TgAb and/or TPOAb positive)
(b) Non-autoimmune (TgAb and TPOAb negative)
2. Postpartum thyroiditis
3. Gestational thyroiditis
Drug-induced painless thyroiditis
1. Immunomodulator (interferon alpha, interleukin 2, etc.)
2. GnRH analogues (leuprorelin, goserelin)
3. Tyrosine kinase inhibitor (sunitinib, sorafenib)
4. Immune checkpoint inhibitor (nivolumab, pembrolizumab, ipilimumab)
5. Others (lithium, amiodarone, potassium iodide)
Others
Mechanical destruction-induced painless thyroiditis such as external radiation, trauma, massage, post-^{131}I therapy for Graves' disease

6.3 Sporadic Painless Thyroiditis

6.3.1 Definitions

"Thyroiditis" is any disorder caused by inflammation of the thyroid tissue, resulting in the release of preformed thyroid hormone leading to thyrotoxicosis followed by hypothyroidism [3]. "Subacute lymphocytic thyroiditis" (painless/silent thyroiditis) is characterized by an autoimmune-mediated lymphocytic inflammation of the thyroid gland resulting in a destructive thyroiditis with release of thyroid hormone and transient thyrotoxicosis (hyperthyroidism). This is frequently followed by a hypothyroid phase before recovery of normal thyroid function. Thus, it classically presents with a tri-phasic course, including a thyrotoxic phase, a hypothyroid phase, and then a euthyroid phase [1].

The term "silent" refers to the absence of thyroid pain and tenderness in contrast with subacute thyroiditis (De Quervain's), which usually causes thyroid pain and tenderness.

6.3.2 Synonyms

Synonyms of this disorder include "silent thyroiditis," "silent sporadic thyroiditis," "painless thyroiditis," "painless sporadic thyroiditis," "painless lymphocytic thyroiditis," "subacute lymphocytic thyroiditis," "lymphocytic thyroiditis with spontaneously resolving hyperthyroidism," and "painless post-partum thyroiditis" (in the first year post-partum).

6.3.3 Epidemiology

6.3.3.1 Geographic Distribution

Painless (silent) thyroiditis is most prevalent in areas with higher dietary iodine intake such as Japan [2].

6.3.3.2 Demography

Painless (silent) thyroiditis is more common in women than men with a reported ratio of 4:1 [1, 2]. The majority of cases of painless thyroiditis are diagnosed in adults with an age ranging between 30 and 40 years [2].

6.3.3.3 Incidence/Prevalence

Painless (silent) thyroiditis is reported to account for 0%–30% of thyrotoxicosis cases worldwide, including 30% in Japan, 22% in Wisconsin (USA), and 6% in Toronto (Canada) [1, 2]. The prevalence of painless thyroiditis diagnosed by thyroid scintigraphy in patients presenting with thyrotoxicosis in Denmark was reported to be 0.5% [6].

Painless thyroiditis may be sporadic. It accounts for approximately 0.5%–5% of cases of hyperthyroidism. However, it causes most cases of post-partum thyroid dysfunction as it occurs in approximately 5%–10% of post-partum women. It has many similarities with post-partum thyroiditis, but by definition excludes women who have a painless thyroiditis syndrome within 1 year after a delivery, abortion, or pregnancy loss, i.e., painless thyroiditis that occurs within 1 year post-partum is called "post-partum thyroiditis" [1–3].

6.3.4 Etiology/Pathogenesis

Silent thyroiditis can occur post-partum, during radiation therapy, or as the result of bacterial or viral infection. It can also occur secondary to certain medications, such as lithium, immune checkpoint inhibitors, tyrosine kinase inhibitors, amiodarone, and cytokine therapy (interferon-alpha) [1, 3].

Painless thyroiditis is part of the spectrum of autoimmune thyroid disease, as evidenced by the presence of anti-thyroid antibodies (reported in approximately 50% of patients) and pathological findings of lymphocytic infiltration of the thyroid gland [1–3]. It is considered by many to be a variant presentation of Hashimoto's thyroiditis (chronic lymphocytic or chronic autoimmune thyroiditis). This is because individuals with painless thyroiditis may progress to permanent hypothyroidism, which is a characteristic feature of Hashimoto's thyroiditis. The two disorders have some pathological similarities, and many patients with painless thyroiditis have high serum concentrations of anti-thyroid peroxidase (TPO) and anti-thyroglobulin (Tg) antibodies, many have a family history of thyroid autoimmune disease, and some develop overt chronic autoimmune thyroiditis several years later.

Painless thyroiditis is associated with specific human leukocyte antigen (HLA) haplotypes, most often HLA-DR3, findings that suggest an inherited susceptibility.

However, the association is considerably weaker than that between HLA-B35 and subacute thyroiditis.

6.3.5 Clinical Presentation

Silent lymphocytic thyroiditis is characterized by a variable degree of painless thyroid enlargement [1, 2] with a classic tri-phasic course (thyrotoxicosis, hypothyroidism, and recovery to euthyroid state) [2, 3]. The initial thyrotoxic phase typically persists for 3–4 months; however, only about 5%–20% of patients present in this phase as it may be mild or asymptomatic. Following the thyrotoxic phase, patients may progress to transient hypothyroidism lasting up to 6 months due to a depletion of thyroid hormone stores and synthesis (most patients present in this phase). The majority of patients recover to euthyroid state after a total duration of 12 months; however, about 10%–20% of patients are reported to progress to chronic autoimmune thyroiditis with persistent hypothyroidism (Hashimoto thyroiditis). Eye signs and pretibial myxedema do *not* occur.

History and physical examination diagnostic findings during the thyrotoxic [7] hypothyroid [8] phases, as well as risk factors [9] of silent thyroiditis, are summarized in Table 6.2.

6.3.6 History-Taking

6.3.6.1 History of Present Illness

- Recent pregnancy (within the past year) [3]
- History of thyroid disorders, including post-partum thyroiditis [9]
- Autoimmune disorders, including (but not limited to) type-1 diabetes mellitus (DM) and systemic lupus erythematosus (SLE) [9]

Table 6.2 Diagnostic and risk factors of silent (painless) thyroiditis

Thyrotoxic phase	Hypothyroid phase	Risk factors
Heat intolerance	Cold intolerance	Post-partum period
Nervousness	Dry skin	Female gender
Irritability	Generalized aches and pains	Thyroid peroxidase (TPO) antibodies
Anxiety	Impaired concentration or memory	Immunomodulatory therapy
Tremors	Fatigue	Type 1 diabetes mellitus (DM).
Palpitations	Constipation	Systemic lupus erythematosus (SLE)
Weight loss	Difficulty losing weight	
Excessive fatigue	Parasthesia	
Bloating	Irregular menses	
Irregular menses		

6.3.6.2 Medication (Drug) History

Medications that increase the risk of thyroid disorders include amiodarone, lithium, cytokines (interferon-alpha [IFN-α]), immune checkpoint inhibitors (most commonly ipilimumab and nivolumab), and tyrosine kinase inhibitors [3].

6.3.6.3 Family History

Positive family history of thyroid autoimmunity or other autoimmune diseases [3].

6.3.7 Physical Examination

6.3.7.1 General Physical Examination

- In the thyrotoxic phase, findings may include tachycardia and arrhythmia, systolic hypertension, and weight loss [10].
- In the hypothyroid phase, findings may include bradycardia, hypopnea, and increase in body mass index (BMI) [11].

6.3.7.2 Skin

- Warm, moist skin may suggest thyrotoxicosis [10].
- Coarse, dry, cold skin may suggest hypothyroidism [11].

6.3.7.3 Head and Neck

- Puffy eyelids (may suggest hypothyroidism) [11].
- Ophthalmopathy consistent with Graves' disease (a differential diagnosis) includes exophthalmos (proptosis), peri-orbital edema, conjunctival erythema and edema (chemosis), corneal opacity, incomplete eyelid closure with cornea still visible (may lead to corneal ulceration and vision loss), ophthalmoplegia, head tilt to compensate for double vision, and papilledema [12].
- Small, painless goiter [1, 2].

6.3.7.4 Cardiac Examination

Cardiac findings that may indicate thyrotoxicosis include sinus tachycardia, extrasystoles, atrial flutter, atrial fibrillation, and heart failure [10].

6.3.7.5 Extremities

Peripheral edema may indicate hypothyroidism [11].

6.3.7.6 Neurological Assessment

- Neurological findings that may indicate thyrotoxicosis include fine tremors, proximal muscle weakness, and hyper-reflexia [10].
- Neurological and psychiatric manifestations that may indicate hypothyroidism include impaired cognitive function and delayed relaxation of tendon reflexes. Rare signs include depression, dementia, and ataxia [11].

6.3.8 Diagnosis

6.3.8.1 History and Physical Examination

The diagnosis of painless thyroiditis depends on the disease phase, as the signs and symptoms change throughout the course of the disease. Silent lymphocytic thyroiditis is frequently undiagnosed. Suspicion of the diagnosis generally depends on clinical findings, typically once hypothyroidism has occurred [1–3]. Commonly, there is no history of recent pregnancy (within the past year) or use of medications associated with thyroid dysfunction, and no pathognomonic signs and symptoms of Graves' disease such as Graves' ophthalmopathy.

6.3.8.2 Laboratory Tests

- Thyroid function test results vary depending on the phase of illness. Initially, serum T4 and T3 are elevated and TSH is suppressed. In the hypothyroid phase, these findings are reversed [2].
- Thyroid peroxidase (TPO) auto-antibodies (reported in 50% of cases) and, less commonly, anti-thyroglobulin (Tg) antibodies are almost always positive during pregnancy and the post-partum period in these patients [1–3]. Thus, this disorder would appear to be a variant of Hashimoto's thyroiditis.
- In patients with thyrotoxicosis with an unclear etiology, measurement of thyroid receptor antibodies (TRAb) can help differentiate painless thyroiditis from Graves' disease (presence of TRAb confirms diagnosis of Graves' disease) [1].
- Recently, Kamijo (2019) [5] reported a rare case of a 41-year-old woman with painless thyroiditis who was positive for thyrotropin (TSH) receptor-blocking (TBAbs) and receptor-stimulating auto-antibodies (TSAbs) in the thyrotoxic phase. Her serum thyroid hormone levels were high, and TSH was undetectable. The low uptake of 99mTc led to the diagnosis of painless thyroiditis. M22-TRAb, TBAb, and TSAb were detectable in the thyrotoxic phase. Three months later, she became severely hypothyroid. M22-TRAb and TBAb were still strongly positive, although the TSAb levels had decreased to just above the reference range. In this case, TBAb led to hypothyroidism.
- Blood tests to differentiate painless thyroiditis from subacute thyroiditis (SAT) are rarely needed, as the presence or absence of thyroid pain can typically differentiate between these entities. White blood cell (WBC) count, erythrocyte sedimentation rate (ESR), and C-reactive protein (CRP) are normal in painless thyroiditis [1].

6.3.8.3 Imaging Studies

Radioactive Iodine Uptake (RAIU) Scan (Scintigraphy)

Radioactive iodine uptake (RAIU) scan may be useful for diagnosing painless thyroiditis, but results will vary depending on disease phase [1, 2]. During the thyrotoxic phase, RAIU is low or absent. Diagnosis can be confirmed by a 4-, 6-, or 24-h RAIU of $<1\%$ during the hyperthyroid phase of the illness. During the hypothyroid phase, RAIU is normal or elevated [1, 2].

Radioactive iodine uptake (RAIU) scan can also be used to distinguish painless thyroiditis from Graves' disease [2]. RAIU is elevated in Graves' disease and low or absent in painless thyroiditis during the thyrotoxic phase. RAIU may be transiently increased during the hypothyroid phase of thyroiditis, so it is not informative once thyrotoxicosis has resolved.

Thyroid Ultrasound (US)

Thyroid ultrasound is *not* routinely performed for diagnosis of painless thyroiditis, but may be performed in patients with irregularities or suspected thyroid nodules. In patients with painless thyroiditis, the thyroid gland may have an inhomogeneous hypo-echogenic texture on US examination and may show a decreased blood flow on Doppler examination [1, 2].

6.3.8.4 Needle Biopsy

Needle biopsy provides definitive diagnosis, but is usually unnecessary. It is *not* routinely performed, but may help distinguish between Hashimoto's thyroiditis and painless thyroiditis. Thyroid biopsy commonly reveals diffuse lymphocytic infiltration in painless thyroiditis as in Hashimoto's thyroiditis, but without lymphoid follicles and fibrosis [1, 2].

6.3.9 Differential Diagnosis

6.3.9.1 Differential Diagnosis During the Thyrotoxic Phase

Graves' Disease

The main differential diagnosis of painless (silent) thyroiditis in the thyrotoxic stage is Graves' disease as follows [1, 2]:

- Patients with Graves' disease present with a diffuse goiter and may have ophthalmopathy, dermatopathy, acropachy, or a thyroid bruit.
- Higher serum triiodothyronine (T3) and T3 to thyroxin (T4) ratios are commonly found in Graves' disease compared with painless thyroiditis.
- Thyroid receptor antibodies (TRAb) or thyroid-binding inhibitory immunoglobulins are typically found in Graves' disease, but not in painless thyroiditis.
- Radioactive iodine uptake (RAIU) is low in painless thyroiditis in the thyrotoxic stage and high in Graves' disease; care must be taken to ensure RAIU is measured during thyrotoxicosis because uptake increases during the hypothyroid phase.
- Higher blood flow on Doppler ultrasound is seen in Graves' disease compared to painless thyroiditis.

Thyrotoxicosis Factitia

Thyrotoxicosis factitia may also present in a similar manner to painless thyroiditis in the thyrotoxic phase [1]:

- It is caused by excess ingestion of thyroid hormone.
- It is similar to thyrotoxic phase of painless thyroiditis, except that the patients with thyrotoxicosis factitia lack a goiter.
- Diagnostic tests may help distinguish between thyrotoxicosis factitia and painless thyroiditis. Serum thyroglobulin (Tg) is elevated in painless thyroiditis, but low in thyrotoxicosis factitia, and on thyroid US, thyroid has a normal echo-texture in thyrotoxicosis factitia compared to a heterogeneous echo-texture in painless thyroiditis.

Other Causes of Thyrotoxicosis

Other causes of thyrotoxicosis (without hyperthyroidism) include radiation-induced thyroiditis and thyroid adenoma infarction [3].

6.3.9.2 Differential Diagnosis During the Hypothyroid Phase

Hashimoto's Thyroiditis

The main differential diagnosis during the hypothyroid phase is Hashimoto's thyroiditis, which can be difficult to distinguish from silent thyroiditis [2].

- It may be distinguished by histology, as certain histological features common in Hashimoto's thyroiditis are absent from painless thyroiditis, including oncocytic (Hürthle) cells, germinal center formation, and fibrosis.
- Measuring anti-thyroid antibodies is not diagnostic, as they can be present in both conditions.
- If definitive diagnosis is not possible, monitor and temporarily treat patients to see if hypothyroidism will resolve over time.

Other Causes of Hypothyroidism

Other causes of hypothyroidism that should be differentiated from silent thyroiditis include iodine deficiency and central hypothyroidism due to pituitary–hypothalamic mass, pituitary–hypothalamic infiltration/infection, or traumatic brain injury, or another cause.

6.3.9.3 Other Causes of Triphasic Thyroid Disease

Other causes of triphasic thyroid disease (thyrotoxicosis, hypothyroidism, recovery) include the following [1]:

- Post-partum thyroiditis (painless thyroiditis that occurs in the first-year post-partum)
- Drug-induced thyroiditis (painless thyroiditis caused by certain medications)
- Subacute thyroiditis (characterized by a hard, painful goiter and an ESR > 50 mm/h)
- Acute (suppurative) thyroiditis (painful goiter typically present)
- Palpation (traumatic) thyroiditis

6.3.10 Management

Screening is indicated for silent lymphocytic thyroiditis in post-partum patients who have no symptoms if they have had silent lymphocytic thyroiditis in previous pregnancies. Management of painless thyroiditis depends on patient presentation and disease phase. In general, treatment is *not* necessary for asymptomatic or mildly symptomatic patients. Because silent lymphocytic thyroiditis lasts only a few months, treatment is conservative. Anti-thyroid medications are *not* used as they are ineffective. Surgery and radioactive iodine (RAI) therapy are contraindicated [1, 2].

6.3.10.1 Management in Thyrotoxic Phase

Treatment may *not* be necessary if the patient is asymptomatic or has mild symptoms only [2]. "Beta-blockers" are recommended for management of symptomatic thyrotoxicosis in patients with painless thyroiditis (ATA Strong recommendation) [1]. Propranolol is the most commonly used with a suggested dose of 10–40 mg orally 3–4 times daily. It is preferred for pregnant or breast-feeding patients. Atenolol may also be used with a suggested dose of 25–100 mg orally once or twice daily. It is avoided during pregnancy. Rarely, "corticosteroids" can be used to treat severe symptoms of thyrotoxicosis due to painless thyroiditis [1].

6.3.10.2 Management in Hypothyroid Phase

Treatment is *not* necessary in asymptomatic or mildly symptomatic patients in the hypothyroid phase of painless thyroiditis [1, 2]. In symptomatic patients, thyroid hormone replacement therapy with levothyroxine may be needed in those with moderate-to-severe symptoms [1, 2]. In patients considering pregnancy, levothyroxine is administered regardless of symptoms [2]. In general, the suggested initial dose is 1.6 μg/kg orally once daily (the dose is adjusted by 12.5- to 25-μg increments every 4–6 weeks until the patient is clinically euthyroid and TSH is normal). Levothyroxine treatment is continued for 12 months after the onset of painless thyroiditis, and discontinued or tapered thereafter. If hypothyroidism persists for more than 12 months, permanent thyroid replacement therapy may be required.

6.3.10.3 Management of Recurrent Painless Thyroiditis

This disorder usually recurs after subsequent pregnancies. Recurrent disease is treated in the same manner as the initial occurrence, though patients with "multiple" recurrences may opt for surgery or RAI ablation of the thyroid (after recovering from the thyrotoxic phase) [1, 2].

6.3.10.4 Follow-Up/Monitoring

Most patients recover normal thyroid function, although some remain permanently hypothyroid. Therefore, patients with painless thyroiditis should be monitored for 12 months, with periodic follow-up thereafter, to determine if hypothyroidism resolves over time or progresses to Hashimoto's thyroiditis [1, 2]. Thyroid function should be re-evaluated after 9–12 months of thyroxin therapy; replacement is stopped for 5 weeks, and TSH is remeasured. It is noteworthy that TSH levels should be monitored 6–8 weeks after any change in dosage.

6.3.11 Complications

Most cases of painless thyroiditis are mild and self-limiting, and not associated with long-term complications [2, 3].

Untreated or inadequately treated thyrotoxicosis may be associated with the following complications: weight loss, osteoporosis and increased bone turnover, cardiac arrhythmias, embolic events, muscle weakness, tremors, neuro-psychiatric symptoms, rarely, cardiovascular collapse and heart failure.

Untreated or inadequately treated hypothyroidism may be associated with the following: cardiac complications, gastrointestinal complications (such as constipation), musculo-skeletal complications (such as weakness, cramps, and arthralgias), hematological complications (such as anemia and increased risk for bleeding), as well as renal failure and myxedema coma in severe cases [8].

6.3.12 Prognosis

Most cases of painless thyroiditis are mild and self-limiting, resolving within 12 months of onset [1, 2]. About 5%–10% of patients are reported to have recurrence of painless thyroiditis after resolution, and 10%–20% are reported to develop persistent hypothyroidism after 12 months (Hashimoto's thyroiditis) [1, 2].

6.4 Post-partum Thyroiditis

6.4.1 Introduction

Post-partum thyroiditis (PPT) is a destructive autoimmune subacute painless thyroiditis that presents as new-onset, painless hypothyroidism, transient thyrotoxicosis, or thyrotoxicosis followed by hypothyroidism within 1-year post-partum and can also occur after a miscarriage at 5–20 weeks gestation [13]. It is found in approximately 5% of mothers in the general population, with a higher frequency (25%) in women with type-1 diabetes mellitus (DM). Three clinical presentations have been suggested for PPT: (1) transient hyperthyroidism (32% of patients), (2) transient hypothyroidism (43% of patients), and (3) transient hyperthyroidism followed by hypothyroidism and then recovery, which is the classic form of PPT (25% of patients).

Post-partum thyroiditis is associated with the presence of antibodies to thyroid peroxidase (TPO). The chance of developing PPT in pregnant women who have positive TPO antibodies early in pregnancy ranges from 30% to 52% [14]. During pregnancy, the level of TPO antibodies (TPO-Ab) naturally decreases due to the immunosuppressed state of pregnancy. Women who remain positive for TPO-Ab in the third trimester of pregnancy will have an 80% chance of developing PPT [15]. Screening of high-risk women for developing PPT, such as a positive test for anti-TPO antibody, history of PPT, and type-1 DM, is recommended by the Endocrine Society clinical guidelines. High-risk women should be evaluated for serum TSH levels at 3- and 6-month post-partum [13].

6.4.2 Epidemiology

The prevalence and frequency of post-partum thyroiditis (PPT) are 8% and 1.1%–16.7% of pregnancies, respectively. Different rates have been reported worldwide. Multiple factors are affecting the rates, such as length of follow-up in the post-partum period and iodine status of the studied population. In Thailand, for example, the reported rate of PPT is 1.1%, whereas the incidence rate in Brazil is 13.3%. Both of these regions have low iodine intake. Prevalence of PPT in the high-risk group, including women with positive thyroid antibodies or other autoimmune diseases, type-1 DM, and positive family history, is reported to be approximately 20% [16, 17]. Up to 50% of all women with TPO-Ab or TG-Ab positivity in the first trimester of pregnancy develop post-partum thyroiditis [18, 19]. The risk of "recurrence" of PPT in a patient with a previous history of PPT is reported to be approximately 42.4% [20, 21].

6.4.3 Etiology

Post-partum thyroiditis is an autoimmune disease that is associated with the presence of antibodies to thyroid peroxidase (TPO). It is also known as destructive thyroiditis with lymphocytic infiltration within the thyroid gland. Histological features of PPT are similar to Hashimoto's thyroiditis, and both are associated with HLA-D and HLA-B haplotypes. These findings indicate the importance of inherited risk factors [22, 23].

The presence of TPO antibodies is seen in other autoimmune thyroid diseases such as Graves' disease and Hashimoto's thyroiditis. The level of TPO antibodies reflects the severity of the infiltration of lymphocytes within the thyroid gland. TPO antibodies are complement-fixing, which subsequently induce antibody-dependent cell-mediated cytotoxicity [15].

6.4.4 Pathophysiology

The inflammatory process in post-partum thyroiditis initiates with the presence of thyroid antibodies (TPOAb and TgAb), activation of the complement cascade, increased levels of IgG1, lymphocyte abnormalities, increased activity of NK cells, and specific HLA haplotypes. The inflammatory process activates the proteolysis of the thyroglobulin (Tg) within the thyroid follicles resulting in their destruction and the release of significant amounts of thyroxin (T4) and tri-iodothyronine (T3) into the blood, and subsequently hyperthyroidism. This hyperthyroid state is transient and lasts until all Tg storages are released into circulation and no more Tg is left behind. During the hyperthyroid state, the synthesis of new hormones is shut down because excessive T4/T3 in circulation causes down-regulation of TSH secretion. Synthesis of thyroid hormones will be resumed once the inflammatory process subsides.

6.4.5 Pathology

Histopathological examination of the thyroid gland in cases with post-partum thyroiditis reveals prominent infiltration of lymphocytes, including associated germinal centers, and the collapse of thyroid follicles. Fine-needle aspiration (FNA) of the thyroid gland shows thyroid follicular cells, lymphocytes, and accumulation of colloid. During the recovery phase, follicles are seen to be "normal," but some degree of fibrosis and lymphocytic infiltration could be seen.

6.4.6 Clinical Presentation

Post-partum thyroiditis (PPT) is a painless condition. Most of the patients with PPT are symptom-free or show mild symptoms during the thyrotoxic state, including irritability, palpitation, fatigue, and heat intolerance. The hypothyroid state of PPT is mostly symptomatic, resulting in constipation, dry skin, fatigue, impaired concentration, cold intolerance, and parasthesia. A study by Alexander et al. (2017) reported that patients with PPT and positive TPO antibodies were more symptomatic than those who had negative TPO antibodies [9].

6.4.7 Investigations

The diagnosis of post-partum thyroiditis requires a high clinical index of suspicion and is confirmed by documenting abnormal serum levels of TSH and T4 in a previously euthyroid patient. Patients with PPT have similar biochemical findings that can be detected in patients with painless thyroiditis: high or upper limit of normal serum free T4 and T3 levels and low serum TSH level in the hyperthyroid phase, which could be subclinical or overt. In patients with hyperthyroid state followed by hypothyroid state, serum T4 level could be low for days to weeks before serum TSH level rises beyond the normal range, as a result of prolonged suppressed TSH, which had occurred in the hyperthyroid state. Serum levels of anti-TPO antibody are high in 60%–85% of patients with PPT and are highest in the hypothyroid state or soon thereafter. Some of the patients may have a slight increase in C-reactive protein (CRP) and/or erythrocyte sedimentation rate (ESR) [24–26]. Clinicians in charge of women after pregnancy have to be aware of the possible post-partum thyroid dysfunction, which can result in different symptoms during the post-partum period.

Scintigraphy with ^{123}I or technetium scans is preferable to ^{131}I scans in breastfeeding women, due to the shorter half-life.

6.4.8 Differential Diagnosis

The differential diagnosis of post-partum thyroiditis (PPT) includes Graves' disease, Hashimoto's thyroiditis, and post-partum mood disorder. Differentiating PPT from Graves' disease can be challenging. Thyroid receptor antibodies are often positive in Graves' disease, but usually are negative in PPT, and radioactive iodine uptake (RAIU) is elevated or normal in Graves' disease and low in PPT.

6.4.9 Management

There have not been any prospective studies to evaluate when and how to treat PPT. A prospective study that evaluated 605 asymptomatic pregnant women and women in the post-partum period showed that none of the cases with thyrotoxicosis and 40% of cases with hypothyroid state needed treatment. If treatment is necessitated, it could usually be tapered over 1 year [27]. Several studies have shown that long-term treatment would be required in up to 20% of cases with PPT; however, a prospective study of 169 women with PPT reported a much higher rate of 54% of women with persistent hypothyroidism after 1 year [28]. Women with the highest levels of TSH, high TPO antibody titers, multiparous women, older women, and those with a history of miscarriage have the highest risk for developing permanent hypothyroidism [28].

Management of the thyrotoxic state is guided by its transitory nature. Antithyroid medications (methimazole and propyl-thiouracil) have been ineffective in the treatment of the thyrotoxic state of PPT as it is a "destructive thyroiditis" in which there is no increase in the synthesis of thyroid hormones. Symptoms are usually mild. In a few cases with clinically significant symptoms, a low dose of betablockers (propranolol) may be helpful.

When the thyrotoxic state of PPT has resolved, serum TSH level should be measured in about 4–8 weeks (or in case of development of new symptoms) in order to screen for the hypothyroid state. In patients who develop significant symptoms, and currently lactating or those who want to get pregnant, treatment should be initiated. Treatment with levothyroxine (L-T4) should be considered in the hypothyroid state of PPT if the patient has mild symptoms or plans to get pregnant again. If treatment is delayed, thyroid function must be evaluated every 4–8 weeks until the patient becomes euthyroid. In addition, women must be counselled to use contraception. The duration that the patient should continue to take L-T4 has not been evaluated. Based on the ATA guidelines (2017), the euthyroid state should be maintained in those who are pregnant or want to get pregnant. To assess if the hypothyroid state of

PPT is permanent or transient, L-T4 doses can be tapered starting 12 months after delivery. The dose should be tapered gradually, and serum TSH level monitored every 6–8 weeks [9].

Both L-T4 and iodine treatment during pregnancy have been investigated as a potential strategy to prevent PPT in women with anti-thyroid antibodies, but neither intervention was effective. On the other hand, a prospective placebo-controlled study by Negro et al. (2007) [29] evaluating the efficacy of selenium in preventing PPT in TPOAb-positive women reported that selenium decreased both the incidence of PPT and permanent hypothyroidism. Selenium administration was also associated with a significant decrease in post-partum TPOAb titers [29]. Given that studies demonstrating benefit are limited, there is insufficient evidence at this time to recommend selenium supplementation during pregnancy in TPOAb-positive women.

Even in women whose thyroid function returns to normal, the risk of recurrent post-partum thyroiditis in a subsequent pregnancy is approximately 70% [30]. Women with a prior history of PPT should thus have annual TSH screening to evaluate for permanent hypothyroidism.

6.4.10 Prognosis

The clinical course of PPT is variable. Only 30% of patients with PPT will remain in hypothyroid state 1 year post-partum [16].

6.4.11 Recommendations [17]

- Women with post-partum depression should have TSH, FT4, and TPO-Ab tests performed.
- During the thyrotoxic phase of post-partum thyroiditis (PPT), symptomatic women may be treated with beta-blockers. Propranolol at the lowest possible dose to alleviate symptoms is the treatment of choice. Therapy is typically required for a few months.
- Treatment with anti-thyroid drugs (ATDs) is *not* recommended for the thyrotoxic phase of PPT.
- Following the resolution of the thyrotoxic phase of PPT, TSH should be tested every 2 months (or if symptoms are present) until 1 year post-partum to screen for the hypothyroid phase.
- Women who are symptomatic with hypothyroidism in PPT should either have their TSH level retested in 4–8 weeks or be started on L-T4 (if symptoms are severe, if conception is being attempted, or if the patient desires therapy). Women who are asymptomatic with hypothyroidism in PPT should have their TSH level retested in 4–8 weeks.
- Women who are hypothyroid with PPT and attempting pregnancy should be treated with L-T4.

- If L-T4 is initiated for PPT, future discontinuation of therapy should be attempted. Tapering of treatment can be begun 6–12 months after its initiation. Tapering of L-T4 should be avoided when a woman is actively attempting pregnancy, is breast-feeding, or is pregnant.
- Women with a prior history of PPT should have an annual TSH test performed to evaluate for permanent hypothyroidism.
- Treatment of euthyroid pregnant woman with either L-T4 or iodine to prevent PPT is ineffective and is *not* recommended.

6.5 Drug-Induced Thyroiditis

6.5.1 Overview

Various medications can cause the development of subacute painless (silent) thyroiditis, especially amiodarone, immune checkpoint inhibitors, lithium, interferon-alpha (IFN-α), interleukin-2 (IL-2), and tyrosine kinase inhibitors. Investigations include measurement of serum levels of TSH, T4/T3, and TPOAb, in addition to TRAb/thyroid scintigraphy, in differential diagnostic suspicion of Graves' disease. The conditions are most often self-limiting, but can have very variable courses. Treatment is conservative and includes beta-blockers for symptoms of thyrotoxicosis and levothyroxine (L-T4) for hypothyroidism, following the same principles as for subacute thyroiditis (SAT).

6.5.2 Amiodarone

Amiodarone is a Vaughan-Williams Class III anti-arrhythmic drug. It is approved by the US Food and Drug Administration (FDA) specifically for the treatment of life-threatening ventricular arrhythmias. However, this drug is also widely used for anti-angina purposes and to treat supra-ventricular tachyarrhythmias, such as atrial fibrillation, and to prevent ventricular tachyarrhythmias in high-risk patients. Amiodarone is often considered the most effective anti-arrhythmic drug from the point of view of effectiveness, but its use is essentially limited by its long-term side effects, making it a second-line treatment. However, it has the advantage of being a low depressant of the heart muscle (unlike other anti-arrhythmic drugs) and remains the anti-arrhythmic of choice in case of heart failure [31]. Amiodarone is contraindicated in hypersensitivity to the drug, bradycardia and cardiac conduction disorders, as well as thyroid dysfunction, pregnancy and breast-feeding.

Administration of amiodarone may lead bradycardia with QT prolongation and a relatively low risk of "torsades de pointes" (the French term for "twisting of points"), which refers to the heart's ventricles beating faster than its atria [32]. Amiodarone may induce other extra-cardiac side effects, especially if used in high doses or for a prolonged period of time. These include the following:

- *Interstitial lung disease:* It is one of the most common side effects occurring in approximately 5% of treated individuals [33].
- *Thyroid dysfunction:* Treatment with amiodarone reduces the peripheral conversion of thyroxin (T4) to tri-iodothyronine (T3) and increases the formation of reverse-T3. The plasma concentration of T4 is therefore increased, while that of T3 is decreased. Plasma TSH concentration may increase moderately at the start of treatment, but spontaneously normalizes in less than 3 months. These changes are not accompanied by any clinical manifestations and their observation should therefore not lead to any change in treatment. However, thyroid abnormalities have been noted in up to 14%–18% of patients receiving long-term amiodarone therapy, but a meta-analysis suggested that with lower doses of amiodarone (150–330 mg), the incidence of thyroid dysfunction is 3.7%. The effects range from abnormal thyroid function test findings to overt thyroid dysfunction, which may be either amiodarone-induced hypothyroidism (common) or amiodarone-induced thyrotoxicosis (less common) [34–37]. Both can develop in apparently normal thyroid glands or in glands with pre-existing abnormalities. Some authors describe two types of hyperthyroidism due to amiodarone, one with an inflammatory component and the other is non-inflammatory and attributed to an excess of iodine; the differential diagnosis is difficult. Hyperthyroidism due to amiodarone may be irreversible and require total thyroidectomy followed by life-long thyroid hormone replacement therapy. Treatment of hyperthyroidism due to amiodarone may be initiated with corticosteroids, potassium perchlorate [38, 39], and synthetic anti-thyroid drugs (ATDs). In practice, annual monitoring of blood TSH levels should be done. Discontinuation of amiodarone is a rule in cases of hyperthyroidism. The medication can be continued without any problems in case of hypothyroidism, possibly with thyroid hormone replacement therapy.
- *Hepatic toxicity:* Moderate increases in serum transaminases are common (15%–20% of treated subjects), usually asymptomatic and transient despite continued treatment. However, progression to fibrosis and cirrhosis has been reported in some cases.
- *Eye disorders:* These are yellowish-brown corneal deposits located in the sub-pupillary area. They are almost constant in adults, but are usually asymptomatic [40]. Their finding during an ophthalmological examination therefore does not require modification of the treatment with amiodarone. These deposits are completely reversible after discontinuation of treatment.
- *Photo-sensitization and skin pigmentation:* The damage is very frequent, requiring protection against sun exposure.
- *Cancer*: Amiodarone treatment is correlated with an increased risk of cancer [41], but there is no evidence of a causal link.
- *Disruption of lipid metabolism:* Amiodarone treatment leads to hypercholesterolemia in a way that is not related to the thyroid [42]. In particular, it decreases the expression of the low-density lipid (LDL) receptor, disrupting the elimination of LDL [43]. In addition, amiodarone may block the conversion of desmosterol into cholesterol, which may play a role in its liver toxicity [44].

6.5.3 Immune Checkpoint Inhibitors (ICIs)

Therapy with immune checkpoint inhibitors (ICIs) is a form of cancer immunotherapy that targets immune checkpoints, key regulators of the immune system that when stimulated can dampen the immune response to an immunological stimulus. Some cancers can protect themselves from attack by stimulating immune checkpoint targets. Checkpoint therapy can block inhibitory checkpoints, restoring immune system function [45]. The first anti-cancer drug targeting an immune checkpoint was "ipilimumab," a CTLA4 blocker approved in the United States in 2011 [46]. More recently, in 2022, "tremelimumab" was also approved.

Cancers treated with checkpoint inhibitors include, among others, metastatic melanoma, renal cell carcinoma, colorectal cancer, hepatocellular carcinoma, non-small cell lung cancer, malignant pleural mesothelioma, and esophageal squamous carcinoma.

Immune-related adverse events may be caused by checkpoint inhibitors. Altering checkpoint inhibition can have diverse effects on most organ systems of the body. Colitis occurs commonly. The precise mechanism is unknown, but it differs in some respects based on the molecule targeted [47]. Infusion of ICIs has also been associated with acute sero-negative myasthenia gravis [48]. Thyroiditis with resulting hypothyroidism is a common immune-related adverse event especially with the use of combinations of different ICIs [49]. The underlying mechanism of ICI-induced thyroiditis may differ from other forms of thyroiditis [50].

In a recent systematic review and meta-analysis by Yang et al. (2024) [51], the final analysis of 3226 patients from 19 studies was included. The total incidence of all-grade hypothyroidism induced by the combination of ICIs and chemotherapy in treating triple-negative breast cancer (12%) was higher than that of hyperthyroidism (5%). Pembrolizumab combined with chemotherapy caused the highest incidence of all grades of hypothyroidism (13%), while durvalumab combined with chemotherapy caused the highest incidence of all grades of hyperthyroidism (7%). ICIs combined with chemotherapy caused a higher incidence of all grades of hypothyroidism in advanced triple-negative breast cancer (15%) than in early-stage disease (10%) [51].

A lower incidence of hypothyroidism was observed in a trial of combined B-cell depletion and ICI treatment compared with studies of ICI mono-therapy [52]. This holds promise for combining checkpoint inhibitor therapy with immune-suppressive drugs to achieve anti-cancer effects with less toxicity.

Clinical and para-clinical findings consistent with thyroiditis in a patient on ICI therapy suggest the diagnosis of ICI-induced thyroiditis. The use of L-T4 replacement therapy is indicated in hypothyroidism. Beta-blocker therapy is used in thyrotoxic cases.

6.5.4 Lithium

Certain lithium compounds, also known as lithium salts, are classified as mood stabilizers and used as psychiatric medications primarily for bipolar disorder and for major depressive disorder [53]. Lithium is taken orally, and its mechanism of action is not known [53].

Common side effects include increased urination, shakiness of the hands, and increased thirst [53]. Serious side effects include hypothyroidism, diabetes insipidus, and lithium toxicity [53]. Blood level monitoring is recommended to decrease the risk of potential toxicity [53]. If levels become too high, diarrhea, vomiting, poor coordination, sleepiness, and tinnitus may occur [53]. Lithium is teratogenic and can cause birth defects at high doses, especially during the first trimester of pregnancy. The use of lithium while breast-feeding is controversial; however, many international health authorities advise against it, and the long-term outcomes of perinatal lithium exposure have not been studied [54]. The American Academy of Pediatrics lists lithium as contraindicated for pregnancy and lactation [55].

Lithium treatment results in goiter in approximately 40% of patients, hypothyroidism in 20% of patients, and thyrotoxicosis in between 0.6% and 3.0% [56]. Destructive thyroiditis is the most common cause of lithium-associated thyrotoxicosis in these patients. The annual incidence of hypothyroidism in individuals who do not harbor auto-antibodies is 0.8%, and in individuals with thyroid-associated autoantibodies, it is 6.4%.

Clinical and para-clinical findings consistent with thyroiditis in a patient on lithium therapy suggest the diagnosis of lithium-induced thyroiditis. Onset is often more than a year after initiation of lithium. The need for L-T4 treatment is increased long-term in hypothyroidism. Continued lithium treatment is *not* contraindicated [56].

6.5.5 Interferon-alpha (IFN-α)

Interferon-alpha (IFN-α) is used in a variety of treatments, including certain forms of leukemia, malignant melanoma, non-Hodgkin lymphoma (NHL) [57], metastatic renal cell carcinoma, hepatitis B, and hepatitis C [58]. It is typically administered as a subcutaneous injection.

Common side effects may occur in ≥10% of people and include increased risk of infection due drop in white blood cells (WBCs), insomnia, mood changes including irritability, excitement, restlessness, or depression, headache and dizziness, dry mouth, blurred vision, feeling or being sick, abdominal pain, diarrhea, sore mouth; taste changes; hair loss; sweating; joint and/or muscle pain; injection site reactions, fatigue, flu-like symptoms, and loss of appetite and weight loss. The US FDA has issued a "black box" warning regarding the potential for "causing" or "aggravating" fatal or life-threatening neuro-psychiatric, autoimmune, ischemic, and infectious disorders.

Thyroid dysfunction can present as silent thyroiditis, Hashimoto's thyroiditis, or Graves' disease [59]. Thyroiditis occurs in approximately 5% of patients treated with INF-α and can result in permanent hypothyroidism. The risk of developing thyroid dysfunction, especially hypothyroidism, is higher in patients with pre-existing thyroid autoimmunity [60]. Thyroid dysfunction is often seen after 3 months of treatment, but can be seen as long as patients are on INF-α and also for several years after treatment has stopped [61, 62].

Clinical and para-clinical findings consistent with thyroiditis in a patient receiving INF-α or interleukin-2 therapy suggest INF-α-induced thyroiditis. Measurement of TRAb should be considered in patients on interferon who develop thyrotoxicosis. Beta-blocker therapy is sufficient in most cases, and INF-α therapy can be continued as thyrotoxic symptoms are usually mild. If thyrotoxic symptoms *cannot* be controlled with beta-blockers, consideration should be given to withholding INF-α until the patient is euthyroid or hypothyroid [59]. Up to half of the patients on INF-α treatment who develop thyrotoxicosis have Graves' disease and should be treated accordingly.

6.5.6 Interleukin-2 (IL-2)

Interleukin-2 (IL-2) is an interleukin, a type of cytokine signaling molecule in the immune system. It is a 15.5–16 kDa protein [63] that regulates the activities of WBCs (leukocytes, often lymphocytes) that are responsible for immunity. It is part of the body's natural response to microbial infection, and in discriminating between foreign ("non-self") and "self". Interleukin-2 IL-2 mediates its effects by binding to IL-2 receptors, which are expressed by lymphocytes. The major sources of IL-2 are activated CD4+ T-cells and activated CD8+ T-cells [64].

In brief, the function of IL-2 is to stimulate the growth of helper, cytotoxic, and regulatory T-cells. IL-2 has essential roles in key functions of the immune system, tolerance and immunity, primarily via its direct effects on T-cells. In the thymus, where T-cells mature, it prevents autoimmune diseases by promoting the differentiation of certain immature T-cells into regulatory T-cells, which suppress other T cells that are otherwise primed to attack normal healthy cells in the body. IL-2 enhances activation-induced cell death (AICD) [63]. IL-2 also promotes the differentiation of T-cells into effector T-cells and into memory T-cells when the initial T-cell is also stimulated by an antigen, thus helping the body fight off infections [64]. Together with other polarizing cytokines, IL-2 stimulates naive CD4+ T-cell differentiation into Th1 and Th2 lymphocytes while it impedes differentiation into Th17 and follicular Thl lymphocytes [65, 66]. IL-2 increases the cell-killing activity of both natural killer (NK) cells and cytotoxic T-cells [66].

Systemic IL-2 has a narrow therapeutic window, and the level of dosing usually determines the severity of the side effects [67]. In the case of local IL-2 application, the therapeutic window spans several orders of magnitude [68]. Common side effects of systemic IL-2 include flu-like symptoms (fever, headache, muscle and joint pain, fatigue), nausea/vomiting, dry, itchy skin or rash, weakness or shortness of breath, diarrhea, hypotension, drowsiness or confusion, and loss of appetite. More serious and dangerous side effects sometimes are seen, such as breathing problems, serious infections, seizures, allergic reactions, heart problems, and renal failure. The most common adverse effect of high-dose IL-2 therapy is vascular leak syndrome (VLS; also known as "capillary leak syndrome"). It is caused by lung endothelial cells expressing high-affinity IL-2R. These cells, as a result of IL-2 binding, cause increased vascular permeability. Thus, intra-vascular fluid extravasates into organs, predominantly lungs, which leads to life-threatening pulmonary or brain edema [69]. Other drawbacks of IL-2 cancer immunotherapy are its short half-life in circulation and its ability to predominantly expand regulatory T-cells at high doses [34, 63].

Interleukin-2 (IL-2) is used mainly to treat some forms of metastatic cancer and leukemia. Silent thyroiditis may be seen in up to 2% of these patients [70]. Clinical and para-clinical findings consistent with thyroiditis in a patient receiving IL-2 therapy suggest the diagnosis of IL-2-induced thyroiditis. Measurement of TRAb should be considered in patients on IL-2 who develop thyrotoxicosis.

6.5.7 Tyrosine Kinase Inhibitors (TKIs)

Tyrosine kinase inhibitors (TKIs) are a group of pharmacological agents that disrupt the signal transduction pathways of protein kinases by several modes of inhibition. They are primarily used as anti-neoplastic therapy for renal cell carcinoma, gastrointestinal stromal tumors, medullary and differentiated follicular thyroid tumors, endocrine pancreatic tumors, and non-small cell lung cancer. Nearly all TKIs are effective when taken orally. Tyrosine kinase inhibitors (especially Sunitinib, Sorafenib, and Nilotinib) can cause thyroiditis. The incidence of hypothyroidism is between 60% and 85% with treatment with Sunitinib and less frequently with treatment with Sorafenib (approximately 20%), Pazopanib, and Tivozanib (approximately [71–73]). The risk of hypothyroidism increases after multiple courses [71].

Tyrosine kinase inhibitors (TKIs) are generally well-tolerated, especially when compared to non-targeted cancer therapy. However, only a few of these drugs are selective for only one target. Due to the ubiquitous physiological role protein kinases play in the body, toxicities affecting various organs can occur. Organs commonly affected include the heart, lungs, liver, gastrointestinal tract, kidneys, thyroid, blood, and skin [74].

Adverse events of TKIs are usually dose-based, with broad side effect profiles unique to each drug. However, due to similarities in drug targets, different classes of TKIs can have similar side effect profiles. Common adverse events related to TKIs are listed in Table 6.3. Not all adverse events are associated with every TKI, occurring at different frequencies depending on the drug [74].

Clinical and para-clinical findings consistent with thyroiditis in a patient receiving TKI treatment suggest TKI-induced thyroiditis. Replacement therapy with levothyroxine (L-T4) is sufficient in most cases of hypothyroidism.

6.5.8 Alemtuzumab

Alemtuzumab is a monoclonal antibody that binds to CD52 (cluster of differentiation 52), a protein present on the surface of mature lymphocytes rendering these CD52-bearing lymphocytes targeted for destruction. Alemtuzumab is used to treat chronic lymphocytic leukemia, cutaneous T-cell lymphoma, peripheral T-cell lymphoma, and multiple sclerosis [75]. It is contraindicated in patients who have active infections, underlying immunodeficiency, or known type-I hypersensitivity or anaphylactic reactions to the substance.

Very common adverse reactions associated with alemtuzumab infusion in people with multiple sclerosis include upper respiratory tract and urinary tract infections, herpes virus infections, lymphopenia, leucopenia, thyroid dysfunction, tachycardia, skin rash, pruritus, pyrexia, and fatigue. Thyroiditis is seen in approximately 3% of patients receiving alemtuzumab treatment. Hyperthyroidism is by far the most common [76].

Table 6.3 Common adverse effects of tyrosine kinase inhibitors

System	Adverse effects
General	Fatigue, fevers/chills, weight loss/gain
Gastrointestinal	Abdominal pain, diarrhea, dysgeusia, constipation, nausea/vomiting, hepatotoxicity, stomatitis
Cardiovascular	Hypertension, hypotension, congestive heart failure, thrombosis, cardiac, ischemia, myocardial infarction, strokes, intestinal hemorrhage, QT-interval prolongation
Dermatological	Stevens–Johnson syndrome, toxic epidermal necrolysis, drug rash with eosinophilia and systemic symptoms, acute generalized exanthematous pustulosis, palmar-plantar erythro-dysesthesia, maculo-papular rashes, cheilitis, facial edema, eczema, pruritis, photosensitivity, xerosis, alopecia, hair color changes, paronychia
Endocrine	Hypokalemia, thyroid dysfunction, lacrimation
Hematological	Anemia, thrombocytopenia, neutropenia, bruising
Musculo-skeletal	Myalgias, arthralgia
Ophthalmic	Central serous retinopathy, retinal pigment epithelial detachment, TKI keratitis
Renal	Kidney dysfunction, proteinuria
Respiratory	Interstitial pulmonary disease, pneumonia, upper respiratory tract infection, dyspnea, epistaxis, rhinorrhea
Neurological	Cognitive impairment, peripheral neuropathy, headache, dizziness

Other adverse reactions that have been reported include serious opportunistic nocardial infections and cytomegalovirus (CMV) syndrome [77–79]. Alemtuzumab can also precipitate autoimmune disease in 30%–40% of patients, predominantly affecting thyroid, kidney, and thrombocytic function [80], through the suppression of regulatory T-cell populations and/or the emergence of auto-reactive B-cells [81, 82]. Cases of multiple sclerosis reactivation/relapse have also been reported [83].

Clinical and para-clinical findings consistent with thyroiditis in a patient receiving Alemtuzumab therapy suggest Alemtuzumab-induced thyroiditis. Treatment with beta-blockers thyrotoxicosis is sufficient in most cases.

6.6 Subacute Post-operative Necrotizing Thyroiditis

6.6.1 Introduction

Post-operative necrotizing thyroiditis is one cause of iatrogenic thyrotoxicosis. It is a rare surgical complication owing to the very rich vascular supply of the thyroid gland. It is related to glandular trauma by vigorous manipulation at surgery such as laryngectomy or parathyroid surgery, or through repeated FNA. Such manipulation could result in a painless subacute thyroiditis-like picture, which in turn may lead to thyrotoxicosis or to a necrotizing thyroiditis [84–86]. No predictive marker or factor has been identified for this condition. Histologically, the specimen typically shows post-operative granulomas, as found in other organs (bladder, prostate) following surgery.

6.6.2 Post-parathyroidectomy Thyroiditis

6.6.2.1 Overview

Various clinical manifestations of thyroiditis after parathyroidectomy have been reported in the literature, ranging from mild symptoms to tachyarrhythmias and myocardial infarction [87]. Parathyroidectomy, typically performed for hyperparathyroidism (HPT), is a common procedure associated with favorable outcomes. However, certain patients may develop post-surgical thyroiditis, as a transient complication, presenting with characteristic clinical features and laboratory findings.

Recently, in 2024, Kwayess et al. reported two patients with post-parathyroidectomy thyroiditis; both had primary hyperparathyroidism (HPT) and underwent parathyroidectomy for a solitary parathyroid adenoma. They subsequently developed symptoms of hyperthyroidism, including palpitations and heat intolerance. Laboratory investigations demonstrated a suppressed TSH level with elevated free T4 levels and low uptake on thyroid radioiodine scan, confirming the diagnosis of thyroiditis. The patients were managed conservatively, and their symptoms gradually resolved with normalization of thyroid hormone levels. In addition, Kwayess et al. (2024) conducted a literature review of post-parathyroidectomy thyroiditis in an attempt to understand its pathogenesis and predictors and ultimately identify measures to prevent this intriguing clinical phenomenon. They retrieved 22 case-reports publications, with a total of 27 cases, excluding their 2 cases (Table 6.4), and reported that this condition is mostly attributed to manipulation of the thyroid during parathyroid surgery and that it occurs more frequently in patients who undergo 4-gland parathyroidectomy for secondary or tertiary HPT and is self-limited within a few weeks [87]. The case reports highlight the importance of recognizing thyroiditis as a potentially under-recognized complication of parathyroid surgery.

Table 6.4 Cases of post-parathyroidectomy thyroiditis reported in the literature

Author [Reference]	Year	Country	Indication of parathyroidectomy	*N*	Age/ gender
Walfish et al. [88]	1992	Canada	Primary HPT	3	16 Y/F 23 Y/M 43 Y/F
Musi et al. [89]	2000	USA	Secondary HPT	1	48 Y/F
Lim et al. [90]	2003	Korea	Secondary HPT	1	26 Y/F
Hamada et al. [91]	2007	Japan	Secondary HPT	1	51 Y/M
Sato et al. [92]	2008	Japan	Secondary HPT	1	59 Y/F
Lederer and Schiffl [93]	2008	Germany	Secondary HPT	2	27 Y/M 49 Y/M
Rudofsky et al. [94]	2009	Germany	Tertiary PHT	1	33 Y/F
Naber et al. [95]	2010	USA	Tertiary PHT	1	51 Y/F
Parker et al. [96]	2010	USA	Primary PTH	1	59 Y/M
Espiritu and Dean [84]	2010	USA	Primary PTH	2	84 Y/F 55 Y/F
Asmar and Ross [97]	2011	USA	Secondary HPT	1	62 Y/M
Kauffels et al. [98]	2012	Germany	Secondary HPT	1	55 Y/F
Upadhyay and Trivedi [99]	2014	USA	Primary PTH	1	70 Y/F
Hakami [100]	2015	Saudi Arabia	Tertiary PHT	1	33 Y/M
Madill et al. [101]	2016	Australia	Tertiary PHT	1	37 Y/M
Xu et al. [102]	2017	China	Secondary PHT	1	35 Y/M
Chan et al. [103]	2017	Hong Kong	Secondary PHT	1	75 Y/F
Rahman et al. [104]	2019		Secondary PHT	1	31 Y/F
Pinxterhuis et al. [105]	2019	Netherlands	Tertiary HPT	1	32 Y/M
Ashorobi et al. [106]	2021	USA	Primary HPT	1	68 Y/F
Boeder et al. [107]	2022	Korea	Tertiary HPT	1	68 Y/M
Mordechay-Heyn et al. [108]	2022	Israel	Primary HPT	2	38 Y/M 66 Y/F
Kwayess et al. [87]	2024	Lebanon	Primary HPT	2	60 Y/F 53 Y/F

N number of post-operative thyroiditis, *USA* United States of America, *HPT* hyperparathyroidism, *Y* year, *F* female, *M* male

6.6.2.2 Incidence

Because of the potentially subtle presentation and the paucity of large prospective studies, it is not possible to speculate on the incidence of post-operative thyroiditis. However, despite the infrequent reported occurrence of thyrotoxicosis, the recognition of post-parathyroidectomy thyroiditis is of paramount importance due to its potential adverse impact on post-operative outcomes [96].

Stang et al. (2005) [109] included 125 patients with primary HPT who had normal pre-operative TSH levels. Most surgeries included unilateral rather than bilateral exploration. They reported that 31% of the patients exhibited TSH suppression 7–10 days after the surgery, with half being symptomatic, with or without an elevated thyroxin level, versus 16% who had subclinical hyperthyroidism in the absence of symptoms. They concluded that the risk of thyrotoxicosis might be under-appreciated in patients undergoing parathyroidectomy due to lack of symptoms and routine testing [109]. In another prospective study, Lindblom et al. (2008) [110] aimed to study the effect of surgeries other than parathyroidectomy on the development of post-operative thyroiditis. They compared 20 patients undergoing surgery for primary HPT to 11 patients undergoing breast cancer surgery. Post-operative levels of T4 and T3 were higher after parathyroidectomy than after breast surgery, with mean serum free T4 levels increasing from 1.24 to 1.63 ng/dL in patients undergoing parathyroidectomy 4 days after the surgery, but no manifestations of hyperthyroidism were seen. In patients undergoing breast cancer surgery, thyroid function tests 4 days after surgery were unchanged from the baseline pre-operative levels. This confirms that the changes in thyroid function post-parathyroidectomy are related to the manipulation of the thyroid gland, rather than the stress of surgery, as the most likely factor contributing to post-operative thyroiditis [110].

In another study by Bergenfelz and Ahren (1994) [111], the rate of post-operative hyperthyroidism after parathyroidectomy was 20%. Kobayashi et al. (1992) reported a type of thyrotoxicosis that occurred after needle aspiration of thyroid cysts. The incidence of post-aspiration thyrotoxicosis was only 0.9% (1 of 115) [112].

In general, several studies have reported biochemical hyperthyroidism, defined as full TSH suppression, occurring after parathyroidectomy in as many as 31%–42% of patients, whereas only 15% are symptomatic [88]. The variability in incidence rates may be accounted for by (1) the primary indication for surgery; (2) varying operative techniques used for primary, secondary, and tertiary HPT; (3) the extent of intra-operative gland manipulation; and (4) variations in thyroid shape, size, and pre-operative function [88].

6.6.2.3 Pathophysiology

The exact pathophysiology of post-parathyroidectomy thyroiditis is unclear and remains largely elusive. In the past, hyperthyroidism arising after PTH surgery has been thought to be transient and relate to retraction of the thyroid gland for exposure during surgery. In 1975, Carney et al. described an association between vigorous thyroid lobe palpations under pentobarbital anesthesia with the histological finding of granulomatous thyroid folliculitis in massaged thyroid lobes in dogs. Similar multifocal inflammatory changes were usually present in resected human thyroid lobes. It is suggested that manipulation of the thyroid gland was sufficient to cause transient inflammatory reactions in both humans and dogs, which they termed as "palpation thyroiditis" and "multifocal granulomatous folliculitis" [113]. Histologically, this is characterized by an infiltrate with histiocytes, plasma cells, lymphocytes, and hemosiderin-laden macrophages [113].

It is postulated that post-operative thyroiditis arises from thyroid gland trauma because of intra-operative manipulation with vigorous palpation of the gland and rupture of thyroid follicles [94, 96, 103, 110]. In 1992, Walfish et al. reported on three patients who underwent resection of PTH adenoma and developed thyrotoxicosis post-operatively. They concluded that the thyroid disruption caused post-operative hyperthyroidism. They were the first to suggest evidence of a clinical syndrome of "trauma-induced thyroiditis" in those patients [88]. On the contrary, in Stang et al.'s study (2005), they treated the thyroid gland as gently as possible, but their data supported a causative role of operative trauma to the thyroid lobe, since bilateral neck exploration was associated with the development of post-operative hyperthyroidism [109].

In Kobayashi et al.'s (1992) study, the mechanism of post-aspiration thyrotoxicosis is unknown; however, they speculated that the combination of thyroiditis and leakage of thyroid contents into the cyst might have triggered thyroid hormone release into circulation after needle aspiration of thyroid cysts [112]. Bergenfelz et al. (1994) conducted a prospective study on 20 patients undergoing operation for primary HPT, compared with 6 patients undergoing laparoscopic cholecystectomy (controls). They reported that four patients (20%) who underwent parathyroidectomy developed biochemical hyperthyroidism, but serum anti-thyroid antibody levels did not increase. Control patients experienced a slight increase in mean TSH post-operatively, and the authors concluded that post-parathyroidectomy hyperthyroidism was related to metabolic derangement intrinsic to the primary hyperparathyroidism itself [111]. Moreover, Calle and Cohen (1993) reported on a patient who developed transient thyroiditis following total laryngo-pharyngo-esophagectomy with gastric pull-up for a right hypopharynx tumor with preservation of the thyroid gland [8].

Stang et al. (2005) [109] reported that the incidence of post-operative hyperthyroidism was independent of age, gender, the pre-operative and intra-operative PTH levels, and adenoma weight. There was no relationship between the type of PTH pathology, whether multi-glandular disease or a solitary adenoma, the presence of goiter, or prior thyroiditis. None of the following indicators of operative trauma were predictive of post-operative thyroiditis: operative time, incision length, difficulty in making the dissection, thyroidectomy for intra-thyroidal PTH adenoma, retro-pharyngeal adenoma, concurrent cervical thymectomy, the degree of peri-thyroidal inflammation, or whether or not a drain was placed [109]. However, The authors identified three surgical variables associated with post-parathyroidectomy hyperthyroidism: bilateral neck exploration, the absence of concurrent thyroid lobectomy, and performance of the operation at community hospitals. When patients were cared for at the community hospitals, exploration had to be done bilaterally because the intra-operative PTH could not be monitored. The use of lithium was observed to be an independent risk factor for post-operative hyperthyroidism. This may be because lithium provides a persistent toxic insult to thyroid tissue, rendering it more sensitive to manipulation during neck surgery. Patients who underwent complete thyroid lobectomy were less likely to have post-operative thyroiditis [109].

In 2016, Madil and Back reported a case of a 37-year-old man with tertiary HPT who developed unexplained hyperthyroidism 1 day after subtotal parathyroidectomy. They postulated that palpation of the thyroid gland may impair the physical integrity of the follicular basement membrane, with consequent development of an inflammatory response leading to post-operative thyroiditis [101].

6.6.2.4 Epidemiology and Clinical Presentation

Post-operative thyroiditis has a wide clinical presentation spectrum, ranging from asymptomatic hyper-thyroxinemia in the majority of cases to severe hyperthyroidism in the minority. In addition, a few cases of thyroiditis following neck surgery that caused the onset of atrial fibrillation have been reported [86, 114]. McDermott et al. (2002) reported a case of transient thyroiditis secondary to surgical manipulation of the thyroid in a 76-year-old man, which caused significant tachyarrhythmia following total laryngectomy for a subglottic tumor with preservation of the thyroid gland [112].

The manifestations of post-operative thyroiditis can mimic other pathologies. The clinical picture might resemble sepsis, and delayed diagnosis may lead to increased morbidity and unnecessary laboratory investigations and inadequate treatment. Therefore, accurate diagnosis is essential to avoid unnecessary investigations and interventions. The diagnostic work-up typically reveals suppressed serum TSH, elevated serum thyroxin levels, and low radionuclide uptake by the thyroid gland [90].

Post-parathyroidectomy thyroiditis was first described in three patients by Walfish et al. in 1992 where hyperthyroidism appeared within 2 weeks of surgery. It was characterized by minor symptoms, and resolved within 4–6 weeks [88]. Analysis of the 27 cases reported in the review reported by Kwayess et al. (2024) [87] revealed that the average age of patients was 47.9 years, with a slight female predominance of 55.5% (15/27). However, prospective studies did not find any association between gender or age and an increased risk of post-parathyroidectomy thyroiditis [115]. Renal disease was the most common co-morbidity, with 74.1% (20/27) of the patients having chronic kidney disease, renal failure, or nephrolithiasis. Only 1 patient had previous thyroid surgery with excision of thyroid follicular adenoma 20 years prior to parathyroid surgery [115], and only 11.1% (3/27) of the patients did not have any other co-morbidities. Thyroiditis was more frequent in patients undergoing 4-gland parathyroidectomy for secondary or tertiary HPT [66.6% (18/27)] compared to primary HPT [33.4% (9/27)]. This is consistent with the hypothesis of manipulation-induced thyroiditis. Indeed, surgery in secondary and tertiary HPT is more extensive, and the parathyroid glands tend to be larger, thus necessitating more intra-operative exploration and manipulation.

In addition, the recent (2024) Kwayess et al. review [87] showed that two-thirds of patients developed post-parathyroidectomy thyroiditis after bilateral neck exploration (BNE) without pre-operative localization (18/27). In both cases reported recently by Kwayess et al. (2024), bilateral neck exploration was also performed. Thus, BNE, with longer exploration of the neck, might be one of the risk factors for developing thyroiditis after parathyroidectomy. The intra-operative localization of the parathyroid glands was reported to be difficult in 18.5% (5/27) of the cases, two of whom necessitated excision of part of the thyroid gland [87].

6.6.2.5 Diagnosis

Post-operative thyroiditis is usually diagnosed 2–3 days after surgery, and rarely on the same day of surgery or more than 2 weeks post-operatively [87]. Diagnosis is based on the laboratory findings of suppressed TSH with elevated T4 and T3 and/or a low thyroidal radionuclide uptake. The free T3/free T4 ratio is an effective, simple method to differentiate destructive thyroiditis (painless and subacute thyroiditis) from Graves' thyrotoxicosis with some overlap, as this ratio is influenced by thyroid binding globulin. A free T3/free T4 ratio less than 0.3 has a sensitivity of 52.4% and specificity of 91.3% for diagnosing destruction-induced thyrotoxicosis in all thyrotoxic patients [115]. Thyroglobulin (Tg) levels greater than 90 ng/mL have been suggestive of post-operative palpation thyroiditis and are attributed to the leakage from thyroid gland during manipulation [84].

6.6.2.6 Treatment

In most cases, the treatment of post-operative thyroiditis includes beta-blockers and supportive measures. Some patients may require propyl-thiouracil or glucocorticoids in addition [87]. Thyroid function tests are normalized eventually between 2 weeks and 9 months after the initial presentation. It has been reported that spontaneous resolution can be expected by 6 weeks in the vast majority of patients given that the half-life of circulating thyroxin is 1 week [84].

6.6.2.7 Conclusions

In summary, it may be concluded that (1) thyroiditis after parathyroid surgery should be suspected in patients with typical symptoms of hyperthyroidism; the consequences may be serious and include cardiac events; (2) post-parathyroidectomy thyroiditis is attributed to the palpation of thyroid during the surgery and is more common in secondary and tertiary HPT; (3) the diagnosis of post-parathyroidectomy thyroiditis is confirmed by the presence of suppressed serum TSH, with elevated T4, and low radionuclide uptake on thyroid scan; an elevated serum Tg level further supports the diagnosis; (4) the lack of routine testing for thyroid abnormalities after parathyroid surgery may contribute to an under-appreciation of post-parathyroidectomy thyroiditis, especially since many patients remain asymptomatic; (5) post-parathyroidectomy thyroiditis is self-limited, and normalization of thyroid function occurs within weeks in the majority of patients; (6) further research is warranted to better understand the underlying pathophysiology and to establish potential risk factors for the development of post-parathyroidectomy thyroiditis; and (7) continued efforts to minimize the extent of PTH exploration surgery, if possible, may reduce the potential morbidity of thyrotoxicosis after surgery.

References

1. Ross DS, Burch HB, Cooper DS, Greenlee C, Laurberg P, Maia AL. American Thyroid Association guidelines for diagnosis and management of hyperthyroidism and other causes of thyrotoxicosis. Thyroid. 2016;26(10):1343–421.
2. Samuels MH. Subacute, silent, postpartum thyroiditis. Med Clin North Am. 2012;96(2):223–33.
3. Sharma A, Stan MN. Thyrotoxicosis: diagnosis and management. Mayo Clin Proc. 2019;94(6):1048–64.
4. Kamijo K. A case report of gestational painless thyroiditis. J Autoimmune Dis. 2018;4:1–3.
5. Kamijo K. Novel classification of painless thyroiditis including potassium iodide-induced painless thyroiditis. Am J Otolaryngol Head Neck Surg. 2019;2:1–2.
6. Carle A, Pedersen IB. Silent/painless thyroiditis diagnosis. Scand J Clin Lab Invest. 2013;73(3):240–4.
7. Cooper DS, Biondi B. Subclinical thyroid disease. Lancet. 2012;379(9821):1142–54.
8. Chaker L, Bianco AC, Jonklaas J, Peeters RP. Subclinical hypothyroidism. Lancet. 2017;390(10101):1550–62.
9. Alexander EK, Pearce EN, Brent GA, Brown RS, Chen H, Dosiou C, et al. 2017 Guidelines of the American Thyroid Association for the diagnosis and management of thyroid disease during pregnancy and the postpartum. Thyroid. 2017;27(3):315–89.
10. Franklyn JA, Boelaert K. Thyrotoxicosis. Lancet. 2012;379(9821):1155–66.
11. McDermott MT. Hypothyroidism. Ann Intern Med. 2020;173(1):ITC1–ITC16.
12. Smith TJ, Hegedüs L. Graves' disease. N Engl J Med. 2016;375(16):1552–65.
13. Muller AF, Drexhage HA, Berghout A. Postpartum thyroiditis and autoimmune thyroiditis in women of childbearing age: recent insights and consequences for antenatal and postnatal care. Endocr Rev. 2001;22(5):605–30.
14. De Groot L, Abalovich M, Alexander EK, Amino N, Barbour L, Cobin RH, et al. Management of thyroid dysfunction during pregnancy and postpartum: an Endocrine Society clinical practice guideline. J Clin Endocrinol Metab. 2012;97(8):2543–65.
15. Prummel MF, Wiersinga WM. Thyroid peroxidase autoantibodies in euthyroid subjects. Best Pract Res Clin Endocrinol Metab. 2005;19(1):1–15.
16. Stagnaro-Green A. Clinical review 152: postpartum thyroiditis. J Clin Endocrinol Metab. 2002;87(9):4042–7.
17. Stagnaro-Green A, Abalovich M, Alexander E, et al. Guidelines of the American Thyroid Association for the diagnosis and management of thyroid disease during pregnancy and postpartum. Thyroid. 2011;21(10):1081–125.
18. Ramezani Tehrani F, Aghaee M, Asefzadeh S. The comparison of thyroid function tests in cord blood following cesarean section or vaginal delivery. Int J Endocrinol Metab. 2003;1:22–6.
19. Smyth PP, Hetherton AM, Smith DF, Radcliff M, O'Herlihy C. Maternal iodine status and thyroid volume during pregnancy: correlation with neonatal iodine intake. J Clin Endocrinol Metab. 1997;82(9):2840–3.
20. Stagnaro-Green A. Postpartum thyroiditis. Best Pract Res Clin Endocrinol Metab. 2004;18(2):303–16.
21. Nicholson WK, Robinson KA, Smallridge RC, Ladenson PW, Powe NR. Prevalence of postpartum thyroid dysfunction: a quantitative review. Thyroid. 2006;16(6):573–82.
22. LiVolsi VA. Postpartum thyroiditis. The pathology slowly unravels. Am J Clin Pathol. 1993;100(3):193–5.

23. Kologlu M, Fung H, Darke C, Richards CJ, Hall R, McGregor AM. Postpartum thyroid dysfunction and HLA status. Eur J Clin Investig. 1990;20(1):56–60.
24. Nikolai TF, Turney SL, Roberts RC. Postpartum lymphocytic thyroiditis. Prevalence, clinical course, and long-term follow-up. Arch Intern Med. 1987;147(2):221–4.
25. Lazarus JH, Hall R, Othman S, Parkes AB, Richards CJ, McCulloch B, et al. The clinical spectrum of postpartum thyroid disease. QJM. 1996;89(6):429–35.
26. Gerstein HC. How common is postpartum thyroiditis? A methodologic overview of the literature. Arch Intern Med. 1990;150(7):1397–400.
27. Lucas A, Pizarro E, Granada ML, Salinas I, Foz M, Sanmarti A. Postpartum thyroiditis: epidemiology and clinical evolution in a non-selected population. Thyroid. 2000;10(1):71–7.
28. Stagnaro-Green A, Schwartz A, Gismondi R, Tinelli A, Mangieri T, Negro R. High rate of persistent hypothyroidism in a large-scale prospective study of postpartum thyroiditis in Southern Italy. J Clin Endocrinol Metab. 2011;96(3):652–7.
29. Negro R, Greco G, Mangieri T, Pezzarossa A, Dazzi D, Hassan H. The influence of selenium supplementation on postpartum thyroid status in pregnant women with thyroid peroxidase autoantibodies. J Clin Endocrinol Metab. 2007;92(4):1263–8.
30. Lazarus JH, Ammari F, Oretti R, Parkes AB, Richards CJ, Harris B. Clinical aspects of recurrent postpartum thyroiditis. Br J Gen Pract. 1997;47:305–8.
31. van Erven L, Schalij MJ. Amiodarone: an effective antiarrhythmic drug with unusual side effects. Heart. 2010;96(19):1593–600.
32. Kaufman ES, Zimmermann PA, Wang T, Dennish GW 3rd, Barrell PD, Chandler ML, et al. Atrial Fibrillation Follow-up Investigation of Rhythm Management Investigators. Risk of proarrhythmic events in the Atrial Fibrillation Follow-up Investigation of Rhythm Management (AFFIRM) study: a multivariate analysis. J Am Coll Cardiol. 2004;44(6):1276–82.
33. Schwaiblmair M, Erghaus T, Haeckel T, Wagner T, von Scheidt W. Amiodarone-induced pulmonary toxicity: an under-recognized and severe side effect? Clin Res Cardiol. 2010;99:693–700.
34. Ahmed S, Van Gelder IC, Wiesfeld AC, Van Veldhuisen DJ, Links TP. Determinants and outcome of amiodarone-associated thyroid dysfunction. Clin Endocrinol. 2011;75(3):388–94.
35. Mosher MC. Amiodarone-induced hypothyroidism and other adverse effects. Dimens Crit Care Nurs. 2011;30(2):87–93.
36. Moore BM, Cordina RL, McGuire MA, Celermajer DS. Adverse effects of amiodarone therapy in adults with congenital heart disease. Congenit Heart Dis. 2018;13(6):944–51.
37. Rizzo LFL, Mana DL, Serra HA. Drug-induced hypothyroidism. Medicina (B Aires). 2017;77(5):394–404.
38. Godley AF, Stanbury JB. Preliminary experience in the treatment of hyperthyroidism with potassium perchlorate. J Clin Endocrinol Metab. 1954;14(1):70–8.
39. Reichert LJ, De Rooy HA. Treatment of amiodarone induced hyperthyroidism with potassium perchlorate and methimazole during amiodarone treatment. BMJ. 1989;298(6687):1547.
40. Mantyjärvi M, Tuppurainen K, Ikaheimo K. Ocular side effects of amiodarone. Surv Ophthalmol. 1998;42:360–6.
41. Su VY, Hu YW, Chou KT, Ou SM, Lee YC, Lin EY, et al. Amiodarone and the risk of cancer: a nationwide population-based study. Cancer. 2013;119(9):1699–705.
42. Lakhdar AA, Farish E, Hillis WS, Dunn FG. Long-term amiodarone therapy raises serum cholesterol. Eur J Clin Pharmacol. 1991;40:477–80.
43. Hudig F, Bakker O, Wiersinga WM. Amiodarone decreases gene expression of low-density lipoprotein receptor at both the mRNA and protein level. Metabolism. 1998;47:1052–7.
44. Simonen P, Lehtonen J, Lampi A-M, Piironen V, Stenman U-H, Kupari M, et al. Desmosterol accumulation in users of amiodarone. J Intern Med. 2018;283:93–101.
45. Pardoll DM. The blockade of immune checkpoints in cancer immunotherapy. Nat Rev Cancer. 2012;12(4):252–64.
46. Cameron F, Whiteside G, Perry C. Ipilimumab: first global approval. Drugs. 2011;71(8):1093–104.

47. Postow MA, Sidlow R, Hellmann MD. Immune-related adverse events associated with immune checkpoint blockade. N Engl J Med. 2018;378(2):158–68.
48. Butterworth JF. Morgan and Mikhail's clinical anaesthesiology. 6th ed. New York: McGraw-Hill Education; 2018. 638 p.
49. Barroso-Sousa R, Barry WT, Garrido-Castro AC, Hodi FS, Min LK, Ian E, et al. Incidence of endocrine dysfunction following the use of different immune checkpoint inhibitor regimens. JAMA Oncol. 2018;4(2):173–82.
50. Pollack R, Stokar J, Lishinsky N, Gurt I, Kaisar-Iluz N, Shaul ME, et al. RNA sequencing reveals unique transcriptomic signatures of the thyroid in a murine lung cancer model treated with PD-1 and PD-L1 antibodies. Int J Mol Sci. 2023;24(13):10526.
51. Yang P, Shen G, Zhang H, Zhang C, Li J, Zhao F, et al. Incidence of thyroid dysfunction caused by immune checkpoint inhibitors combined with chemotherapy: a systematic review and meta-analysis. Int Immunopharmacol. 2024;133:111961.
52. Risbjerg RS, Hansen MV, Sørensen AS, Kragstrup TW. The effects of B cell depletion on immune related adverse events associated with immune checkpoint inhibition. Exp Hematol Oncol. 2020;9(1):9.
53. Tondo L, Alda M, Bauer M, Bergink V, Grof P, Hajek T, et al. International Group for Studies of Lithium (IGSLi). Clinical use of lithium salts: guide for users and prescribers. Int J Bipolar Disord. 2019;7(1):16.
54. Poels EM, Bijma HH, Galbally M, Bergink V. Lithium during pregnancy and after delivery: a review. Int J Bipolar Disord. 2018;6(1):26.
55. Armstrong C. ACOG guidelines on psychiatric medication use during pregnancy and lactation. Am Fam Physician. 2008;78(6):772–8.
56. Carle A, Pedersen IB, Knudsen N, Perrild H, Ovesen L, Rasmussen LB, et al. Epidemiology of subtypes of hyperthyroidism in Denmark: a population-based study. Eur J Endocrinol. 2011;164(5):801–9.
57. Williams CD, Linch DC. Interferon alfa-2a. Br J Hosp Med. 1997;57(9):436–9.
58. Woo MH, Burnakis TG. Interferon alfa in the treatment of chronic viral hepatitis B and C. Ann Pharmacother. 1997;31(3):330–7.
59. Carella C, Mazziotti G, Amato G, Braverman LE, Roti E. Clinical review 169: interferon-alpha-related thyroid disease: pathophysiological, epidemiological, and clinical aspects. J Clin Endocrinol Metab. 2004;89(8):3656–61.
60. Roti E, Minelli R, Giuberti T, Marchelli S, Schianchi C, Gardini E, et al. Multiple changes in thyroid function in patients with chronic active HCV hepatitis treated with recombinant interferon-alpha. Am J Med. 1996;101(5):482–7.
61. Jacobs EL, Clare-Salzler MJ, Chopra IJ, Figlin RA. Thyroid function abnormalities associated with the chronic outpatient administration of recombinant interleukin-2 and recombinant interferon-alpha. J Immunother. 1991;10(6):448–55.
62. Carella C, Mazziotti G, Morisco F, Manganella G, Rotondi M, Tuccillo C, et al. Long-term outcome of interferon-alpha-induced thyroid autoimmunity and prognostic influence of thyroid autoantibody pattern at the end of treatment. J Clin Endocrinol Metab. 2001;86(5):1925–9.
63. Arenas-Ramirez N, Woytschak J, Boyman O. Interleukin-2: biology, design and application. Trends Immunol. 2015;36(12):763–77.
64. Liao W, Lin JX, Leonard WJ. IL-2 family cytokines: new insights into the complex of roles of IL-2 as a broad regulator of T helper cell differentiation. Curr Opin Immunol. 2011;23(5):598–604.
65. Liao W, Lin JX, Leonard WJ. Interleukin-2 at the crossroads of effector responses, tolerance, and immunotherapy. Immunity. 2013;38(1):13–25.
66. Spolski R, Li P, Leonard WJ. Biology and regulation of IL-2: from molecular mechanisms to human therapy. Nat Rev Immunol. 2018;18(10):648–59.
67. Shaker MA, Younes HM. Interleukin-2: evaluation of routes of administration and current delivery systems in cancer therapy. J Pharm Sci. 2009;98(7):2268–98.
68. Den Otter W, Jacobs JJ, Battermann JJ, Hordijk GJ, Krastev Z, Moiseeva EV, et al. Local therapy of cancer with free IL-2. Cancer Immunol Immunother. 2008;57(7):931–50.

69. Correction for Krieg C, et al. Improved IL-2 immunotherapy by selective stimulation of IL-2 receptors on lymphocytes and endothelial cells. Proc Natl Acad Sci USA. 2012;109(1):345. Erratum for: Proc Natl Acad Sci USA. 107:11906. PMCID: PMC3252892.
70. Vialettes B, Guillerand MA, Viens P, Stoppa AM, Baume D, Sauvan R, et al. Incidence rate and risk factors for thyroid dysfunction during recombinant interleukin-2 therapy in advanced malignancies. Acta Endocrinol. 1993;129(1):31–8.
71. Desai J, Yassa L, Marqusee E, George S, Frates MC, Chen MH, et al. Hypothyroidism after sunitinib treatment for patients with gastrointestinal stromal tumors. Ann Intern Med. 2006;145(9):660–4.
72. Rini BI, Tamaskar I, Shaheen P, Salas R, Garcia J, Wood L, et al. Hypothyroidism in patients with metastatic renal cell carcinoma treated with sunitinib. J Natl Cancer Inst. 2007;99(1):81–3.
73. Malhotra A, Gupta R, Mahajan S. Tyrosine kinase inhibitors induced thyroid dysfunction: myth or reality? Rep Pract Oncol Radiother. 2023;28(4):463–7.
74. Fujita KI, Ishida H, Kubota Y, Sasaki Y. Toxicities of receptor tyrosine kinase inhibitors in cancer pharmacotherapy: management with clinical pharmacology. Curr Drug Metab. 2017;18(3):186–98.
75. Havrdova E, Horakova D, Kovarova I. Alemtuzumab in the treatment of multiple sclerosis: key clinical trial results and considerations for use. Ther Adv Neurol Disord. 2015;8:31–45.
76. Scappaticcio L, Castellana M, Virili C, Bellastella G, Centanni M, Cannavò S, et al. Alemtuzumab-induced thyroid events in multiple sclerosis: a systematic review and meta-analysis. J Endocrinol Investig. 2020;43(2):219–29.
77. Sheikh-Taha M, Corman LC. Pulmonary Nocardia beijingensis infection associated with the use of alemtuzumab in a patient with multiple sclerosis. Mult Scler. 2017;23(6):872–4.
78. Clerico M, De Mercanti S, Artusi CA, Durelli L, Naismith RT. Active CMV infection in two patients with multiple sclerosis treated with alemtuzumab. Mult Scler. 2017;23(6):874–6.
79. Brownlee WJ, Chataway J. Opportunistic infections after alemtuzumab: new cases of nocardial infection and cytomegalovirus syndrome. Mult Scler. 2017;23(6):876–7.
80. Menge T, Stuve O, Kieseier BC, Hartung HP. Alemtuzumab: the advantages and challenges of a novel therapy in MS. Neurology. 2014;83:87–97.
81. Costelloe L, Jones J, Coles A. Secondary autoimmune diseases following alemtuzumab therapy for multiple sclerosis. Expert Rev Neurother. 2012;12(3):335–41.
82. Aranha AA, Amer S, Reda ES, Broadley SA, Davoren PM. Autoimmune thyroid disease in the use of alemtuzumab for multiple sclerosis: a review. Endocr Pract. 2013;19(5):821–8.
83. Wehrum T, Beume LA, Stich O, Mader I, Mäurer M, Czaplinski A, et al. Activation of disease during therapy with alemtuzumab in 3 patients with multiple sclerosis. Neurology. 2018;90(7):e601–5.
84. Espiritu RP, Dean DS. Parathyroidectomy-induced thyroiditis. Endocr Pract. 2010;16(4):656–9.
85. McDermott A, Onyeaka CV, Macnamara M. Surgery-induced thyroiditis: fact or fiction? Ear Nose Throat J. 2002;81(6):408–10.
86. Blenke EJ, Vernham GA, Ellis G. Surgery-induced thyroiditis following laryngectomy. J Laryngol Otol. 2004;118(4):313–4.
87. Kwayess R, Cooper DS, Fuleihan GE. Thyroiditis after parathyroidectomy. JCEM Case Rep. 2024;2:1–12.
88. Walfish PG, Caplan D, Rosen IB. Postparathyroidectomy transient thyrotoxicosis. J Clin Endocrinol Metab. 1992;75(1):224–7.
89. Musi N, Braverman LE, Norris CM Jr. Severe thyrotoxicosis after parathyroid surgery for hyperparathyroidism. Am J Med. 2000;108(6):519–20.
90. Lim W, Luxton G, Hutchison B. Acute thyroiditis following parathyroidectomy for secondary hyperparathyroidism in a chronic renal failure patient. Intern Med J. 2003;33(3):131–3.
91. Hamada C, Tanaka Y, Sakamoto T, Kaneko K, Shou S, Fukui M, et al. Transient thyrotoxicosis after parathyroidectomy in a hemodialysis patient with secondary hyperparathyroidism. Hong Kong J Nephrol. 2007;9(1):45–9.

92. Sato H, Miyamoto Y, Inagaki M, Kanai G, Suzuki H, Tanaka R, et al. Atrial fibrillation induced by post-parathyroidectomy transient thyrotoxicosis. Intern Med. 2008;47(20):1807–11.
93. Lederer SR, Schiffl H. Transient hyperthyroidism after total parathyroidectomy for tertiary hyperparathyroidism: a report of two cases. Wien Klin Wochenschr. 2008;120(13–14):432–4.
94. Rudofsky G Jr, Grafe IA, Metzner C, Leowardi C, Fohr B. Transient post-operative thyrotoxicosis after parathyroidectomy. Med Sci Monit. 2009;15(3):CS41–3.
95. Naber TH, Jhaveri KD, Sachdeva M. Reactive thyrotoxicosis: under diagnosed complication of parathyroidectomy in the dialysis population. Am J Kidney Dis. 2010;55(4):A82.
96. Parker G, Brand WW 3rd, Dyess E, Webster SA. Acute thyroiditis complicating parathyroidectomy. Am J Med Sci. 2010;339(5):491–2.
97. Asmar A, Ross EA. Post-parathyroidectomy thyrotoxicosis and atrial flutter: a case for caution. NDT Plus. 2011;4(2):117–9.
98. Kauffels A, Lee IO, Schilling MK, Slotta JE. Thyrotoxicosis after parathyroidectomy mimicking myocardial infarction: a case report and review of the literature. Clin Res Cardiol. 2012;101(8):687–90.
99. Upadhyay J, Trivedi N. Transient thyrotoxicosis following minimally invasive radio-guided parathyroidectomy. Endocr Pract. 2014;20(1):e1–3.
100. Hakami YA. Transient thyroiditis after surgery for tertiary hyperparathyroidism: a case report. Front Endocrinol (Lausanne). 2015;6:123.
101. Madill EM, Cooray SD, Bach LA. Palpation thyroiditis following subtotal parathyroidectomy for hyperparathyroidism. Endocrinol Diabetes Metab Case Rep. 2016;2016:16–0049.
102. Xu Z, Wu YT, Li X, Wu H, Chen HR, Shi YL, et al. Thyrotoxicosis occurring in secondary hyperparathyroidism patients undergoing dialysis after total parathyroidectomy with autotransplantation. Chin Med. 2017;130(16):1995–6.
103. Chan GC, Lee PC, Kwan LP, Yip TP, Tang SC. Acute thyroiditis: an under-recognized complication of parathyroidectomy in end-stage renal failure patients with secondary hyperparathyroidism. Nephrology (Carlton). 2017;22(7):572.
104. Rahman O, Naqvi K, Saeed Z, Adnan S, Shah U. Thyroid storm due to palpation thyroiditis after parathyroidectomy: a rare form of thyrotoxicosis. Crit Care Med. 2019;47(1):132.
105. Pinxterhuis TH, Out M, van den Broek RWF, Wouters RSME, van der Kleij FGH. Transient thyroiditis after parathyroidectomy for tertiary hyperparathyroidism. Neth J Med. 2019;77(3):119–21.
106. Ashorobi D, Mandal K, Liao H, Rosenthal D, Kumar S. A case of transient thyrotoxicosis postparathyroidectomy. Thyroid. 2021;31(Suppl 1):A69–70.
107. Boeder S, Choe C, Mao J. Altered mental status, hypercalcemia, and atrial fibrillation induced by post-parathyroidectomy thyroiditis. J Endocr Soc. 2022;6(Suppl 1):A823–4.
108. Mordechay-Heyn T, Mazeh H, Elitzur Y, Szalat A. Atrial fibrillation and thyrotoxicosis following parathyroidectomy. Isr Med Assoc J. 2022;24(1):64–6.
109. Stang MT, Yim JH, Challinor SM, Bahl S, Carty SE. Hyperthyroidism after parathyroid exploration. Surgery. 2005;138(6):1058–65.
110. Lindblom P, Valdemarsson S, Westerdahl J, Tennvall J, Bergenfelz A. Hyperthyroidism after surgery for primary hyperparathyroidism. Langenbecks Arch Surg. 1999;384(6):568–75.
111. Bergenfelz A, Ahren B. Hyperthyroxinemia after surgery for primary hyperparathyroidism. Langenbecks Arch Chir. 1994;379:178–81.
112. Kobayashi A, Kuma K, Matsuzuka F, Hirai K, Fukata S, Sugawara M. Thyrotoxicosis after needle aspiration of thyroid cyst. J Clin Endocrinol Metab. 1992;75:21–4.
113. Carney JA, Moore SB, Northcutt RC, Woolner LB, Stillwell GK. Palpation thyroiditis (multifocal granulomatous folliculitis). Am J Clin Pathol. 1975;64:639–47.
114. Mai VQ, Glister BC, Clyde PW, Shakir KM. Palpation thyroiditis causing new-onset atrial fibrillation. Thyroid. 2008;18(5):571–3.
115. Izumi Y, Hidaka Y, Tada H, et al. Simple and practical parameters for differentiation between destruction-induced thyrotoxicosis and Graves' thyrotoxicosis. Clin Endocrinol. 2002;57(1):51–8.

Chronic Thyroiditis: Overview

7

7.1 Etiology of Chronic Thyroiditis

7.1.1 Autoimmune Thyroiditis

Autoimmune thyroiditis includes Hashimoto's thyroiditis and post-partum thyroiditis, and its association with HLA-DR3, HLA-DR4, and HLA-DR5 has been reported in White races [1–3].

7.1.1.1 Hashimoto's Thyroiditis

Hashimoto's thyroiditis is the most common cause of hypothyroidism in the United States of America (USA). It is presumed to be due to a viral infection, with the viral structure being similar to thyroid protein, leading to the production of antibodies against the thyroid gland. Approximately 10% of the general population in the USA has a high concentration of these antibodies, but the majority of them have normal thyroid function tests [4]. However, there is a risk of progression to overt hypothyroidism in such individuals.

7.1.1.2 Post-partum Thyroiditis

Post-partum thyroiditis is an autoimmune phenomenon where antibodies formed against fetal thyroid cells accumulate in the mother's thyroid gland [5]. It occurs in post-partum women within 1 year of childbirth. The maternal presence of positive thyroid peroxidase (TPO) antibody or other autoimmune diseases is a risk factor.

7.1.2 Drug-Induced Thyroiditis

The most common drugs causing thyroid dysfunction are amiodarone, lithium, tyrosine kinase inhibitors, immune checkpoint inhibitors, interferon-alpha (IFN-α), and interleukin-2 (IL-2). The conditions are most often self-limiting but can have very

M. Sakr, *Thyroiditis*, https://doi.org/10.1007/978-3-032-19513-5_7

variable courses. Treatment is conservative and includes beta-blockers for symptoms of thyrotoxicosis and levothyroxine (L-T4) for hypothyroidism.

7.1.2.1 Amiodarone

Amiodarone can cause both hyper- and hypothyroidism. In euthyroid individuals, amiodarone can cause transient changes in thyroid function tests (TFTs), followed by normalization. Pregnant women and patients who have underlying Hashimoto's disease are at risk of developing worsening hypothyroidism. It is thought to be secondary to the anti-thyroid effect of the iodine in amiodarone. Amiodarone can induce hyperthyroidism in two ways. In type 1, there is increased synthesis and release of thyroid hormone, whereas in type 2, there is destructive thyroiditis leading to the release of preformed T4 and T3 from the damaged thyroid gland [6].

7.1.2.2 Lithium

Lithium, used as a psychiatric medication primarily for bipolar disorder and for major depressive disorder, is known to cause hypothyroidism by decreasing the secretion of thyroid hormones. This causes a rise in TSH and eventually goiter in approximately 40% of patients, hypothyroidism in 20% of patients, and thyrotoxicosis in between 0.6 and 3.0%. Clinical and para-clinical findings consistent with thyroiditis in a patient on lithium therapy suggest the diagnosis of lithium-induced thyroiditis. Onset is often more than a year after initiation of lithium [7].

7.1.2.3 Tyrosine Kinase Inhibitors (TKIs)

Thyroiditis with thyroid abnormalities, including both hyper- and hypothyroidism, can be seen in patients on tyrosine kinase inhibitors, especially Sunitinib, Sorafenib, Nilotinib, and Lenvatinib. The incidence of hypothyroidism is between 60 and 85% with treatment with Sunitinib and approximately 20% with Sorafenib. The risk of hypothyroidism increases after multiple courses [8–10].

7.1.2.4 Checkpoint Inhibitors

Checkpoint inhibitors are a type of immunotherapy with anti-neoplastic properties and include several drugs such as Nivolumab, Ipilimumab, Pembrolizumab, and Atezolizumab. They are associated with endocrinopathies, especially hypothyroidism secondary to destructive thyroiditis [6]. Patients usually present with vague symptoms of hypothyroidism like fatigue and weight gain. It should be distinguished from secondary hypothyroidism as these drugs also cause hypophysitis. Hyperthyroidism, though very rare, is also occasionally encountered.

7.1.2.5 Interferon-Alfa (IFN-α)

About 15% of patients on interferon-alfa (IFN-α) therapy can develop thyroid dysfunction, and approximately 5% can develop permanent hypothyroidism [7]. Up to half of the patients on INF-α treatment who develop thyrotoxicosis have Graves' disease and should be treated accordingly. Thyroid dysfunction is often seen after 3 months of treatment, but can be seen as long as patients are on INF-α and also for several years after treatment has stopped.

7.1.2.6 Interleukin-2 (IL-2)

Interleukin-2 (IL-2) is a type of cytokine signaling molecule in the immune system that regulates the activities of WBCs (leukocytes, often lymphocytes) that are responsible for immunity. Clinical and para-clinical findings consistent with silent thyroiditis in a patient receiving IL-2 therapy suggest the diagnosis of IL-2-induced thyroiditis. Measurement of TRAb should be considered in patients on IL-2 who develop thyrotoxicosis [11].

7.1.3 Riedel's Thyroiditis

Riedel's thyroiditis is a rare disorder characterized by progressive fibrosis of the thyroid gland. The exact etiology is still unclear, but recent data indicate that it is closely related to IgG-4-related sclerosing disease. The fibrosis of the thyroid gland may or may not be associated with progressive fibrosis of other organs [12].

7.2 Clinical Manifestations

7.2.1 History-Taking

For chronic thyroiditis, a detailed history is of paramount importance in order to narrow the possible etiologies. Medication history is important to diagnose underlying drug-induced thyroiditis. Personal history and family history of autoimmune disease can help discover any increased risk of autoimmune thyroid disease.

Symptoms related to local compressive symptoms in the neck, including dysphagia, choking sensation, or hoarseness of voice, could indicate underlying large goiter or large thyroid nodule, or Riedel's thyroiditis. Patients with Riedel's thyroiditis usually present with dysphagia, odynophagia, and respiratory distress due to compression of the trachea, esophagus, and also because of the extension of the fibrosis [13].

Patients with thyroiditis due to checkpoint inhibitors usually present with vague symptoms of hypothyroidism like fatigue and weight gain [14]. Autoimmune/Hashimoto's thyroiditis usually presents with a painless goiter. Post-partum thyroiditis usually presents with symptoms of thyrotoxicosis like tachycardia, nervousness, and diarrhea with a history of recent childbirth [15].

7.2.2 Physical Examination

Physical examination should include a detailed thyroid examination to evaluate any enlargement, tenderness on palpation, any abnormality in the texture, or any palpable nodules.

Drug-induced thyroiditis can be clinically benign on examination. Symptoms of hypothyroidism like weight gain, fatigue, constipation, and dry skin in patients on amiodarone should raise the suspicion of drug-induced thyroiditis. Amiodarone can also cause hyperthyroidism, and clinical manifestations may be masked initially because amiodarone has beta-adrenergic blocking activity. Patients with Riedel's thyroiditis can have a fixed, hard, painless goiter on physical examination. Most of the patients are euthyroid but can develop hypothyroidism [16].

7.3 Evaluation/Diagnosis

Diagnostic tests for autoimmune/Hashimoto's thyroiditis include thyroid peroxidase (TPO) antibody, which is present in 90% of patients, and thyroglobulin (Tg) antibody, which is present in 20% to 50%. Thyroid function tests show a hypothyroid picture with high TSH and low T3 and T4. It has been reported to be associated with HLA-DR3, HLA-DR4, and HLA-DR5 in Whites [17, 18].

Post-partum thyroiditis presents with symptoms of hyperthyroidism and history of recent pregnancy and should be evaluated with TSH, free T4, and free T3. It can be distinguished from Graves' disease by 24-h iodine uptake scan, and the uptake is low in post-partum thyroiditis [15].

Patients who are on drugs like amiodarone, lithium, interferon, interleukin 2, and checkpoint inhibitors should have baseline TSH at the commencement of treatment [14, 19]. TSH, free T4, and free T3 should be obtained in case of the development of symptoms of thyroid dysfunction. Thyroid ultrasound (US) with an iodine uptake scan can be obtained to distinguish drug-induced destructive inflammatory thyroiditis from Graves' disease. Uptake is low in drug-induced inflammatory thyroiditis and high in Graves' disease.

In Riedel's thyroiditis, biopsy is necessary for definitive diagnosis. Fine-needle aspiration (FNA) may not be sufficient for diagnosis and may require an open biopsy for definitive diagnosis of this disease [13, 20].

7.4 Treatment

7.4.1 Autoimmune Thyroiditis

Hashimoto's thyroiditis with normal thyroid function can be monitored without treatment with levothyroxine (L-T4) [17]. Hyperthyroidism or Graves' disease can be treated with anti-thyroid drugs (ATDs) such as methimazole or propyl-thiouracil. Methimazole is the drug of choice, but propyl-thiouracil is preferred during the first trimester of pregnancy and for treatment of thyroid storm. Permanent treatment of Graves' disease includes radioactive iodine (RAI) treatment and thyroidectomy [21].

Postpartum thyroiditis: It is usually transient, and 80% of patients eventually become euthyroid. Hypothyroid patients can be treated with levothyroxine (L-T4) and monitored with regular thyroid function [15].

7.4.2 Drug-Induced Thyroiditis

Amiodarone-induced thyroiditis can cause both hypothyroidism and hyperthyroidism [22]. Hypothyroidism: Once diagnosed, amiodarone is usually continued along with T-L4 replacement. If amiodarone is stopped for a different reason, individuals without previous thyroid dysfunction usually progress to euthyroid state with the withdrawal of amiodarone [22].

Hyperthyroidism: Treatment of type I hyperthyroidism is treated with beta-blockers and methimazole. For type 2 thyroiditis, the use of glucocorticoids is recommended to alleviate the hyperthyroid symptoms.

For lithium-induced thyroiditis, treatment is to continue lithium and start treatment with L-T4. It can also cause hyperthyroidism and Graves' disease secondary to goiter formation [7].

References

1. Tandon N, Zhang L, Weetman AP. HLA associations with Hashimoto's thyroiditis. Clin Endocrinol. 1991;34(5):383–6.
2. Jenkins D, Penny MA, Fletcher JA, Jacobs KH, Mijovic CH, Franklyn JA, Sheppard MC. HLA class II gene polymorphism contributes little to Hashimoto's thyroiditis. Clin Endocrinol. 1992;37(2):141–5.
3. Vargas MT, Briones-Urbina R, Gladman D, Papsin FR, Walfish PG. Antithyroid microsomal autoantibodies and HLA-DR5 are associated with postpartum thyroid dysfunction: evidence supporting an autoimmune pathogenesis. J Clin Endocrinol Metab. 1988;67(2):327–33.
4. Pearce EN, Farwell AP, Braverman LE. Thyroiditis. N Engl J Med. 2003;348(26):2646–55.
5. Imaizumi M, Pritsker A, Unger P, Davies TF. Intrathyroidal fetal microchimerism in pregnancy and postpartum. Endocrinology. 2002;143(1):247–53.
6. Garon-Czmil J, Petitpain N, Rouby F, Sassier M, Babai S, Yelehe-Okouma M, Weryha G, Klein M, Gillet P. Thyroiditis and immune check point inhibitors: the post-marketing experience using the French National Pharmacovigilance database. Fundam Clin Pharmacol. 2019;33(2):241–9.
7. Miller KK, Daniels GH. Association between lithium use and thyrotoxicosis caused by silent thyroiditis. Clin Endocrinol. 2001;55(4):501–8.
8. Desai J, Yassa L, Marqusee E, George S, Frates MC, Chen MH, et al. Hypothyroidism after sunitinib treatment for patients with gastrointestinal stromal tumors. Ann Intern Med. 2006;145(9):660–4.
9. Rini BI, Tamaskar I, Shaheen P, Salas R, Garcia J, Wood L, et al. Hypothyroidism in patients with metastatic renal cell carcinoma treated with sunitinib. J Natl Cancer Inst. 2007;99(1):81–3.
10. Malhotra A, Gupta R, Mahajan S. Tyrosine kinase inhibitors induced thyroid dysfunction: myth or reality? Reports Pract Oncol Radiother J Gt Cancer Cent Pozn Polish Soc Radiat Oncol. 2023;28(4):463–7.
11. Vialettes B, Guillerand MA, Viens P, Stoppa AM, Baume D, Sauvan R, et al. Incidence rate and risk factors for thyroid dysfunction during recombinant interleukin-2 therapy in advanced malignancies. Acta Endocrinol. 1993;129(1):31–8.
12. Umehara H, Okazaki K, Masaki Y, Kawano M, Yamamoto M, Saeki T, et al. Comprehensive diagnostic criteria for IgG4-related disease (IgG4-RD), 2011. Mod Rheumatol. 2012;22(1):21–30.
13. Fatourechi MM, Hay ID, McIver B, Sebo TJ, Fatourechi V. Invasive fibrous thyroiditis (Riedel thyroiditis): the Mayo Clinic experience, 1976-2008. Thyroid. 2011;21(7):765–72.

14. Muller I, Moran C, Lecumberri B, Decallonne B, Robertson N, Jones J, et al. 2019 European Thyroid Association guidelines on the management of thyroid dysfunction following immune reconstitution therapy. Eur Thyroid J. 2019;8(4):173–85.
15. Ide A, Amino N, Kang S, Yoshioka W, Kudo T, Nishihara E, et al. Differentiation of postpartum Graves' thyrotoxicosis from postpartum destructive thyrotoxicosis using antithyrotropin receptor antibodies and thyroid blood flow. Thyroid. 2014;24(6):1027–31.
16. De Groot L, Abalovich M, Alexander EK, Amino N, Barbour L, Cobin RH, et al. Management of thyroid dysfunction during pregnancy and postpartum: an Endocrine Society clinical practice guideline. J Clin Endocrinol Metab. 2012;97(8):2543–65.
17. Peng CC, Huai-En Chang R, Pennant M, Huang HK, Munir KM. A literature review of painful Hashimoto thyroiditis: 70 published cases in the past 70 years. J Endocr Soc. 2020;4(2):bvz008.
18. Ruchala M, Szczepanek E, Sowinski J. Sonoelastography in de Quervain thyroiditis. J Clin Endocrinol Metab. 2011;96(2):289–90.
19. Iyer PC, Cabanillas ME, Waguespack SG, Hu MI, Thosani S, Lavis VR, et al. Immune-related thyroiditis with immune checkpoint inhibitors. Thyroid. 2018;28(10):1243–51.
20. Harigopal M, Sahoo S, Recant WM, DeMay RM. Fine-needle aspiration of Riedel's disease: report of a case and review of the literature. Diagn Cytopathol. 2004;30(3):193–7.
21. Ross DS, Burch HB, Cooper DS, Greenlee MC, Laurberg P, Maia AL, et al. 2016 American Thyroid Association guidelines for diagnosis and management of hyperthyroidism and other causes of thyrotoxicosis. Thyroid. 2016;26(10):1343–421.
22. Benjamens S, Dullaart RPF, Sluiter WJ, Rienstra M, van Gelder IC, Links TP. The clinical value of regular thyroid function tests during amiodarone treatment. Eur J Endocrinol. 2017;177(1):9–14.

8 Chronic Thyroiditis: Riedel's Fibrosing Thyroiditis

8.1 Introduction

Riedel's thyroiditis is a chronic sclerosing (fibrosing) thyroiditis, occurring especially in women, that tends to progress inexorably to complete destruction of the thyroid gland and frequently causes pressure symptoms in the neck [1–3]. Initially described by Semple in 1864 and Bolby in 1888 [4], the condition was later reported in 1896 by Riedel as an "eisenharte Struma" (iron-hard goiter), characterized by a fixed and usually painless enlargement of the thyroid gland [1, 5, 6]. Physical examination, laboratory analysis, cytology, and imaging features are not useful for differentiating between Riedel's thyroiditis and neoplastic diseases or the fibrotic variant of Hashimoto's thyroiditis. Histological examination is necessary to establish the final diagnosis [7].

8.2 Epidemiology

Riedel's thyroiditis is exceedingly rare with an estimated incidence of 1.06 cases per 100,000 population and 37/57,000 (0.06%) of thyroid surgical outcomes over a 64-year period [8]. In the Mayo Clinic series [8], it occurred approximately one-fiftieth as frequently as Hashimoto's thyroiditis. It is more frequent in women (F:M 3.1:1) [1, 9–12] who were recently reported to represent 81% of those with confirmed Riedel's in a Mayo clinic series and further confirmed in a meta-analysis [12, 13]. Riedel's thyroiditis is principally reported to occur in the 30- to 50-year age group and has a reported median age of 47 years [9, 11–13].

M. Sakr, *Thyroiditis*, https://doi.org/10.1007/978-3-032-19513-5_8

8.3 Pathology

8.3.1 Gross Appearance

In Riedel's thyroiditis, the thyroid gland is normal in size or enlarged, focally or symmetrically involved, and extremely (woody) hard. The gland is replaced by the inflammatory process which may extend into adjacent structures including parathyroid glands, skeletal muscle, nerves, blood vessels, and trachea [14]. Gross observation of the mass reveals a pale gray appearance similar to a malignant lesion [15]. There are no tissue planes visible, and the cut-surface of the mass is stark white due to the hypo-vascularity of the tissue [16].

8.3.2 Histological Features

Histologically, normal tissue is replaced by inflammatory cells, predominantly lymphocytes, plasma cells, eosinophils [11, 17], and small amounts of colloid [18–20] in a dense matrix of hyalinized connective tissue (Fig. 8.1). Characteristically, an inflammatory reaction of the venous vascular structures has been described by Balach et al. (2005) [15]. An oft-stated criterion useful in assuring the pathological diagnosis is to note the absence of granulomatous tissue and malignancy [11, 15, 16]. A potentially difficult differential diagnostic decision may be encountered with diffuse sclerosing variant of papillary thyroid carcinoma (PTC) and the nodular sclerosing variant of Hodgkin's disease [12], rare sarcomas of the thyroid region [21], or with the pauci-cellular variant of anaplastic thyroid cancer, both of which, although similar in gross appearance, will have distinctive histopathological immuno-histochemical findings [22].

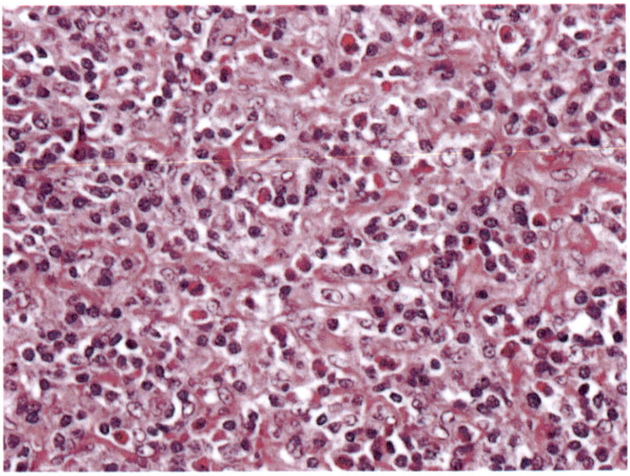

Fig. 8.1 Microscopy of Riedel's thyroiditis showing inflammatory infiltrate with numerous plasma cells, lymphocytes, and eosinophils. Thyroid parenchyma is replaced by hyalinized fibrous tissue. H&E stain

8.4 Etiology

Although the etiology remains unclear, Riedel's thyroiditis has been described as the cervical manifestation of a systemic fibrosing disorder with an identical histopathological appearance [23]. Further, Riedel's thyroiditis has been called a "variant of Hashimoto's thyroiditis," a "primary infiltrative disease of the thyroid," and even a "manifestation of end-stage de Quervain's thyroiditis" [2, 18, 24, 25].

Riedel's thyroiditis has been reported following subacute thyroiditis (SAT) [25]. A case of concurrent Riedel's, Hashimoto's, and acute thyroiditis has also been reported by Pirola et al. (2009) [26]. The report of a case of Graves' disease following Riedel's thyroiditis [27] and the observation that the B-cell proliferation observed in the course of these diseases has been shown to be polyclonal [28] supports the notion of "autoimmune mechanisms" in the etiology of Riedel's disease. The occurrence of marked tissue eosinophilia and the extra-cellular deposition of eosinophil granule major basic protein suggests a role for eosinophils and their products in the development of fibrosis in Riedel's thyroiditis [307]. Fibrosis may also be related to the action of transforming growth factor-beta1 (TGF-β1), as seen in murine thyroiditis [29]. Moreover, links between Hashimoto's, IgG4-related systemic disease (IgG4-RSD), and Riedel's thyroiditis have recently been reported by several authors [30–32]. Supporting evidence is the presence of IgG4-bearing plasma cells in thyroidectomy specimens and other affected organs [12, 32, 33]. A comprehensive review of potential etiology has been published by Hennessey in 2011 [14].

IgG4-related disease (IgG4-RD) was first described in 1961 as a distinctive presentation of pancreatitis, which was observed to be associated with hypergammaglobulinemia [34]. A specific association with IgG4 was published by Hamano et al. in 2001 [35], and eventually an international consensus was established to define the criteria for recognizing IgG4-RD [36, 37]. Through this understanding of pathophysiology, the term IgG4-RD has been adopted to describe a common underlying pathology found in a variety of fibrosing disorders that over the years have been designated in various ways, primarily based on the organ of involvement and the names of the initial authors of reports describing their occurrence. Under the umbrella of IgG4-RD, newer nomenclature captures entities such as "Mikulicz syndrome" as IgG4-related dacryoadentis and sialadenitis, and "Riedel's thyroiditis" as IgG4-related thyroid disease (IgG4RTD) [38, 39]. More recently, IgG4-related thyroid disease has included Riedel's thyroiditis, fibrosing variant of Hashimoto's thyroiditis, and few patients of Graves' orbitopathy to represent IgG4-related thyroid disease [40].

One or several organs may be involved at the time of diagnosis or subsequent to the identification of IgG4-RD in a particular organ. The most frequently involved organs include the pancreas, bile ducts, salivary glands, lachrymal glands and kidneys [38]. The majority of cases are identified by the presence of characteristic fibrosing pathology and it is expected that serum IgG4 levels be elevated in most cases.

The diagnosis if IgG4-RD is based on the identification of a (1) mass in one or more organs associated with an (2) elevated serum IgG4 level (>1.35 g/L) and (3) histopathology demonstrating marked lymphocytic and plasma cell infiltration, more than 10 IgG4 positive plasma cells per high powered field (>40% IgG4/IgG ratio) and storiform fibrosis [36, 41]. Definitive diagnosis is assured when all three criteria are present; the diagnosis is probable when the first and third criteria are met and possible when only the first and second criteria are present [38].

Based on these criteria, the position of Riedel's thyroiditis among the IgG4-RDs would be considered "probable" as the vast majority of cases reported thus far are *not* associated with elevated serum IgG4 levels although the typical histopathological criteria are met when applied. A recent review of 10 cases studied in Japan confirmed the IgG4-RD connection in histopathological data and noted a paucity of serum IgG4 levels in their summary of the published literature [42]. Most recent cases specifically noting this association and including the association with IgG4-RD in their titles document the first and third diagnostic criteria [32, 42–45], while only a few have documented an elevated serum IgG4 level [46, 47]. A recent series of cases from Sweden, where serum IgG4 levels were measured in 66% of the subjects, indicated that none of the four evaluated had elevated serum IgG4 levels [48]. The most recent meta-analysis does not detail any serum IgG4 data among the 212 subjects reviewed in published reports from 1925 to 2019 [12].

8.5 Clinical Presentation

Riedel's thyroiditis usually presents as a hard thyroid mass, frequently associated with compressive symptoms including dyspnea, stridor, hoarse voice, dysphagia for months before diagnosis [1, 2, 8, 9, 11, 13] and historically has been diagnosed by a surgeon faced with an inflammatory mass of fibro-sclerosing tissue [49, 50] when expecting a thyroid tumor [29]. Intra-operative diagnostic confusion with anaplastic thyroid carcinoma (ATC) [22], sarcoma of the thyroid [21], thyroid lymphoma [51], or fibrosing Hashimoto's thyroiditis [52] has been reported.

A case of asymptomatic Riedel's associated with a benign follicular adenoma has also been reported [53]. Riedel's thyroiditis may occur in a multinodular goiter (MNG) or as a rapidly growing hard neck mass in a previously normal gland mimicking thyroid cancer [50, 54, 55].

As the extent of the fibrosis increases, or concomitant Hashimoto's is present, involvement of a critical mass of the thyroid tissue results in primary hypothyroidism in 25-80% of cases [2, 13, 19, 30, 56]. Anti-thyroid antibodies may be present in 36-90% of reported cases [3, 12, 13]. A detailed breakdown of antibodies encountered has recently been reported in the context of systemic review of documented Riedel's thyroiditis reports, where thyroid peroxidase (TPO) was positive in 43% of those tested, thyroglobulin (Tg) antibodies were detected in 27% of those evaluated, and thyrotropin receptor antibodies were considered present in 20% when they were drawn [12].

Extension of the inflammatory process into the underlying parathyroid glands may result in non-surgical hypoparathyroidism [56–61] in up to 14% cases encountered [13]. The fibrosis may remain relatively stable or progress, resulting in local complications by compressing the trachea or esophagus and resulting in symptoms of local pressure, dyspnea, dysphagia, as well as stridor out of proportion to the size of the mass [62, 63], with subsequent hoarseness, and aphonia, with involvement of the recurrent laryngeal nerves (RLNs) [52, 59]. Further extension of the inflammatory process involving other neck structures can result in Tolosa-Hunt syndrome (severe and unilateral peri-orbital headache associated with painful and restricted eye movements). Synonyms include "painful ophthalmoplegia," "recurrent ophthalmoplegia," and "ophthalmoplegia syndrome" [64], Horner's syndrome [59], or occlusive phlebitis of cervical vessels [65–67]. The occurrence of cerebral sinus thrombosis suggests that Riedel's thyroiditis may cause venous stasis, vascular damage, and possibly hyper-coagulability [68].

Estimates as high as 38% associate Riedel's thyroiditis with similar fibrosclerotic processes in other areas [13]. Subcutaneous fibrosclerosis has also been reported, but it is very rare [69]. The lesions appear in the lacrimal glands, orbits [70], parotid glands [71], mediastinum [8, 13, 15, 19], coronary arteries [13], retroperitoneal tissues [2, 8, 56, 72, 73], bile ducts [11, 14], and pancreas [74] in varying combinations in the syndrome of multifocal fibro-sclerositis [75, 76].

8.6 Evaluation

8.6.1 Laboratory Tests

Initially, the patient with a thyroid mass will need an assessment of thyroid function and may benefit from screening thyroid antibodies [77]. A complete blood count (CBC) reveals normal to elevated white blood cell (WBC) counts. The erythrocyte sedimentation rate (ESR) is usually moderately elevated [18, 19]. Due to the potential of hypo-parathyroidism, an assessment of calcium status is prudent [14].

8.6.2 Imaging Studies

8.6.2.1 Ultrasonography (US)/Sono-Elastography

Ultrasonography (US) of the thyroid typically reveals a diffuse, hypoechoic, hypovascular appearance due to the extensive fibrosing process [50, 56, 78–80]. Unique to the findings in Riedel's thyroiditis is an encasement of the carotid arteries, *not* typically seen in other forms of multinodular goiter (MNG) or Hashimoto's thyroiditis [13, 81]. Sonographic elastography demonstrates significant stiffness of the tissue compared to normal thyroid [81].

8.6.2.2 Computed Tomography (CT) Scan

In patients with significant obstructive symptomatology, a neck computed tomography (CT) scan may be ordered to assess tracheal integrity. Characteristically, CT images demonstrate hypo-dense tissue which does *not* enhance with iodinated contrast in the affected area [79]. The CT images readily reveal extra-thyroidal extension of the inflammatory process [79, 82], and have been reported to document arterial encasement in about 50% of subjects and jugular involvement in approximately 33% of cases [13].

8.6.2.3 Magnetic Resonance Imaging (MRI)

Magnetic resonance imaging (MRI) can be expected to show hypo-intense images on both T1 and T2 weighted images [79] and variable enhancement patterns after gadolinium enhancement [79, 80, 82–84].

8.6.2.4 Positron Emission Tomography (PET) Scan

Unlike the hypo-intense images produced by CT scan and MRI, 18FDG-PET images have shown metabolic activity *not* only in extra-thyroidal masses associated with the systemic inflammatory process, but also increased glucose metabolism in the Riedel's thyroid, likely as a result of active inflammation involving lymphocytes, plasma cells, and fibroblast proliferation [81, 85, 86]. The FDG metabolic activity can also be used to assess a patient's response to therapy [85, 86], but not all reports of this phenomenon have documented the usefulness of this effect [81].

8.6.2.5 Radionuclide Scanning

Although not typically indicated in the evaluation of a eu- or hypo-thyroid individual with a thyroid mass, ^{99m}Tc-pertechnetate or $^{123/131}$I scanning in Riedel's thyroiditis is typically compromised due to low uptake and patchy images typical of other forms of chronic thyroiditis [11, 18, 19]. An exception to the utility of radionuclide scanning is found in the thyrotoxic patient presenting with a thyroid mass. In those with Graves' disease or a toxic thyroid nodule, the hyper-functioning portion of the thyroid is indeed well visualized, while the portion involved with Riedel's thyroiditis typically demonstrates no uptake [27]. Finally, it has been documented that gallium scanning may, as expected, also demonstrate significant uptake in the Riedel's lesion [87].

8.6.3 Fine-Needle Aspiration (FNA)

A fine-needle aspiration (FNA) of the thyroid mass is usually obtained. Results of FNA are typically non-diagnostic due to the lack of thyroid follicular cells [9, 11, 13, 16] but may contain evidence of the inflammatory process [13], fibrous tissue and myofibroblasts [88], or even cytopathology findings consistent with follicular neoplasm [58]. A novel case reported by Iacconi et al. (2012) illustrates a potential use of FNA to obtain protein used in proteomic analysis, which was successful in differentiating the tissue of a patient with Riedel's thyroiditis from the tissue profile of anaplastic thyroid carcinoma (ATC) [89].

8.6.4 Histopathology

Establishing the diagnosis of Riedel's thyroiditis requires histopathological confirmation at the present time. Biopsy material may be obtained by Tru-cut needle biopsy [90], open biopsy [9], or at the time of decompressive thyroidectomy. Histopathological findings required to establish this diagnosis include: (1) the presence of an inflammatory process in the thyroid with extension into surrounding tissue, (2) the inflammatory infiltrate should contain no giant cells, lymphoid follicles, oncocytes, or granulomas, (3) there should be evidence of occlusive phlebitis, and (4) there should be no evidence of thyroid malignancy [91].

More recent work has suggested that the IgG4+ plasma cells per high-powered field (HPF) and an IgG4+/IgG+ > 40% criteria for IgG4-Related Disease (IgG4-RD) is seldom met in the thyroid and a more modest finding of 10 IgG4+ plasma cells/HPF, and an IgG4+/IgG ratio of 20% would be a more appropriate diagnostic threshold [92]. In light of recent work defining Riedel's thyroiditis as a potential manifestation of the IgG4-related systemic sclerosing disease, the role of incorporating immuno-histochemical (IHC) assessment of tissue lymphocytes and the measurement of serum IgG4 levels into working diagnostic criteria is very supportive but remains to be defined.

8.7 Management

8.7.1 Surgical Treatment

Although there is no specific therapy for Riedel's thyroiditis, several management strategies are available dependent on the clinical features of the disease in the individual patient. Patients commonly undergo surgery for relief of obstructive symptoms. Histopathology then allows for the definitive establishment of the diagnosis. Most are then treated medically for associated hormone deficiencies with levothyroxine (L-T4) and/or calcium along with calcitriol as indicated [55]. This supplementation is *not* thought to influence the course of the disease. Finally, anti-inflammatory treatment aimed at diminishing the inflammatory tissue mass is applied and may even result in resolution of limited biochemical findings such as primary hypoparathyroidism [61].

Surgical therapy for debulking and symptom relief should usually be limited to isthmusectomy [9, 11, 58, 93] when total thyroidectomy (TT) is not possible. Due to the obliteration of tissue planes, there is an enhanced danger of hypoparathyroidism and recurrent laryngeal nerve (RLN) injury even when limited surgery is performed by experienced surgical specialists as documented in a series from the Mayo clinic where 39% of patients with Riedel's thyroiditis suffered surgical complications [13]. Previous and contemporary experience therefore recommends that extensive surgical procedures be considered inappropriate [9, 13, 16, 58]. Microscopic surgery has recently been attempted by Jung (2017) to minimize complications [94].

8.7.2 Medical Therapy

8.7.2.1 Corticosteroid Therapy

Medical therapy to arrest progression of symptomatic disease should be pursued after the establishment of diagnosis. Corticosteroid therapy has been reported by many authors to be effective in some cases [3, 12, 57, 61, 68, 75, 83, 90, 95–100], probably most in those with active inflammation [32, 99]. Initial doses of up to 100 mg/day of prednisone have been used [11], but sustained improvement has been reported with lower doses of 15-60 mg/day for about 3 months [12, 51, 59, 75, 95, 98, 100]. There are no controlled trials of steroid therapy in Riedel's disease, and a variety of medications have been used including most frequently prednisone, prednisolone, dexamethasone, methylprednisolone, and betamethasone [12]. Although some patients obtain long-term benefit after steroid withdrawal [23, 75, 99], others may relapse, usually leading to re-introduction of glucocorticoids or the addition of alternative anti-inflammatory therapy [59, 101, 102]. The reasons for this variation are unclear, but inflammatory activity and duration of disease may be relevant factors. More recently, the observation that smoking history may play a role in the responsiveness of Riedel's pathology to glucocorticoid therapy has been published [13].

8.7.2.2 Tamoxifen Therapy

In those who fail to respond to glucocorticoid therapy, or relapse after withdrawal, tamoxifen therapy is the next most common therapy reported to have been tried. Many reports have described an encouraging response with this agent when administered in doses of 20 mg/day for an average of 8 months, admittedly in only a small number of patients [103, 104, 61, 101, 105–110]. It is possible that tamoxifen acts in Riedel's disease by inhibition of fibroblast proliferation through the stimulation of TGF-β [111–113]. Tamoxifen as monotherapy or in combination with prednisone has been reported to be effective [59, 101, 108, 110]. There appears to be a persistent benefit of tamoxifen therapy during continued application in most but *not* all cases [13, 102].

8.7.2.3 Other Immunosuppressive Agents

Limited data on effective therapy with other immunosuppressive agents indicate that responses to azathioprine in doses ranging from 40 to 150 mg/day have recently been reported by Zala et al. (2020) in 4 patients [12]. A combination of mycophenolate mofetil (inosine mono-phosphate dehydrogenase inhibitor) and prednisone has also been observed to have successfully treated an individual who failed a prednisone and tamoxifen combination [102], and three cases of rituximab (anti-CD20 monoclonal antibody) use have also been reported to be useful [44, 114, 115]. The potential usefulness and relative effectiveness of these interventions await confirmation by further studies.

References

1. Riedel BM. Die chronische zur Bildung eisenharter Tumoren fuehrende Entzuendung der Shilddruese. Verh Ges Chir. 1896;25:101–5.
2. de Lange WE, Freling NJ, Molenaar WM, Doorenbos H. Invasive fibrous thyroiditis (Riedel's struma): a manifestation of multifocal fibrosclerosis? A case report with review of the literature. Q J Med. 1989;72(268):709–17.
3. Zimmermann-Belsing T, Feldt-Rasmussen U. Riedel's thyroiditis: an autoimmune or primary fibrotic disease? J Intern Med. 1994;235(3):271–4.
4. Goodman HI. Riedel's thyroiditis: a review and report of two cases. Am J Surg. 1941;54(2):472–8.
5. Riedel BM. Vorstellung eines Kranken mit chronischer Strumitis. Verh Ges Chir. 1896;26:127–9.
6. Riedel BM. Ueber Verlauf und Ausgang der chronischer Strumitis. Munch Med Wochenschr. 1910;57:1946–7.
7. Papi G, LiVolsi VA. Current concepts on Riedel thyroiditis. Am J Clin Pathol. 2004;121:S50–63.
8. Hay ID. Thyroiditis: a clinical update. Mayo Clin Proc. 1985;60(12):836–43.]
9. Singer PA. Thyroiditis. Acute, subacute, and chronic. Med Clin North Am. 1991;75(1):61–77.
10. Kabalak T, Ozgen AG. Familial occurrence of subacute thyroiditis. Endocr J. 2002;49(2):207–9.
11. Guimaraes VC. Subacute and Reidel's thyroiditis. In: Jameson JL, De Groot LJ, editors. Endocrinology: adult and pediatric. 6th ed. Philadelphia: Elsevier; 2010. p. 1600–3.
12. Zala A, Berhane T, Juhlin CC, Calissendorff J, Falhammar H. Riedel thyroiditis. J Clin Endocrinol Metab. 2020;105(9):468.
13. Fatourechi MM, Hay ID, McIver B, Sebo TJ, Fatourechi V. Invasive fibrous thyroiditis (riedel thyroiditis): the Mayo clinic experience, 1976-2008. Thyroid. 2011;21(7):765–72.
14. Hennessey JV. Clinical review: Riedel's thyroiditis: a clinical review. J Clin Endocrinol Metab. 2011;96(10):3031–41.
15. Balach ZW, LiVolsi VA. Pathology. In: Braverman LE, Utiger RE, editors. Werner & Ingbar's the thyroid; a fundamental and clinical text. 9th ed. Philadelphia: Lippincott Williams & Wilkins; 2005. p. 427.
16. Lee SL, Ananthakrishnan S. Infiltartive thyroid disease. In: Rose BD, Mulder JE, editors. UpToDate. Wellesley: BDR, Inc.; 2011. p. 1–21.
17. Heufelder AE, Goellner JR, Bahn RS, Gleich GJ, Hay ID. Tissue eosinophilia and eosinophil degranulation in Riedel's invasive fibrous thyroiditis. J Clin Endocrinol Metab. 1996;81(3):977–84.
18. Volpe R. Subacute and Sclerosing thyroiditis. In: De Groot LJ, editor. Endocrinology. 3rd ed. Philadelphia: WB Saunders; 1995. p. 742–51.
19. Schwaegerle SM, Bauer TW, Esselstyn CB Jr. Riedel's thyroiditis. Am J Clin Pathol. 1988;90(6):715–22.
20. Beahrs OH, McConahey WM, Woolner LB. Invasive fibrous thyroiditis (Riedel's struma). J Clin Endocrinol Metab. 1957;17(2):201–20.
21. Torres-Montaner A, Beltran M, Romero de la Osa A, Oliva H. Sarcoma of the thyroid region mimicking Riedel's thyroiditis. J Clin Pathol. 2001;54(7):570–2.
22. Wan SK, Chan JK, Tang SK. Paucicellular variant of anaplastic thyroid carcinoma. A mimic of Reidel's thyroiditis. Am J Clin Pathol. 1996;105(4):388–93.
23. Katsikas D, Shorthouse AJ, Taylor S. Riedel's thyroiditis. Br J Surg. 1976;63(12):929–31.
24. LiVolsi VA, LoGerfo P, editors. Thyroiditis. Boca Raton: CRC Press; 1981.

25. Cho MH, Kim CS, Park JS, Kang ES, Ahn CW, Cha BS, et al. Riedel's thyroiditis in a patient with recurrent subacute thyroiditis: a case report and review of the literature. Endocr J. 2007;54(4):559–62.
26. Pirola I, Morassi ML, Braga M, De Martino E, Gandossi E, Cappelli C. A case of concurrent Riedel's, Hashimoto's and acute Suppurative thyroiditis. Case Rep Med. 2009;2009:535974.
27. McIver B, Fatourechi MM, Hay ID, Fatourechi V. Graves' disease after unilateral Riedel's thyroiditis. J Clin Endocrinol Metab. 2010;95(6):2525–6.
28. Kojima M, Nakamura S, Yamane Y, Shimizu K, Sugiharal S, Masawa N. Riedel's thyroiditis containing cytologically atypically appearing B-cells: a case report. Pathol Res Pract. 2003;199(7):497–501.
29. Chen K, Wei Y, Sharp GC, Braley-Mullen H. Characterization of thyroid fibrosis in a murine model of granulomatous experimental autoimmune thyroiditis. J Leukoc Biol. 2000;68(6):828–35.
30. Li Y, Bai Y, Liu Z, Ozaki T, Taniguchi E, Mori I, Nagayama K, Nakamura H, Kakudo K. Immunohistochemistry of IgG4 can help subclassify Hashimoto's autoimmune thyroiditis. Pathol Int. 2009;59(9):636–41.
31. Neild GH, Rodriguez-Justo M, Wall C, Connolly JO. Hyper-IgG4 disease: report and characterisation of a new disease. BMC Med. 2006;4:23.
32. Dahlgren M, Khosroshahi A, Nielsen GP, Deshpande V, Stone JH. Riedel's thyroiditis and multifocal fibrosclerosis are part of the IgG4-related systemic disease spectrum. Arthritis Care Res (Hoboken). 2010;62(9):1312–8.
33. Yamamoto M, Takahashi H, Shinomura Y. IgG4-related systemic disease/systemic IgG4-related disease. Rinsho Byori. 2010;58(5):454–65.
34. Sarles H, Sarles JC, Muratore R, Guien C. Chronic inflammatory sclerosis of the pancreas—an autonomous pancreatic disease? Am J Dig Dis. 1961;6:688–98.
35. Hamano H, Kawa S, Horiuchi A, Unno H, Furuya N, Akamatsu T, et al. High serum IgG4 concentrations in patients with sclerosing pancreatitis. N Engl J Med. 2001;344(10):732–8.
36. Umehara H, Okazaki K, Masaki Y, Kawano M, Yamamoto M, Saeki T, et al. Comprehensive diagnostic criteria for IgG4-related disease (IgG4-RD). Mod Rheumatol. 2012;22(1):21–30.
37. Umehara H, Okazaki K, Masaki Y, Kawano M, Yamamoto M, Saeki T, et al. A novel clinical entity, IgG4-related disease (IgG4RD): general concept and details. Mod Rheumatol. 2012;22(1):1–14.
38. Palazzo E, Palazzo C, Palazzo M. IgG4-related disease. Joint Bone Spine. 2014;81(1):27–31.
39. Dutta D, Ahuja A, Selvan C. Immunoglobulin G4 related thyroid disorders: diagnostic challenges and clinical outcomes. Endokrynol Pol. 2016;67(5):520–4.
40. Stan MN, Sonawane V, Sebo TJ, Thapa P, Bahn RS. Riedel's thyroiditis association with IgG4-related disease. Clin Endocrinol. 2017;86(3):425–30.
41. Deshpande V, Zen Y, Chan JK, Yi EE, Sato Y, Yoshino T, et al. Consensus statement on the pathology of IgG4-related disease. Mod Pathol. 2012;25(9):1181–92.
42. Takeshima K, Inaba H, Ariyasu H, Furukawa Y, Doi A, Nishi M, et al. Clinicopathological features of Riedel's thyroiditis associated with IgG4-related disease in Japan. Endocr J. 2015;62(8):725–31.
43. Pusztaszeri M, Triponez F, Pache JC, Bongiovanni M. Riedel's thyroiditis with increased IgG4 plasma cells: evidence for an underlying IgG4-related sclerosing disease? Thyroid. 2012;22(9):964–8.
44. Soh SB, Pham A, O'Hehir RE, Cherk M, Topliss DJ. Novel use of rituximab in a case of Riedel's thyroiditis refractory to glucocorticoids and tamoxifen. J Clin Endocrinol Metab. 2013;98(9):3543–9.
45. Sakai Y, Imamura Y. Case report: IgG4-related mass-forming thyroiditis accompanied by regional lymphadenopathy. Diagn Pathol. 2018;13(1):3.
46. Oriot P, Amraoui A, Rousseau E, Malvaux P, Dechambre S, Delcourt A. Fibrosis of the thyroid gland caused by an IgG4-related sclerosing disease: three years of follow-up. Acta Clin Belg. 2014;69(6):446–50.

47. Ghys C, Depierreux M, Ozalp E, Velkeniers B. Cervical lymph nodes, thyroiditis and ophthalmopathy: the pleomorphic face of an immunoglobulin g4-related disease. Eur Thyroid J. 2014;3(4):252–7.
48. Falhammar H, Juhlin CC, Barner C, Catrina SB, Karefylakis C, Calissendorff J. Riedel's thyroiditis: clinical presentation, treatment and outcomes. Endocrine. 2018;60(1):185–92.
49. Lu L, Gu F, Dai WX, Li WY, Chen J, Xiao Y, et al. Clinical and pathological features of Riedel's thyroiditis. Chin Med Sci J. 2010;25(3):129–34.
50. Annaert M, Thijs M, Sciot R, Decallonne B. Riedel's thyroiditis occurring in a multinodular goiter, mimicking thyroid cancer. J Clin Endocrinol Metab. 2007;92(6):2005–6.
51. Vigouroux C, Escourolle H, Mosnier-Pudar H, Thomopoulos P, Louvel A, Chapuis Y, et al. Riedel's thyroiditis and lymphoma. Diagnostic difficulties. Presse Med. 1996;25(1):28–30.
52. Sheu SY, Schmid KW. Inflammatory diseases of the thyroid gland. Epidemiology, symptoms and morphology. Pathologe. 2003;24(5):339–47.
53. Ozgur T, Gokce H, Ustun I, Yaldiz M, Akin MM, Gokce C. A case of asymptomatic riedel thyroiditis with follicular adenoma in a patient with a multinodular goiter: an unusual association. Eur Thyroid J. 2012;1(3):204–7.
54. Shahi N, Abdelhamid MF, Jindall M, Awad RW. Riedel's thyroiditis masquerading as anaplastic thyroid carcinoma: a case report. J Med Case Rep. 2010;4:15.
55. Kumar SS, Fraser S, Scarsbrook A, Maclennan K, Lansdown M, Murray RD. Atypical presentation of Riedel's thyroiditis: multifocal nodular fibrosis and resolution with Levothyroxine. Eur Thyroid J. 2012;1(4):259–63.
56. Best TB, Munro RE, Burwell S, Volpe R. Riedel's thyroiditis associated with Hashimoto's thyroiditis, hypoparathyroidism, and retroperitoneal fibrosis. J Endocrinol Investig. 1991;14(9):767–72.
57. Chopra D, Wool MS, Crosson A, Sawin CT. Riedel's struma associated with subacute thyroiditis, hypothyroidism, and hypoparathyroidism. J Clin Endocrinol Metab. 1978;46(6):869–71.
58. Marin F, Araujo R, Paramo C, Lucas T, Salto L. Riedel's thyroiditis associated with hypothyroidism and hypoparathyroidism. Postgrad Med J. 1989;65(764):381–3.
59. Yasmeen T, Khan S, Patel SG, Reeves WA, Gonsch FA, de Bustros A, et al. Clinical case seminar: Riedel's thyroiditis: report of a case complicated by spontaneous hypoparathyroidism, recurrent laryngeal nerve injury, and Horner's syndrome. J Clin Endocrinol Metab. 2002;87(8):3543–7.
60. Nazal EM, Belmatoug N, de Roquancourt A, Lefort A, Fantin B. Hypoparathyroidism preceding Riedel's thyroiditis. Eur J Intern Med. 2003;14(3):202–4.
61. Stan MN, Haglind EG, Drake MT. Early hypoparathyroidism reversibility with treatment of Riedel's thyroiditis. Thyroid. 2015;25(9):1055–9.
62. Heufelder AE, Hay ID. Further evidence for autoimmune mechanisms in the pathogenesis of Riedel's invasive fibrous thyroiditis. J Intern Med. 1995;238(1):85–6.
63. Heufelder AE, Bahn RS. Modulation of Graves' orbital fibroblast proliferation by cytokines and glucocorticoid receptor agonists. Invest Ophthalmol Vis Sci. 1994;35(1):120–7.
64. Khan MA, Hashmi SM, Prinsley PR, Premachandra DJ. Reidel's thyroiditis and Tolosa-Hunt syndrome, a rare association. J Laryngol Otol. 2004;118(2):159–61.
65. Meijer S, Hoitsma HF, Scholtmeijer R. Idiopathic retroperitoneal fibrosis in multifocal fibrosclerosis. Eur Urol. 1976;2(5):258–60.
66. Meyer S, Hausman R. Occlusive phlebitis in multifocal fibrosclerosis. Am J Clin Pathol. 1976;65(3):274–83.
67. Geissler B, Wagner T, Dorn R, Lindemann F. Extensive sterile abscess in an invasive fibrous thyroiditis (Riedel's thyroiditis) caused by an occlusive vasculitis. J Endocrinol Investig. 2001;24(2):111–5.
68. Vaidya B, Coulthard A, Goonetilleke A, Burn DJ, James RA, Kendall-Taylor P. Cerebral venous sinus thrombosis: a late sequel of invasive fibrous thyroiditis. Thyroid. 1998;8(9):787–90.
69. Natt N, Heufelder AE, Hay ID, Grant CS, Goellner JR. Extracervical fibrosclerosis causing obstruction of a ventriculo-peritoneal shunt in a patient with hydrocephalus and invasive fibrous thyroiditis (Riedel's struma). Clin Endocrinol. 1997;47(1):107–11.

70. Egsgaard Nielsen V, Hecht P, Krogdahl AS, Andersen PB, Hegedus L. A rare case of orbital involvement in Riedel's thyroiditis. J Endocrinol Investig. 2003;26(10):1032–6.
71. Hines RC, Scheuermann HA, Royster HP, Rose E. Invasive fibrous (Riedel's) thyroiditis with bilateral fibrous parotitis. JAMA. 1970;213(5):869–71.
72. Rao CR, Ferguson GC, Kyle VN. Retroperitoneal fibrosis associated with Riedel's struma. Can Med Assoc J. 1973;108(8):1019–21.
73. Julie C, Vieillefond A, Desligneres S, Schaison G, Grunfeld JP, Franc B. Hashimoto's thyroiditis associated with Riedel's thyroiditis and retroperitoneal fibrosis. Pathol Res Pract. 1997;193(8):573–7.
74. Brihaye B, Lidove O, Sacre K, Laissy JP, Escoubet B, Valla D, et al. Diffuse periarterial involvement in systemic fibrosclerosis with Riedel's thyroiditis, sclerosing cholangitis, and retroperitoneal fibrosis. Scand J Rheumatol. 2008;37(6):490–2.
75. Owen K, Lane H, Jones MK. Multifocal fibrosclerosis: a case of thyroiditis and bilateral lacrimal gland involvement. Thyroid. 2001;11(12):1187–90.
76. Hamed G, Tsushima K, Yasuo M, Kubo K, Yamazaki S, Kawa S, et al. Inflammatory lesions of the lung, submandibular gland, bile duct and prostate in a patient with IgG4-associated multifocal systemic fibrosclerosis. Respirology. 2007;12(3):455–7.
77. Cooper DS, Doherty GM, Haugen BR, Kloos RT, Lee SL, Mandel SJ, et al. Revised American Thyroid Association management guidelines for patients with thyroid nodules and differentiated thyroid cancer. Thyroid. 2009;19(11):1167–214.
78. Fukata S, Miyauchi A, Kuma K, Sugawara M. Acute suppurative thyroiditis caused by an infected piriform sinus fistula with thyrotoxicosis. Thyroid. 2002;12(2):175–8.
79. Ozgen A, Cila A. Riedel's thyroiditis in multifocal fibrosclerosis: CT and MR imaging findings. AJNR Am J Neuroradiol. 2000;21(2):320–1.
80. Papi G, Corrado S, Cesinaro AM, Novelli L, Smerieri A, Carapezzi C. Riedel's thyroiditis: clinical, pathological and imaging features. Int J Clin Pract. 2002;56(1):65–7.
81. Slman R, Monpeyssen H, Desarnaud S, Haroche J, Fediaevsky LD, Fabrice M, et al. Ultrasound, elastography, and fluorodeoxyglucose positron emission tomography/computed tomography imaging in Riedel's thyroiditis: report of two cases. Thyroid. 2011;21(7):799–804.
82. Perez Fontan PJ, Cordido Carbillido F, Pompo Felipe F, Mosquera Oses J, Villalba MC. Riedel thyroiditis: US, CT, and MR evaluation. J Comput Assist Tomogr. 1993;17(2):324–5.
83. Lo JC, Loh KC, Rubin AL, Cha I, Greenspan FS. Riedel's thyroiditis presenting with hypothyroidism and hypoparathyroidism: dramatic response to glucocorticoid and thyroxine therapy. Clin Endocrinol. 1998;48(6):815–8.
84. Takahashi N, Okamoto K, Sakai K, Kawana M, Shimada-Hiratsuka M. MR findings with dynamic evaluation in Riedel's thyroiditis. Clin Imaging. 2002;26(2):89–91.
85. Drieskens O, Blockmans D, Van den Bruel A, Mortelmans L. Riedel's thyroiditis and retroperitoneal fibrosis in multifocal fibrosclerosis: positron emission tomographic findings. Clin Nucl Med. 2002;27(6):413–5.
86. Kotilainen P, Airas L, Kojo T, Kurki T, Kataja K, Minn H, et al. Positron emission tomography as an aid in the diagnosis and follow-up of Riedel's thyroiditis. Eur J Intern Med. 2004;15(3):186–9.
87. Yung G, Kannangara K, Bui C, Mansberg R, Champion B. Riedel thyroiditis demonstrated on gallium scintigraphy. Clin Nucl Med. 2010;35(8):614–7.
88. Harigopal M, Sahoo S, Recant WM, DeMay RM. Fine-needle aspiration of Riedel's disease: report of a case and review of the literature. Diagn Cytopathol. 2004;30(3):193–7.
89. Iacconi P, Giusti L, Da Valle Y, Ciregia F, Giannaccini G, Torregrossa L, et al. Proteomic approach used in the diagnosis of Riedel's thyroiditis: a case report. J Med Case Rep. 2012;6:103.
90. Moulik PK, Al-Jafari MS, Khaleeli AA. Steroid responsiveness in a case of Riedel's thyroiditis and retroperitoneal fibrosis. Int J Clin Pract. 2004;58(3):312–5.
91. Papi G, LiVolsi VA. Current concepts on Riedel thyroiditis. Am J Clin Pathol. 2004;121(Suppl):S50–63.

92. Yu Y, Liu J, Yu N, Zhang Y, Zhang S, Li T, et al. IgG4 immunohistochemistry in Riedel's thyroiditis and the recommended criteria for diagnosis: a case series and literature review. Clin Endocrinol. 2021;94(5):851–7.
93. Pearce EN, Farwell AP, Braverman LE. Thyroiditis. N Engl J Med. 2003;348(26):2646–55.
94. Jung K-Y. Surgical treatment for Riedel's thyroiditis: a case report. Int J Thyroidol. 2017;10(1):66–9.
95. Vaidya B, Harris PE, Barrett P, Kendall-Taylor P. Corticosteroid therapy in Riedel's thyroiditis. Postgrad Med J. 1997;73(866):817–9.
96. Tutuncu NB, Erbas T, Bayraktar M, Gedik O. Multifocal idiopathic fibrosclerosis manifesting with Riedel's thyroiditis. Endocr Pract. 2000;6(6):447–9.
97. Hostalet F, Hellin D, Ruiz JA. Tumefactive fibroinflammatory lesion of the head and neck treated with steroids: a case report. Eur Arch Otorrinolaringol. 2003;260(4):229–31.
98. Bagnasco M, Passalacqua G, Pronzato C, Albano M, Torre G, Scordamaglia A. Fibrous invasive (Riedel's) thyroiditis with critical response to steroid treatment. J Endocrinol Investig. 1995;18(4):305–7.
99. Thomson JA, Jackson IM, Duguid WP. The effect of steroid therapy on Riedel's thyroiditis. Scott Med J. 1968;13(1):13–6.
100. Rodriguez I, Ayala E, Caballero C, De Miguel C, Matias-Guiu X, Cubilla AL, Rosai J. Solitary fibrous tumor of the thyroid gland: report of seven cases. Am J Surg Pathol. 2001;25(11):1424–8.
101. Few J, Thompson NW, Angelos P, Simeone D, Giordano T, Reeve T. Riedel's thyroiditis: treatment with tamoxifen. Surgery. 1996;120(6):993–8.
102. Levy JM, Hasney CP, Friedlander PL, Kandil E, Occhipinti EA, Kahn MJ. Combined mycophenolate mofetil and prednisone therapy in tamoxifen- and prednisone-resistant Reidel's thyroiditis. Thyroid. 2010;20(1):105–7.
103. Parida PK, Gopalakrishnan S, Saxena SK. Pediatric recurrent acute suppurative thyroiditis of third branchial arch origin—our experience in 17 cases. Int J Pediatr Otorhinolaryngol. 2014;78(11):1953–7.
104. Nieuwland Y, Tan KY, Elte JW. Miliary tuberculosis presenting with thyrotoxicosis. Postgrad Med J. 1992;68(802):677–9.
105. De M, Jaap A, Dempster J. Tamoxifen therapy in steroid-resistant Riedels disease. Scott Med J. 2002;47(1):12–3.
106. Dabelic N, Jukic T, Labar Z, Novosel SA, Matesa N, Kusic Z. Riedel's thyroiditis treated with tamoxifen. Croat Med J. 2003;44(2):239–41.
107. Erdogan MF, Anil C, Turkcapar N, Ozkaramanli D, Sak SD, Erdogan G. A case of Riedel's thyroiditis with pleural and pericardial effusions. Endocrine. 2009;35(3):297–301.
108. Jung YJ, Schaub CR, Rhodes R, Rich FA, Muehlenbein SJ. A case of Riedel's thyroiditis treated with tamoxifen: another successful outcome. Endocr Pract. 2004;10(6):483–6.
109. Clark CP, Vanderpool D, Preskitt JT. The response of retroperitoneal fibrosis to tamoxifen. Surgery. 1991;109(4):502–6.
110. Pritchyk K, Newkirk K, Garlich P, Deeb Z. Tamoxifen therapy for Riedel's thyroiditis. Laryngoscope. 2004;114(10):1758–60.
111. Butta A, MacLennan K, Flanders KC, Sacks NP, Smith I, McKinna A, et al. Induction of transforming growth factor beta 1 in human breast cancer in vivo following tamoxifen treatment. Cancer Res. 1992;52(15):4261–4.
112. Colletta AA, Wakefield LM, Howell FV, van Roozendaal KE, Danielpour D, Ebbs SR, et al. Anti-oestrogens induce the secretion of active transforming growth factor beta from human fetal fibroblasts. Br J Cancer. 1990;62(3):405–9.
113. Arteaga CL, Tandon AK, Von Hoff DD, Osborne CK. Transforming growth factor beta: potential autocrine growth inhibitor of estrogen receptor-negative human breast cancer cells. Cancer Res. 1988;48(14):3898–904.

114. Falhammar H, Juhlin C, Barner C, Catrina S, Karefylakis C, Calissendorff J. Riedel's thyroiditis: clinical presentation, treatment and outcomes. Endocrine. 2018;60(1):185–92.
115. Hunt L, Harrison B, Bull M, Stephenson T, Allahabadia A. Rituximab: a novel treatment for refractory Riedel's thyroiditis. Endocrinol Diabetes Metab Case Rep. 2018:2018, 17-0132.

Chronic Thyroiditis: Hashimoto's Disease 9

9.1 Overview

Hashimoto's thyroiditis, also known as chronic lymphocytic thyroiditis and struma lymphomatosa, is part of the spectrum of autoimmune thyroid diseases (AITDs), which also include the following variants: atrophic thyroiditis, juvenile thyroiditis, postpartum thyroiditis (PPT), silent thyroiditis, and focal thyroiditis [1].

Hashimoto's disease (or Hashimoto's thyroiditis) is characterized by painless, diffuse enlargement of the thyroid gland occurring predominantly in middle-aged women. The patients are often euthyroid, but hypothyroidism may eventually develop. The thyroid parenchyma is diffusely replaced by a lymphocytic infiltrate and fibrotic reaction. Patients with Hashimoto's thyroiditis have serum antibodies reacting with thyroglobulin (Tg), thyroid peroxidase (TPO), and against an unidentified protein present in colloid leading to destruction of thyroid cells. The increasing use of needle biopsy and serologic tests for antibodies has led to much more frequent recognition of this disease, which is currently the most common cause of hypothyroidism in the United States after age 6 years.

A patient with a small goiter and euthyroidism does not require therapy unless the TSH level is elevated. The presence of a large gland, progressive growth of the goiter, or hypothyroidism indicates the need for replacement thyroid hormone. Surgery is rarely indicated. Development of lymphoma, though very unusual, must be considered if there is growth or pain in the involved gland. With early diagnosis, proper L-T4 replacement therapy, regular patient follow-up care, and attention to early detection and management of complications, the prognosis in Hashimoto's thyroiditis is excellent, with patients leading a normal life. This chapter addresses a wide range of topics related to Hashimoto's disease, including epidemiology, pathology, etiology, pathogenesis, clinical manifestations, diagnosis and differential diagnosis, association with papillary thyroid carcinoma, management, and prognosis.

M. Sakr, *Thyroiditis*, https://doi.org/10.1007/978-3-032-19513-5_9

9.2 Historical Review

By strict criteria, Hashimoto's thyroiditis is a histological diagnosis first described by the Japanese surgeon *Hakaru Hashimoto*, who was born on May 5, 1881, in the village of Midai, Nishitsuge, in Mie Prefecture, Japan. He graduated from Kyushu University Medical School in 1907. Hakaru Hashimoto also studied in England, but with the outbreak of World War I, he was forced to return home to Japan. The year 2013 marked the centennial anniversary of his original description of "struma lymphomatosa" (his observation of unique histological features, including lymphocytic infiltration, eosinophilic change to follicular cells, and interstitial fibrosis that were described in four women with goiters that were treated with thyroidectomy) [1]. His work was published in a German journal in 1912 and went unnoticed for over 40 years. At the time of his original description, Hashimoto realized that some stimulus was responsible for the reactive changes he noticed, but he admitted that he did not know the nature of that stimulus. Due to his sudden death on January 9, 1934 (at the age of 52) because of typhoid fever, he was never able to witness the impact of his discovery.

It was not until 1956 that a link between antibodies to thyroid cells present in the serum of patients and Hashimoto's disease was made. The thyroid gland was the first organ in which an immune etiology to a specific disease process (Hashimoto's thyroiditis) was described. Over time, our understanding of the immunological pathways involved in Hashimoto's thyroiditis has evolved. We now recognize the association of this disease with other autoimmune diseases and thyroid cancer [2].

The disease has been called Hashimoto's thyroiditis, chronic thyroiditis, lymphocytic thyroiditis, lymphadenoid goiter, and recently, autoimmune thyroiditis. Classically, it presents as a painless, diffuse enlargement of the thyroid gland in a young or middle-aged woman. It is often associated with hypothyroidism.

In 1956, Rose and Witebsky [3] showed that immunization of rabbits with extracts of rabbit thyroids produced histological changes in the thyroid glands resembling those seen in Hashimoto's thyroiditis. They also found anti-thyroglobulin antibodies in the blood of the animals. Subsequently, Roitt et al. (1956) [4] observed that a precipitate formed when an extract of human thyroid gland was added to serum from a patient with Hashimoto's thyroiditis. Thus, it appeared that the serum contained antibodies to a constituent of the human thyroid and that these antibodies might be responsible for the disease process. These original observations led directly to entirely new concepts of the causation of disease by auto-immunization.

Hakaru Hashimoto's initial description of this disease was the necessary first step to our current-day understanding of Hashimoto's thyroiditis. His contributions to the fields of endocrinology and autoimmune disease are immense and, unfortunately, frequently under-appreciated.

9.3 Epidemiology

The most common cause of hypothyroidism worldwide is iodine deficiency. However, Hashimoto's thyroiditis, the most frequent autoimmune thyroiditis, remains the most common cause of spontaneous hypothyroidism in areas of adequate iodine intake, such as North America [5].

9.3.1 Incidence

9.3.1.1 Worldwide Incidence

The annual incidence of Hashimoto's thyroiditis observed in clinical practice worldwide is unknown, but it is roughly equal to that of Graves' disease (approximately, 0.3–1.5 cases per 1000 population per year) [6–10]. It is more common in regions of high iodine dietary intake and among people who are genetically susceptible. It is certain that Hashimoto's disease exists with a much higher frequency than is diagnosed clinically, and its frequency seems to be increasing [11].

9.3.1.2 Incidence in the United States

Hashimoto's thyroiditis is the most common cause of hypothyroidism in the United States after age 6 years, with the incidence estimated to be 1.3% in a series of 5000 children aged 11–18 years. In adults, the incidence is estimated to be 3.5 per 1000 per year in women and 0.8 per 1000 per year in men. The incidence may be as high as 6% in the Appalachian region [5].

9.3.1.3 Gender- and Age-Related Demographics

The incidence of Hashimoto's thyroiditis is estimated to be 10–20 times higher in women. The most commonly affected age range is 30–50 years, with the peak incidence in men occurring 10–15 years later, but it may be seen in any age group, including children. In general, the overall incidence of hypothyroidism increases with age in men and women [5].

9.3.2 Prevalence

9.3.2.1 Prevalence of Hashimoto's Disease

The prevalence of Hashimoto's thyroiditis is 4.5% (4.2% subclinical and 0.3% clinical hypothyroidism) based on biochemical analysis, but with cytological diagnosis, the prevalence increases to 13.4% [11]. The prevalence of hypothyroidism and of thyroid disease in general increases with *age*.

Hashimoto's thyroiditis appears to occur in more than 10% of patients presenting with a thyroid nodule. It is associated with other autoimmune disorders such as Addison's disease, diabetes mellitus type-1, rheumatoid arthritis, systemic lupus erythematosus (SLE), or vitiligo. The occurrence of papillary thyroid carcinoma (PTC) in Hashimoto's thyroiditis has been extensively studied, and the association ranges from 0.5 to 30% of cases [11].

9.3.2.2 Prevalence of Thyroid Antibodies

For several decades, a strong genetic predisposition to autoimmune thyroid disease has been recognized, predominantly on the basis of family and twin studies. Many of these persons have thyroglobulin (Tg) and thyroid peroxidase (TPO) antibodies, and most are entirely asymptomatic. Soon after the discovery of thyroid antibodies (T-Abs), Hall and Stanbury reported, in 1967, the presence of T-Abs in 56% of siblings of patients with autoimmune thyroid disease (AITD) [12]. In 1975, Inoue et al. [13] reported that 3% of Japanese children aged 6–18 years have thyroiditis.

This familial clustering of AITD and the presence of T-Abs in up to 60% of first-degree relatives of patients has been later confirmed by many authors [14–18]. When both parents were affected, the prevalence of TPO-Abs and Tg-Abs was 42% in daughters and 33% in sons, compared with 28.9% and 16.7%, respectively, when only one parent was positive for T-Abs [15]. In the National Health and Nutrition Examination Survey (NHANES) III (2003), the prevalence of T-Abs was 18% regardless of age and gender. Moreover, the calculated sibling risk ratio for Hashimoto's thyroiditis was 28, thus confirming the highly significant contribution of genetic factors to the disease development [19]. The prevalence of T-Abs is twice more common in women than in men and higher in whites and Asians than in Blacks or Mexicans. A more recent German study (2011) also indicated a 32-fold increase in risk for developing Hashimoto's thyroiditis in children and 21-fold increased risk in siblings of patients with Hashimoto's thyroiditis, with females being significantly more often affected than males [20].

Several epidemiological studies showed that women present with positive T-Abs up to three times more often than men [21–28]. According to the study of Danish twins, by Hansen et al. (2006) [29], the genetic contribution to TPO-Ab and Tg-Ab susceptibility in females was 72% and 75%, respectively, while in males it was only 61% and 39%, respectively.

A number of small datasets have suggested a potential role for *skewed X-chromosome activation (XCI)*, away from the expected 50:50 parent of origin ratio, as an explanation for the strong female preponderance seen in the common autoimmune thyroid diseases, Graves' disease, and Hashimoto's thyroiditis [28].

A possible role for fetal cell micro-chimerism in triggering an autoimmune process has been repeatedly proposed, based on the evidence that autoimmune diseases have a higher prevalence in females, with peak incidence in women of child-bearing age. Fetal micro-chimeric cells have been found to be significantly more represented within the thyroid gland of women with Hashimoto's thyroiditis and Graves' disease compared to those without thyroid autoimmunity, suggesting a pathogenic role [30–32].

9.4 Pathology

9.4.1 Gross Appearance

In Hashimoto's thyroiditis, the enlarged thyroid gland is generally diffuse and symmetrical, often with a conspicuous pyramidal lobe, a characteristic feature. Consistency is rubbery firm, but not stony hard as in Riedel's thyroiditis. There is no extension of the process outside the gland. The capsule is intact, and the capsular surface is gently lobulated and generally non-adherent to surrounding tissues. Although it may have adhesions, the thyroid gland is easily separated from other structures. The cut surface is distinctly nodular. There is no necrosis or calcification. The tissue involved by Hashimoto's thyroiditis is pinkish-tan to frankly yellowish (Fig. 9.1) in color.

9.4.2 Microscopic Picture

In Hashimoto's thyroiditis, there is a diffuse process consisting of a combination of epithelial cell destruction, lymphoid cellular infiltration, and fibrosis. Lymphocytes are predominantly T-cells and plasma cells (polyclonal). The thyroid cells tend to be slightly larger in size and assume an acidophilic staining character; they are then called "Hürthle, Ashkenazy, oxyphilic, or more recently, oncocytic cells" and are packed with mitochondria. The follicular spaces shrink, and colloid is absent or sparse. Fibrosis may be completely absent or present in degrees ranging from slight to moderate; it may be severe, as observed in subacute or Riedel's thyroiditis, but does not extend beyond the capsule. In contrast to subacute thyroiditis, foreign body

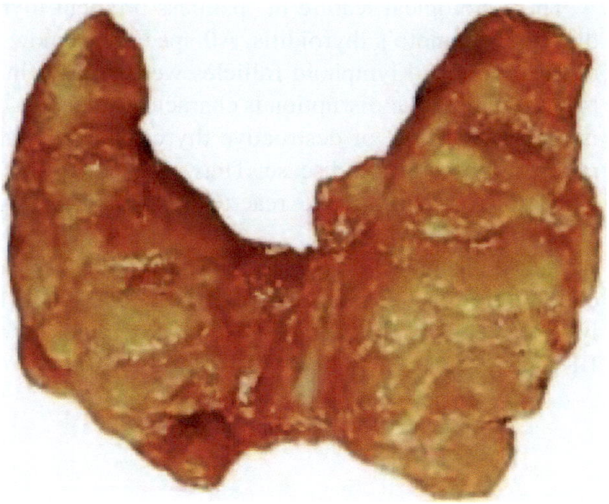

Fig. 9.1 Hashimoto's thyroiditis. Note the symmetrical enlargement of the gland and the yellowish discoloration

giant cells and granulomas are *not* features of Hashimoto's thyroiditis. In children, oxyphilia and fibrosis are less prominent, and hyperplasia of epithelial cells may be marked.

Clusters of macrophage-like cells may be seen within the follicles. The lymphoid infiltration in the interstitial tissue is accompanied by actual follicles and germinal centers [33]. Plasma B-cells are prominent and can often be seen as secondary lymphoid follicles (germinal centers, not to be confused with the normally present colloid-filled follicles that constitute the thyroid). Back in 1977, Totterman et al. [33] studied the characteristics of the lymphocytes in the thyroid and reported that they are made up of equal proportions of T- and B-cells.

Most infiltrating T-cells have α/β T-cell receptors. Gamma/delta T-cells are rare [34] although their proportion in intra-thyroidal lymphocytes is higher than that in peripheral lymphocytes [35]. CD4+/CD8+ cells and CD3lo-TCRα/β-lo/CD4-CD8- cells also are present in the infiltrate in the thyroid [35]. Infiltrating T-cells are considered to be a highly restricted population, based on the study of T-cell receptor Vα [36] and β [37] gene expression. Heuer et al. (1996) [38] studied cytokine mRNA expression in intra-thyroidal T-cells and reported increased expression of IFN-gamma, IL-2, and CD25 cytokines in Hashimoto's thyroiditis. Thyroglobulin-binding lymphocytes were increased in a percentage relative to their occurrence in blood.

The quantity of parenchymal tissue left in the thyroid is variable. In some instances, it is actually increased, perhaps as a compensatory hyperplastic response to inefficient iodide metabolism. Typically, the pathological process involves the entire lobe or gland. Focal thyroiditis, which is microscopically similar, may be found in thyroid glands with diffuse hyperplasia of Graves' disease, in association with thyroid tumors, or in multinodular thyroid glands. The thymus, which is frequently enlarged in thyroiditis as it is in Graves' disease, does not present the picture of enhanced immunological activity [39, 40].

The histological feature in "painless or silent thyroiditis" is almost similar to that of Hashimoto's thyroiditis. All specimens show chronic thyroiditis, focal or diffuse type, and lymphoid follicles were present in about half of the specimen [41]. The follicular disruption is characteristic, and a common histological feature is seen at the time of destructive thyrotoxicosis, but disappears during the late recovery phase of the disease. Thus, painless thyroiditis may be induced by the activation of autoimmune reaction within the thyroid gland in patients with Hashimoto's thyroiditis.

As seen in Table 9.1, Hashimoto's thyroiditis has been graded based on lymphocytic infiltration seen on cytology into Grades 0–III, where "Grade 0" means no lymphoid cells, Grade I is mild (Fig. 9.2), Grade II moderate (Fig. 9.3), and Grade III severe (Fig. 9.4) lymphoid cell infiltration.

Table 9.1 Grading of thyroiditis on cytological material

Grade	Morphological features	%
Grade 0	No lymphoid cell	0
Grade I (Mild)	Few lymphoid cells infiltrating the follicles/increased number of lymphocytes in the background	38.67
Grade II (Moderate)	Moderate lymphocytic infiltration or mild lymphocytic infiltration with Hürthle cell change/giant cells/anisonucleosis	44
Grade III (Severe)	Florid lymphocytic inflammation with germinal center formation, very few follicular cells left	17.33

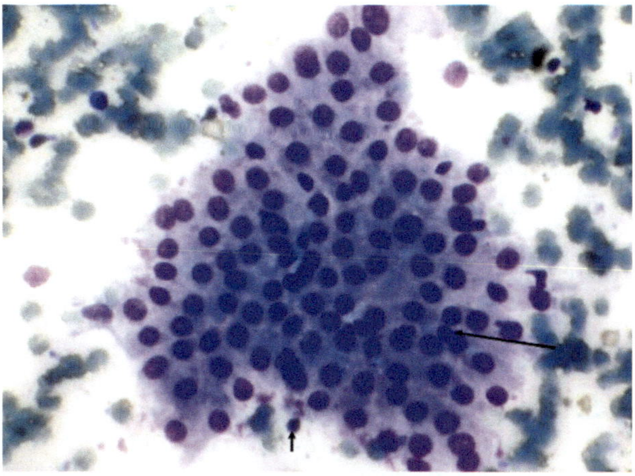

Fig. 9.2 Grade I thyroiditis with mild lymphocytic inflammatory infiltrate (arrows) (May Grünwald Giemsa)

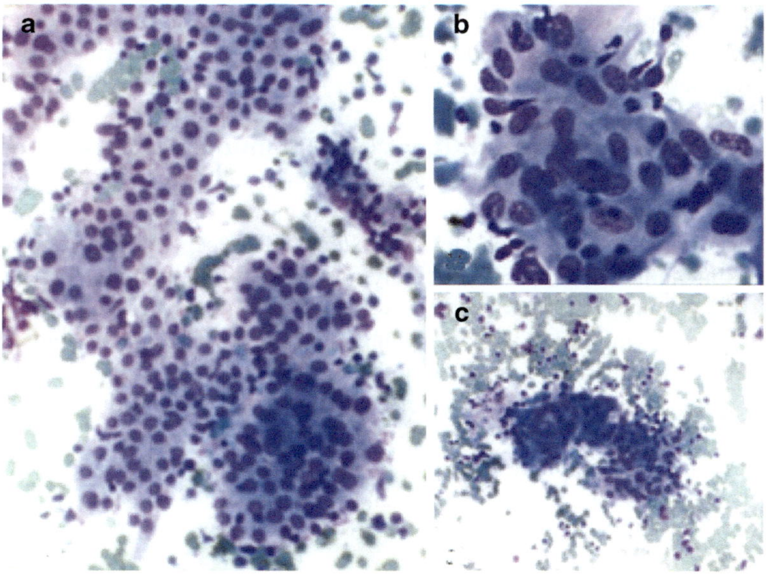

Fig. 9.3 Grade II thyroiditis with (**a**) moderate lymphocytic inflammation; (**b**) epithelioid cell granuloma; (**c**) multi-nucleated giant cell (May Grünwald Giemsa)

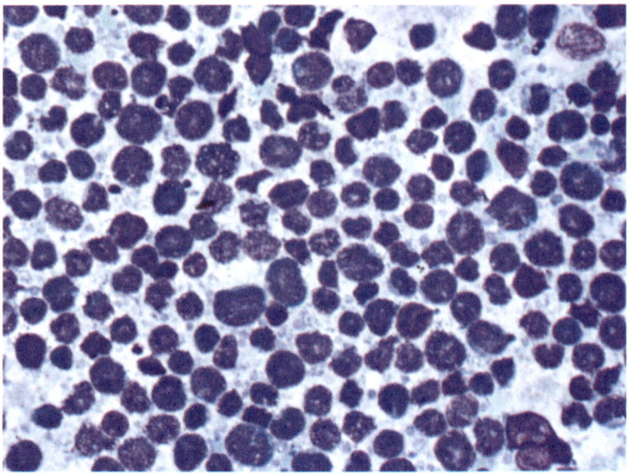

Fig. 9.4 Grade III Hashimoto's thyroiditis, marked inflammation, and germinal center formation as in a reactive node. Note polymorphic population of lymphoid cells in contrast to a lymphoma (May Grünwald Giemsa)

9.5 Etiology/Risk Factors

The etiology of Hashimoto's thyroiditis is multi-factorial, arising from interaction between genetic and non-genetic (environmental, dietary, and demographic) factors.

9.5.1 Genetic Factors

The strong genetic component is borne out in studies on *monozygotic twins*, with a concordance of 38–55%, and an even higher concordance of circulating thyroid antibodies irrespective of clinical presentation (up to 80% in monozygotic twins). Neither result was seen to a similar degree in *dizygotic twins*, offering strong favor for high genetic etiology.

9.5.1.1 Human Leukocyte Antigens (HLA)/Immune Response Genes

Hashimoto's thyroiditis is caused by a breakdown in self-tolerance to thyroid autoantigens. This is exemplified by the presence of circulating autoantibodies against Tg and TPO in most cases, and to a lesser extent, TSH receptors (thyrotropin receptor-blocking antibodies). The genetic polymorphisms of the human leukocyte antigens (HLA), mainly HLA-DR3 and HLA-DR5; T-cell immune response genes such as cytotoxic T-lymphocyte-associated antigen-4 (CTLA-4) and protein tyrosine phosphate-22 (PTPN-22); vitamin D receptor (VDR); and thyroid-specific genes play a major role in the development of Hashimoto's thyroiditis [5]. Single-nucleotide polymorphism at the thyroglobulin promoter site leads to activation of T-cell response, and polymorphism at CD-40 gene leads to proliferation of B-cells, antibody secretion, and generation of memory cells. CTLA-4 down-regulates, i.e., transmits an inhibitory signal to T-cells, so reduced functioning is associated with increased T-lymphocyte activity. Both CTLA-4 and PTPN-22 are major negative regulators of cell-mediated immunity. Thus, depletion of regulatory T-cell (Treg) leads to autoimmunity [42]. The genes implicated vary in different ethnic groups, and the incidence is increased in people with chromosomal disorders, including Turner, Down, and Klinefelter syndromes.

Patients with Hashimoto's thyroiditis have antibodies to various thyroid antigens, most frequently anti-thyroid peroxidase (anti-TPO), anti-thyroglobulin (anti-Tg), and, to a lesser extent, TSH receptor-blocking antibodies (TBII). Nevertheless, a small percentage (approximately 10%–15%) of patients with Hashimoto's thyroiditis may be serum antibody negative. Other anti-thyroid antibodies found in autoimmune thyroid disease (AITD) (including Hashimoto's thyroiditis) include thyroid-stimulating antibody and cytotoxic antibody.

9.5.1.2 The Initiating Events

The inciting events or initiating processes in Hashimoto's thyroiditis are not well understood and have not been elucidated [43–46], but possibilities include abnormalities of regulatory T-cells, or exposure of normally sequestered thyroid antigen. Induction of thyroid autoimmunity is accompanied by a progressive depletion of thyroid epithelial cells by apoptosis and replacement of thyroid parenchyma by mononuclear cell infiltration and fibrosis. Multiple immunological mechanisms may contribute to thyroid cell death, including CD8+ cytotoxic T cell-mediated cell death, cytokine-mediated cell death, and, less likely, binding of anti-thyroid antibodies followed by antibody-dependent cell-mediated toxicity.

The thyroid gland is typically "goitrous" but may be "atrophic" or "normal" in size. Thyrotropin receptor blocking antibodies binding to and blocking the thyroid-stimulating hormone (TSH) receptor thyrotropin receptor blocking antibodies (TBII) have also been described and may contribute to impairment in thyroid function. The result is inadequate thyroid hormone production and secretion, although initially, preformed T4 and T3 may "leak" into the circulation from damaged cells.

9.5.1.3 Other Autoimmune Diseases

Having *other autoimmune diseases* is a risk factor to develop Hashimoto's thyroiditis, and the opposite is also true. Hashimoto's thyroiditis has a markedly higher clustering of other autoimmune diseases, including pernicious anemia, adrenal insufficiency (Addison's disease), celiac disease, type 1-diabetes mellitus (DM), rheumatoid arthritis, Sjogren's syndrome, systemic lupus erythematosus (SLE), vitiligo, and alopecia [47, 48]. A study by Ruggeri et al. (2017) indicated that Hashimoto's thyroiditis is associated with different non-thyroidal autoimmune diseases (NTADs) at different ages. Associated NTADs were significantly more prevalent in adults than in children/adolescents in that study, and more adults than children/adolescents suffered from two or more associated NTADs, with the frequency of arthropathies and connective tissue diseases being greater in adults and the frequency of type 1 diabetes mellitus and celiac disease being higher in children/adolescents [49].

9.5.1.4 Family History

A study by Bothra et al. (2017) reported that, compared with the general population, first-degree relatives of persons with Hashimoto's thyroiditis have a ninefold greater risk of developing the disease [50].

9.5.1.5 Patient Gender

Female gender is associated with an eightfold increased risk for Hashimoto's thyroiditis than male gender; the possible mechanisms being the effects of sex hormones, X-chromosome-encoded susceptibility, skewed X-chromosome inactivation, pregnancy, and fetal micro-chimerism. Thus, a possible explanation for the high female predominance in AITD might be associated with the X-chromosome containing several sex and immune-related genes, which are important for preservation of immune tolerance [51]. The increased immuno-reactivity might be related to genetic defects of the X-chromosome, such as structural abnormalities or monosomy. Accordingly, a higher incidence of AITD was reported in patients with a higher rate of X-chromosome monosomy in peripheral white blood cells [52] or in patients with Turner's syndrome [53].

Another potential mechanism of impaired immuno-tolerance in females is "skewed X-chromosome inactivation" (XCI) leading to the escape of X-linked self-antigens from presentation in thymus with subsequent loss of T-cell tolerance. Skewed XCI was associated with a higher risk of developing AITD [54–57]. Furthermore, a study of Danish twins demonstrated a significant association of skewed XCI with TPO-Ab serum concentrations in dizygotic, but not in monozygotic twin pairs, indicating that shared genetic determinants of XCI pattern and TPO-Ab production are more likely than a causal relationship [58].

9.5.1.6 Pregnancy

The tolerance of the fetal semi-allograft during pregnancy is enabled by the state of immunosuppression, which results from hormonal changes and trophoblast expression of key immunomodulatory molecules. The pivotal players in regulation of the immune response are the regulatory T-cells (Tregs), which rapidly increase during pregnancy. Consequently, both cell-mediated and humoral immune responses are attenuated with a shift toward humoral immune response, resulting in immune tolerance of the conceptus tissues and suppression of autoimmunity [59, 60]. Accordingly, the decrease of both TPO-Ab and Tg-Ab concentrations during pregnancy has been reported, reaching the lowest values in the third trimester [61–64].

In the postpartum period, the rapid decrease of Tregs and re-establishment of the immune response to the pre-pregnancy state may cause or aggravate thyroid autoimmunity [60, 63]. The increase of TPO-Ab concentrations occurred as soon as 6 weeks after delivery, reaching the baseline level at approximately 12 weeks and the maximum level at about 20 weeks after delivery [61, 62]. In up to 50% of women with positive TPO-Abs in early pregnancy, thyroid autoimmunity, in the form of postpartum thyroiditis may occur within the first year after delivery, usually presenting clinically with transient thyrotoxicosis and/or transient hypothyroidism. In about one-third of women permanent hypothyroidism may even develop [64].

Interestingly, a significantly higher secretion of IFN-γ and IL-4 together with a lower median plasma cortisol concentration in 36th week of gestation has been reported in women with postpartum thyroiditis than in euthyroid females, indicating that weaker immunosuppression in the former group of women in late pregnancy could contribute to the postpartum thyroid dysfunction [65].

9.5.1.7 Fetal Micro-chimerism

Fetal micro-chimerism is defined by the "presence of fetal cells in maternal tissues being transferred in the maternal circulation during pregnancy." Several years after the delivery, the chimeric male cells can be detected in the maternal peripheral blood [66, 67] and in maternal tissues, such as thyroid, lung, skin, or lymph nodes [68]. The fetal immune cells, settled in the maternal thyroid gland, may become activated in the postpartum period when the immuno-tolerance ceases, representing a possible trigger that may initiate or exaggerate AITD. In Hashimoto's thyroiditis, fetal micro-chimeric cells were detected in the thyroid gland in 28% to 83% [30, 31, 69, 70], which is significantly higher than that reported in the absence of AITD. A recent study of twins supported the putative role of micro-chimerism in triggering thyroid autoimmunity, showing a significantly higher prevalence of T-Abs in opposite sex twins compared to monozygotic twins [71]. In addition, euthyroid women with previous pregnancy presented significantly more often with positive TPO-Ab as compared to women with no history of pregnancy [72]. However, the relation between parity and AITD was not confirmed by large population-based studies, advocating against the essential contribution of fetal micro-chimerism to the pathogenesis of AITD including Hashimoto's thyroiditis [73–76].

9.5.2 Non-genetic (Environmental) Factors

In genetically susceptible individuals, preventable environmental factors, including high iodine intake [77], selenium and vitamin D deficiency [78], infectious diseases, and certain drugs, have been implicated in the development of autoimmune thyroid disease (may initiate the autoimmune process). These factors may act through epigenetic modifications, like DNA methylation and histone modification at the tissue level, which is evidenced by twin studies.

9.5.2.1 Iodine Intake

More than adequate intake of I_2 induces autoimmunity by various mechanisms including (1) increasing the immunogenicity of thyroglobulin (Tg) molecules exposing cryptic epitopes that facilitate presentation by antigen presenting cell (APC) and subsequent T-cell activation, (2) release of free radicals, which induce elevated expression of intracellular adhesion molecule-1 that attracts immunocompetent cells, (3) free radicals damaging thyrocytes and exposing auto-antigens, (4) promoting follicular cell apoptosis by abnormal expression of tumor necrosis factor-related apoptosis-inducing ligand (TRAIL) and its death receptor, and (5) increased maturation of APC, B-cells and T-cells. A country-wide screening program done by All India Institute of Medical Science (AIIMS), Delhi, revealed that there is increased incidence of "juvenile autoimmune thyroiditis" including Hashimoto's thyroiditis among the goitrous young girls in the post-iodization phase in India [79].

9.5.2.2 Selenium Deficiency

There is some evidence supporting the role of selenium deficiency in the development of thyroid autoimmunity. Selenium deficiency decreases the activity of selenoproteins leading to raised concentrations of hydrogen peroxide, thus promoting inflammation and disease.

9.5.2.3 Vitamin D Deficiency

Vitamin D deficiency has recently been reported by Mazokopakis et al. (2015) [80] to have an association with the development of Hashimoto's thyroiditis. The study, which included 218 patients with Hashimoto's thyroiditis, found serum 25-hydroxy vitamin D levels to be negatively correlated with anti-TPO levels in all patients, with the anti-TPO levels being significantly greater in the 186 patients who were vitamin D deficient. After receiving oral vitamin D3 supplementation of 1200–4000 IU daily for 4 months, serum anti-TPO levels in the vitamin D-deficient patients were significantly reduced.

9.5.2.4 Drugs, Infections, and Chemicals

"Drugs" such as interferon-alpha (INF-α), lithium, and amiodarone; "infections" due to hepatitis C, Rubella, Herpes simplex virus, Epstein-Barr virus, human T-cell lympho-trophic viruses; and exposure to "chemicals" such as poly-aromatic hydrocarbons, poly-halogenated biphenyls, as well as heavy metals like mercury and lead, which can be found in body care products, amalgam fillings, as well as some water and food supplies, can also trigger autoimmune thyroid disease. There is evidence that mercury, in particular, accumulates in the thyroid gland and is one cause of autoimmune thyroid response [81].

9.5.2.5 Lipid Profile

Levels of TSH positively correlate with serum levels of total cholesterol, triglycerides, low-density lipoprotein (LDL), high-density lipoprotein (HDL), and non-HDL, as well as with the ratio of LDL to HDL. Free T4 levels, on the other hand, are negatively correlated with these lipid parameters [82].

9.5.2.6 Age of the Patient

The risk of Hashimoto's thyroiditis and development of hypothyroidism are known to increase with age of the patient. In a study of 830 patients with Hashimoto's thyroiditis, Tagami et al. (2010) [82] reported a slight, but significant increase in TSH serum levels and decrease in free T4 levels with increasing patient age.

9.5.2.7 Physical and Emotional Stress

Stress, physical or emotional, is a known risk factor of autoimmunity. Stress makes it harder for the body to heal itself and perform the necessary immune functions. Stressful situations cause changes in the adrenal system, resulting in the release of hormones stimulated by the pituitary gland: cortisol, aldosterone, and dehydroepiandrosterone. In the event of adrenal fatigue, the pituitary gland could perhaps not function properly. With the thyroid being a part of the endocrine system, understanding the link between various hormones is important to understand autoimmune thyroid disease [81].

9.6 Pathogenesis

9.6.1 Introduction

Hashimoto's thyroiditis is the most prevalent autoimmune thyroid disorder, where lymphocytic infiltration of the thyroid gland may be followed by a gradual destruction and fibrous replacement of the thyroid parenchymal tissue. The thyroid gland may or may not be enlarged. There are multiple suggested mechanisms, though not fully understood, by which the pathology of Hashimoto's thyroiditis develops.

Various autoantibodies may be present against thyroid peroxidase (TPO), thyroglobulin (Tg), and thyroid-stimulating hormone (TSH) receptors, although a small percentage of people may have none of these antibodies present. At the same time, as indicated in various twin studies, a percentage of the population may also have these antibodies without developing Hashimoto's thyroiditis. Nevertheless, antibody-dependent cell-mediated cytotoxicity is a substantial factor behind the apoptotic fall-out of Hashimoto's thyroiditis. Activation of cytotoxic T-lymphocytes (CD8+ T-cells) in response to cell-mediated immune response affected by helper T-lymphocytes (CD4+ T-cells) is central to thyrocyte destruction. As is characteristic of type IV hypersensitivity, recruitment of macrophages is another effect of the helper T-lymphocyte activation, with Thl axis lymphocytes producing certain inflammatory cytokines within the thyroid tissue for further macrophage activation and migration into the thyroid gland for direct effect.

In Hashimoto's thyroiditis, the immunological attack appears to be typically aggressive and destructive, rather than stimulatory as in Graves' disease, and the difference is most likely due to the characteristics of the immune response. Hashimoto's thyroiditis is reported to occur in two varieties: an "atrophic" variety, perhaps associated with human leukocytic antigen-DR3 (HLA-DR3) gene inheritance, and a "goitrous" form associated with HLA-DR5 [83].

Many of the genes associated with autoimmune thyroid disease (AITD) are also associated with other autoimmune diseases, which highlights a key role for disrupted T-cell central tolerance, antigen monitoring, and peripheral immune tolerance in autoimmune onset. In studies of autoimmune hypothyroidism in monozygotic twins, the concordance rate is below 1 and thus, environmental factors are also etiologically important [84].

9.6.2 Susceptibility Genes

9.6.2.1 Human Leukocyte Antigen (HLA) Genes

The first gene locus identified in association with autoimmune thyroid disease (AITD) was major histocompatibility complex (MHC) region on *chromosome 6p21*, which encodes human leukocyte antigens (HLAs). The HLA region, which is highly polymorphic, comprises several immune response genes. The HLA molecule, located on antigen-presenting cells (APCs), binds and presents an antigenic peptide, enabling T-cell recognition and response to an antigen. Presumably, specific HLA alleles have a higher affinity for auto-antigenic thyroidal peptides and are thus likely to contribute to the development of the AITD. However, in order to initiate thyroid autoimmunity, auto-antigen occurrence within the thyroid gland or its draining lymph nodes is needed, followed by HLA presentation. In Hashimoto's thyroiditis, aberrant expression of HLA class II molecules on thyrocytes has been demonstrated. Presumably, such thyrocytes may act as APCs capable of presenting the thyroid auto-antigens and initiating AITD [85].

While in Graves' disease HLA-DR3 was reported by several studies as the primary susceptibility allele, no consistent associations were observed in Hashimoto's thyroiditis. The large United Kingdom Caucasian Hashimoto's Thyroiditis Case Control Cohort Study demonstrated clear differences in association within the HLA class II region between Hashimoto's thyroiditis and Graves' disease. Differences in HLA class II genotype may, in part, contribute to the different immuno-pathological processes and clinical presentation of these related diseases [83]. The MHC class-II molecules expressed on the thyroid follicles of patients with Hashimoto's thyroiditis are induced by viral infections or inflammatory cytokines. They act as non-professional APCs and present themselves as foreign antigens, initiating an autoimmune response. The activated T-helper cell stimulates B-cells and plasma cells to produce anti-thyroid antibodies. Interferon-gamma (INF-γ), tumor necrosis factor-alpha (TNF-α), and interleukin-1 (IL-1) produced by Th1 cells activate macrophages that destroy thyroid follicles.

In Caucasians, different forms of Hashimoto's thyroiditis were reported to be associated with various HLA alleles, including DR3, DR5, DQ7, *DQB1*03* [86], *DQw7* [87], or DRB1*04-DQB1*0301 Haplo-type [88]. In Japanese patients, associations with *DRB4*0101*, *HLA-A2* [89] and *DRw53* [90] were shown, while in Chinese patients, association with *DRw9* was observed [91].

9.6.2.2 Cytotoxic T-Lymphocyte Antigen-4 (CTLA-4) Gene

Cytotoxic T-cell antigen-4 (CTLA-4) gene locus, which lies on *chromosome 2q33*, was reported by Jacobson et al. (2007) to be associated with various autoimmune diseases, including type-1 diabetes mellitus (T1-DM), myasthenia gravis, systemic lupus erythematosus (SLE), systemic sclerosis, Graves' disease, and Hashimoto's thyroiditis [92].

CTLA-4 is the second major negative regulator of T-cell-mediated immune functions. Its expression on the surface of T-cells, induced by the activation of the T-cell receptor, results in suppression of T-cell activation. CTLA-4 gene polymorphisms may reduce expression or function of the CTLA-4 antigen and may therefore contribute to the reduced inhibition of T-cell proliferation and subsequently increase susceptibility to an autoimmune response. Studies on several polymorphisms of the CTLA-4 gene in patients with Hashimoto's thyroiditis showed that (AT)n microsatellite CTLA-4 polymorphism in the 3′-untranslated region (UTR) was associated with Hashimoto's thyroiditis in the Caucasian [93] and in Japanese patients [94], but *not* in the Italian population [88]. In the exon 1 located 49A/G single-nucleotide polymorphism (SNP), resulting in threonine to alanine substitution, was reported by several authors to be associated with Hashimoto's thyroiditis [95–97]; however, this observation was *not* confirmed by several other studies [88, 98–100]. A large meta-analysis of 866 patients with Hashimoto's thyroiditis showed a significant association with 49A/G [101]. The initial observations of the association with Hashimoto's thyroiditis [102, 103] were *not* confirmed by later studies [100, 104]; however, the results of the meta-analysis indicated a significant association with CT60 SNP [101]. Nevertheless, further studies are still needed to determine which CTLA-4 polymorphism is causative.

Apart from being associated with Hashimoto's thyroiditis, CTLA-4 seems to be the major thyroid antibody (T-Ab) susceptibility gene. In 2001, Tomer and colleagues demonstrated a link of the CTLA-4 region to the presence of T-Abs by a whole genome linkage analysis [105]. Later, CTLA-4 was confirmed as a main locus for T-Ab status by other researchers [106, 107]. In 2011, the studies by Zaletel and Gaberscek [108] of Slovenian Hashimoto's thyroiditis patients indicated a strong association between T-Ab production and the three CTLA-4 SNPs, including -318C/T in the promoter, 49A/G, and CT60. In patients carrying one of those three SNPs, evidently higher TPO-Ab concentrations were demonstrated in relation to the polymorphous CTLA-4 gene, while the association with the Tg-Ab concentrations was weaker [109, 110].

9.6.2.3 Protein Tyrosine Phosphatase Nonreceptor-Type 22 (PTPN22) Gene

Functional polymorphism of PTPN22, C1858T (R620W), is associated with susceptibility to several autoimmune disorders including AITD (Graves' disease and Hashimoto's thyroiditis), type-1 diabetes (T1D), rheumatoid arthritis (RA), and SLE [111–116].

PTPN22 was recently identified as an immune-regulatory gene, located on *chromosome 1p13*. Similar to CTLA-4, PTPN22, which is predominantly expressed in lymphocytes, acts as a negative regulator of T-cell activation. 1858C/T SNP of the PTPN22 gene, causing arginine to tryptophan substitution at codon 620 (R620W), was shown to be a risk factor for many autoimmune diseases though the mechanism is still not clear [117]. In 2005, Criswell et al. (2005) reported a significant association of Hashimoto's thyroiditis with 1858C/T SNP [113]. However, this observation was *not* confirmed in German [118], Tunisian [119], or Japanese [120] populations. In a small group of patients with both Hashimoto's thyroiditis and autoimmune diabetes, Dultz and colleagues (2009) reported that T allele was determined in 50% of patients as compared to only 14% in healthy controls [121]; however, 1 year later

(2010), Kordonouri et al., estimating the same polymorphism, did *not* confirm this association [122]. Five other PTPN22 SNPs have been tested by Ban et al. (2010) in Japanese patients and showed no relation with Hashimoto's thyroiditis, but a novel protective haplotype containing those SNPs has been observed [123].

9.6.2.4 Thyroglobulin (Tg) Gene

Thyroglobulin (Tg) is an important thyroid-specific antigen, also present in the circulation, which makes it an easy target of autoimmune response. The gene for Tg is located on *chromosome 8q24*, and the link of this region with Hashimoto's thyroiditis and AITD was first identified by a Japanese [124] and an American [125] whole genome study. A subsequent fine mapping of this region by Tomer et al., in 2002, exposed Tg gene as one of the major thyroid-specific susceptibility genes, linked and associated with the AITD [126]. Later, different alleles of various microsatellite markers and different SNPs of Tg gene were related to Hashimoto's thyroiditis, possibly affecting its expression, antigenicity, iodination, or binding to HLA. The association of Tgms2 microsatellite marker in intron 27 with Hashimoto's thyroiditis was confirmed in both Japanese [127] and Caucasian [128] populations. Sequencing of human Tg revealed 14 SNPs, among which four SNPs, including exon 10–12 SNP cluster and exon 33 SNP, were reported by Ban et al. (2003) to be associated with Hashimoto's thyroiditis [129]. However, this observation was neither confirmed in the UK Caucasian patients [130] nor in Chinese population, although in a later study by Maierhaba et al. (2008), one haplotype was significantly associated with Hashimoto's thyroiditis and Tg-Ab positivity [131].

9.6.2.5 Vitamin D Receptor Gene

Vitamin D, which acts via vitamin D receptor (VDR), possesses immunomodulatory properties, and its deficiency has been implicated in the development of autoimmune diseases. Many immune cells express VDR, particularly dendritic cells, where VDR stimulation has been shown to enhance their tolerogenicity [132]. The VDR gene is located on the *chromosome 12q12*, and its polymorphisms have been related to different autoimmune disorders such as type I diabetes or Addison's disease. In 2001, the association between *VDR-FokI* SNP in exon 2 and Hashimoto's thyroiditis was identified by Ban and colleagues [133] and confirmed later (2006) by Lin et al. in Taiwanese Chinese patients [134]. In the Croatian population, VDR gene 3′ region polymorphisms were related to Hashimoto's thyroiditis, possibly affecting VDR mRNA expression [135]. A significant relation has also been discovered between Hashimoto's thyroiditis and both promoter and intron 6 gene polymorphisms of CYP27B1 hydroxylase, which is located on chromosome 12q13, catalyzing the conversion of 25-hydroxy-vitamin D3 to its active form [136].

9.6.2.6 FCRL3 Gene

The FCRL3 affects B-cell receptor signaling and results in the incomplete induction of energy to auto-reactive B-cells [137], causing an elevated expression of FCRL3 to induce the generation of these cells. The C allele of the -169C/T polymorphism (rs7528684) in the FCRL3 promoter region, which was more closely related to a higher expression of FCRL3 than the -169T allele [138], was found to be associated with the susceptibility to autoimmune diseases, such as rheumatoid arthritis, T1-DM, SLE, multiple sclerosis (MS), and AITDs (Graves' disease and Hashimoto's thyroiditis) [139–142].

9.6.2.7 ZFAT Gene (Zinc Finger and AT-Hook Domain Containing)

The ZFAT gene is expressed on B- and T-lymphocytes and has been shown to be a critical transcriptional regulator [143] and as an anti-apoptotic molecule in lymphocytes [144]. The Ex9b-SNP10 (rs16905194) polymorphism in ZFAT was associated with the susceptibility to AITDs [145]. The T allele of Ex9b-SNP10 was associated with a lower expression of small antisense transcription of ZFAT (SAS-ZFAT) than its A allele. SAS-ZFAT suppresses the expression of 3′UTR of truncated ZFAT (TR-ZFAT), which is strongly expressed on B-cells and monocytes [145]. However, the functions of TR-ZFAT and SAS-ZFAT remain to be determined. The G allele of Ex9b-SNP2 (rs1036819) was also associated with the development of AITD among the Japanese [145] although the function of Ex9b-SNP2 was not determined.

9.6.2.8 Cytokine Genes and Other Immune-Related Genes

Recently, several genes encoding different inflammatory cytokines have been shown to influence the severity of Hashimoto's thyroiditis.

Interferon-Gamma (IFN-γ)

"Interferon-gamma" (IFN-γ), produced by T-helper type 1 (Th1) cells, promotes cell-mediated cytotoxicity, which underlies thyroid destruction in Hashimoto's thyroiditis. Ito et al. (2006) reported that T allele of the +874A/T IFN-γ SNP, causing increased IFN-γ production, was associated with the severity of hypothyroidism in Hashimoto's thyroiditis patients [146].

Interleukin 4 (IL-4) SNP

A higher frequency of severe hypothyroidism was also observed in patients carrying CC genotype of -590C/T "interleukin 4" (IL-4) SNP, leading to a lower production of IL-4, one of the key Th2 cytokines, which suppresses cell-mediated autoimmunity [147].

Transforming Growth Factor-Beta (TGF-β)

Gene polymorphism of "transforming growth factor-beta (TGF-β), inhibitor of cytokine production, was also associated with Hashimoto's thyroiditis. T allele of +369T/C SNP, leading to a lower secretion of TGF-β, was more frequent in severe hypothyroidism than in mild hypothyroidism [148]. Moreover, Inoue et al. reported in 2010 that more severe forms of Hashimoto's thyroiditis were associated with -2383C/T SNP of the gene for forkhead box P3 (FoxP3), an essential regulatory factor for the development of Tregs [149].

Tumor Necrosis Factor-Alpha (TNF-α) -1031T/C SNP. C-Allele
Unlike the severity of hypothyroidism, the development of Hashimoto's thyroiditis itself was associated with C allele of "tumor necrosis factor-alpha" (TNF-α) -1031T/C SNP. C-allele carriers had higher concentrations of TNF-α, which acts as the stimulator of the IFN-γ production, as demonstrated also by Inoue et al. (2009) [150].

Other Susceptibility Genes of AITD
Genome-wide association studies (GWAS) detected other susceptibility genes of AITD [151] including *FOXE1* and *IL-2RA* [152]. Association of polymorphisms in micro-RNA genes (miR499A and miR125A) with autoimmune thyroid diseases has been reported by Cai et al. in 2017 [153]. There is a report that micro-RNAs (miRNAs)—miR-146a1, miR-155-2, and miR-200a1—are altered in autoimmune thyroid diseases (AITD). Accumulating data suggest that miRNAs crucially control innate and adaptive immune responses, and implicate some miRNAs as having an important role in the pathophysiology of immunity and autoimmunity [154]. For example, miR-155-2 was previously shown to possess important functions in the mammalian immune system. MicroRNA-142-5p may contribute to Hashimoto's thyroiditis by targeting CLDN1 [155].

9.6.3 Environmental Factors

Regarding environmental factors, high iodine (I_2) intake, selenium deficiency, pollutants such as tobacco smoke, infectious diseases such as chronic hepatitis C, and certain drugs are implicated in the development of autoimmune thyroiditis [156, 157]. Environmental factors have not yet, however, been sufficiently investigated to clarify their roles in the pathogenesis of Hashimoto's disease, and there is a need to assess their effects on the development of the autoimmune process and the mechanisms of their interactions with susceptibility genes.

9.6.3.1 Increased Iodine Intake

Increased iodine (I_2) intake is a well-established environmental factor for triggering thyroid autoimmunity. Prevalence of T-Abs was 13% in I_2-deficiency areas [21], approximately 18% with sufficient I_2 intake [22], and about 25% in areas with excessive I_2 intake [158]. Moreover, up to fourfold increase in prevalence of T-Abs was shown after higher I_2 intake as I_2 prophylaxis in previously I_2-deficient areas [159–161]. In an interventional study by Kahaly et al. (1998), deliberate exposure to 500 μg of I_2 provoked thyroid autoimmunity in 20% of previously healthy individuals [162]. In 2002, Rose et al., using experimental animal models of autoimmune thyroiditis, reported that the prevalence and severity of thyroid autoimmunity significantly increased when the dietary I_2 was added [163].

Several putative mechanisms by which iodine may promote thyroid autoimmunity have been proposed. *Firstly*, long-term I_2 exposure leads to increased iodination of thyroglobulin (Tg), which increases its antigenicity by creating novel iodine-containing epitopes or exposing cryptic epitopes, and thus initiates the autoimmune process in genetically susceptible individuals by facilitating presentation by APC and enhancing the binding affinity of the T-cell receptor leading to specific T-cell activation [163]. *Secondly*, I_2 exposure increases the level of reactive oxygen species in the thyrocyte, which is generated during TPO oxidation of excessive amounts of iodine. They enhance the expression of the intracellular adhesion molecule-1 (ICAM-1) on the thyroid follicular cells, which could attract the immunocompetent cells into the thyroid gland [164]. *Thirdly*, iodine toxicity to thyrocytes has been reported by Fountoulakis et al. (2007). Highly reactive oxygen species may bind to membrane lipids and proteins, causing release of auto-antigens and thyrocyte damage [161]. *Fourthly*, Yu and colleagues reported in 2011 that I_2 excess promotes follicular cell apoptosis by inducing an abnormal expression of tumor necrosis factor-related apoptosis-inducing ligand (TRAIL) and its death receptor (DR)-5 in thyroid [165]. *Fifthly*, in vitro evidence also suggests an enhancing influence of I_2 on the cells of the immune system, including augmented maturation of dendritic cells, increased number of T-cells, and stimulated B-cell immunoglobulin production [161].

9.6.3.2 Selenium Deficiency

Selenium deficiency decreases the activity of selenoproteins, including glutathione peroxidases, which can lead to raised concentrations of hydrogen peroxide (H_2O_2) and thus promote inflammation and disease. In animal models, selenium has been shown to exert protective effects in cases of excessive iodine ingestion [166]. Similarly, human studies have demonstrated that when addressing iodine deficiency through supplementation, co-administration of selenium is important to maintain adequate glutathione peroxidase (GPx) function [167].

9.6.3.3 Certain Drugs

Certain drugs were reported to initiate or exacerbate thyroid autoimmunity in susceptible individuals.

Interferon-Alpha (IFN-α)

Interferon-alpha (IFN-α), used to treat chronic hepatitis, is frequently associated with AITD since T-Abs were observed in up to 40% and clinical disease in 5–10% of patients treated with IFN-α. Presumably, IFN-α has toxic effects on the thyroid gland with consequent auto-antigen presentation and immune effects, such as switching to Th1 immune response, suppression of Treg function, activation of immune cells, stimulation of cytokine release, and expression of MHC class I on thyroid cells [168].

Interleukin-2 (IL-2)

Interleukin-2 (IL-2), used for treatment of melanoma and renal carcinoma, seems to act also through immune and toxic mechanisms, leading to both T-Ab positivity and hypothyroidism [169].

Lithium

In patients with known AITD, lithium may increase the risk of hypothyroidism. Some studies reported that treatment with lithium increases T-Ab titers and the prevalence of thyroid autoimmunity, although this observation was *not* confirmed by other reports [169, 170]. Among putative mechanisms, direct toxicity of lithium on the thyroid gland or toxicity of increased intra-thyroidal I_2 resulting from lithium treatment were reported by Barbesino et al. (2010) [169].

Amiodarone

Similarly, amiodarone, a frequently prescribed anti-arrhythmic medication, may be cytotoxic leading to thyroid auto-antigen presentation and provoke thyroid autoimmunity [171].

9.6.3.4 Infections

Hepatitis C Virus

Not only the IFN-α treatment, but also *hepatitis C* infection itself has been reported to be associated with thyroid autoimmunity and hypothyroidism. Possible mechanisms include the molecular mimicry between viral and self-antigens, and activation of auto-reactive T-cells by the release of pro-inflammatory mediators caused by the viral infection [167].

Other Putative Triggering Viruses

In Hashimoto's thyroiditis, several other putative triggering viruses have been implicated such as parvovirus, rubella, herpes simplex virus, Epstein-Barr virus, and human T-lymphotropic virus type 1 [172].

Toxoplasma gondii

In 2009, Wasserman et al. reported that the study of sera in pregnant women has also indicated an association between a prior infection with *Toxoplasma gondii* and an increase of TPO-Abs [173]. Nevertheless, the evidences are scarce and further studies are required in order to confirm the role of infections as causative agents.

9.6.3.5 Certain Chemicals

The exposure to environmental toxicants such as polyaromatic hydrocarbons or polyhalogenated biphenyls, both commonly used in a variety of industrial applications, has been shown to provoke thyroid autoimmunity in both experimental animals and humans [164]. Recently, a significantly higher prevalence of Hashimoto's thyroiditis and T-Ab (9.3% and 17.6%, respectively) has been demonstrated in residents living in the area of petrochemical complex of Sao Paolo (Brazil) compared to the control area (3.9% and 10.3%, respectively) [174]. In Slovakia, the exposure to polychlorinated biphenyls was associated with T-Ab and hypothyroidism [175]. Although there is strong evidence attesting the contribution of chemicals to thyroid autoimmunity, the exact mechanisms of their action are yet to be established.

9.6.3.6 Radiation Exposure

An increase in the prevalence of thyroid autoantibodies (AT-Abs) was reported 6–8 years after the Chernobyl accident in radiation-exposed children and adolescents [176]. TPO-Ab prevalence in adolescents exposed to radioactive fallout was still increased in Belarus 13–15 years after the Chernobyl accident [177]. This increase was less evident than previously reported and was not accompanied by thyroid dysfunction. These data suggest that radioactive fallout elicited a "transient" autoimmune reaction, without triggering full-blown thyroid autoimmune disease. Longer observation periods are certainly needed to exclude later effects.

9.6.4 Protection Against Thyroid Autoimmunity

9.6.4.1 Self-Tolerance

Two mechanisms enable the maintenance of self-tolerance. "Central tolerance" refers to thymic deletion of auto-reactive T-cells during fetal life. Cells that escape central tolerance are prevented from triggering autoimmunity by mechanisms of "peripheral tolerance" where the pivotal role is played by Tregs (regulatory T-cells) [178]. They have a suppressive effect on the effector T-cells, APCs, and B-cells, therefore maintaining the immunological unresponsiveness to self-antigens and suppressing the excessive immune response [179]. They may directly suppress target cells or act through secreted suppressor cytokines.

9.6.4.2 Regulatory T-Cells (Tregs)

Tregs derive from thymus as a sub-population of T-cells or from naive T-cells in the periphery and express CD25 (α-chain of IL-2 receptor) and FoxP3. Thus, the critical role in the immune system is played by CD4+CD25+Foxp3+ Tregs [178]. Cells with the highest CD25 expression (CD4+CD25 high) are responsible for regulatory suppressive effects [180]. The role of Tregs in self-tolerance was extensively studied in murine experimental autoimmune thyroiditis, where protection against autoimmunity was mediated by thymically derived CD4+CD25+Foxp3+ Tregs [181]. In humans, CD25 expression was higher in patients with Hashimoto's thyroiditis than in healthy controls [182]. In patients with AITD, the proportion of Tregs was lower intra-thyroidally than in peripheral blood [183]. When compared to controls, a higher proportion of special Tregs with high levels of FoxP3 (termed CD4+CD25 high HLA-DR+ cells) in patients with Hashimoto's thyroiditis was found by three-color flow cytometry [184]. This indicates a compensatory expansion of Tregs sub-population in order to diminish the immune response [185].

The expression of Foxp3 and generation of Treg cells are both induced by TGF-β produced in Tregs, fibroblasts, macrophages, endothelial cells in inflammatory thyroid tissue, and in thyrocytes [186, 187]. Transforming growth factor-beta (TGF-β) is a key regulator of immune tolerance, which stimulates suppressive Tregs and inhibits T-cell differentiation [187]. Accordingly, in patients with Hashimoto's thyroiditis, serum levels of TGF-β were lower than in controls, which did not change after the treatment with levothyroxine. Thus, TGF-β levels seem to be associated with Hashimoto's thyroiditis and not thyroid dysfunction [188]. Suppressive effect of TGF-β was established in the development of experimental autoimmune thyroiditis [189]. At the later stage of the thyroiditis, TGF-β may trigger the development of fibrosis [190].

9.6.5 Development of Thyroid Gland Autoimmunity

The exact mechanisms of initiation and progression of thyroid autoimmunity have not been completely clarified yet. Nevertheless, proper interaction of thyroid cells, APCs, and T-cells is essential for the initiation of thyroid autoimmunity. The result is a secretion of different cytokines leading to Th1 response, a characteristic of Hashimoto's thyroiditis. Cytokines have an important role in AITD and are secreted by the immune cells, thyroid follicular cells, and inflammatory cells [191].

T-lymphocytes proliferate and secrete cytokines after being stimulated by two signals. The "first signal" is the activation of T-cell receptor induced by binding of antigen peptide presented on HLA molecule on the surface of APC. The "second signal" is ligation of CD28 on the surface of the T-cell to B7 ligands (B7.1 and B7.2) expressed on APC, including dendritic cells, activated macrophages, and activated B-cells. Activation of T-cells induces the expression of CTLA-4, which suppresses further T-cell activation by binding and blocking of B7 ligands. In patients with Hashimoto's thyroiditis, but not in Graves' disease or goitrous patients, thyroid follicular cells were positive for B7.1 [192] and may also express MHC class II molecules induced by interferon-gamma (IFN-γ), which is secreted by intra-thyroidal lymphocytes [192]. Colocalization (defined by the presence of two or more different molecules residing at the same physical location in a specimen) of MHC class II and B7.1 antigens on the same thyroid follicular cell indicates that in the pathogenesis of Hashimoto's thyroiditis, follicular cells may act also as APCs and may be capable of inducing or maintaining the autoimmune process [193].

Autoimmune response is predominantly determined by the antigen, nature of APC, and several genetic, endogenous, and environmental triggers [193]. In Hashimoto's thyroiditis, autoimmune response is mediated predominantly by Th1-type cytokines such as TNF-α, IFN-γ and IL-2 [194]. When exposed to a thyroid self-antigen such as human Tg, peripheral blood mononuclear cells from patients with Hashimoto's thyroiditis produced more TNF-α, IL-2, IL-10, and IFN-γ, and less IL-5 than controls. Since higher production was observed with autologous sera than with pooled normal sera, the importance of serum elements, such as the complement and serum anti-Tg activity, was proposed. It was postulated that these two serum elements accelerate Th1/Th2 cell cytokine reaction by increasing the uptake of auto-antigens by APCs [195]. Patients with more severe hypothyroidism presented with a higher Th1/Th2 ratio compared with those with mild hypothyroidism [196]. Furthermore, the correlation between the TPO-Ab levels and the production of TNF-α and IFN-γ has been demonstrated by Karanikas et al. in 2005 [197] and later confirmed by Nielsen et al. in 2009 [198]. In their study, they indicated that TPO-Abs seem to promote TPO-elicited cytokine production, including IFN-γ, TNF-α, and IL-6 [198].

High titers of antibody against thyroglobulin (Tg) and thyroid peroxidase (TPO) are present in most patients with Hashimoto's thyroiditis [199], and TPO antibodies are complement-fixing and may be cytotoxic. However, the evidence of cytotoxicity is scant, especially since normal trans-placental antibody passage of anti-TPO Ab to the human fetus does *not* usually induce thyroid damage. Thus, it is conceivable that cytotoxic T-cells, or killer (K) or natural killer (NK) cells, or regulatory T (Treg) or suppressor T-cells, may play an important role. A few reports do show T-cell line or clone cytotoxicity toward isologous thyroid epithelial cells, and experimental thyroiditis can be transferred by lymphocytes. T-cells from patients with Hashimoto's disease proliferate when exposed to Tg and TPO. These responses are known to be directed to specific sequences in the TPO molecule, including epitopes at aa 110–129, 210–230, 420–439, and 842–861 [200], T-cells from mice immunized to TPO react strongly to TPO sequence 540–559, and when immunized with this peptide, develop hypothyroidism and thyroiditis. This peptide may be a central factor in immunity to TPO [201]. Muixí et al. (2008) [202] identified natural HLA-DR-associated peptides in autoimmune organs that will allow finding peptide-specific T-cells in situ.

In vitro binding identified HLA-DR3 as the allele to which one of these peptides likely associates in vivo. Computer modeling and bioinformatics analysis suggested other HLA-DR alleles for binding of other thyroglobulin peptides. Increased K- and NK-cell function has been reported in Hashimoto's thyroiditis [203]. Dysfunction of regulatory (or suppressor) CD4+ T-cell populations may lead to the development of various organ-specific autoimmune diseases including Hashimoto's thyroiditis [204].

In the past few years, a new subset of (T-helper) Th cells, designated Th17 (T-helper type 17), has been studied. Th17 cells have also been proved highly pro-inflammatory by producing the pro-inflammatory cytokine IL-17, and may lead to autoimmunity in animal models and potentially also in human autoimmune diseases [187]. The possible importance of Th17 in the pathogenesis of Hashimoto's thyroiditis has been indicated by a recent study showing increased levels of Th17 lymphocytes and Th17 cytokines compared with healthy controls [205]. Similarly, when estimating the expression in peripheral blood mononuclear cells, Th17 cells rather than Th1 cells predominated in Hashimoto's thyroiditis patients [206]. Imbalance of Th17/Treg is reported in different subtypes of autoimmune thyroid diseases. Increased Th17 lymphocytes may play a more important role in the pathogenesis of Hashimoto's thyroiditis, while decreased Treg may be involved in Graves' disease [207]. In contrast, a significant decrease in the ratios of CD4+ IL17+/CD4+ CD25+ CD127− ($p < 0.0001$) and CD4+ IL17+/CD4+ CD25+ CD127− FoxP3+ ($p < 0.0001$) T-cells was observed in Hashimoto's thyroiditis in comparison to healthy children [208].

9.6.6 Destruction of the Thyroid Gland

9.6.6.1 Lymphocytic Infiltration

Despite the lack of understanding of the primary cause(s), it is certain that thyroid autoimmunity drives the lymphocyte collection in the thyroid and is responsible for thyroid epithelial cell damage. Progressive thyroid cell damage can change the apparent clinical picture from goitrous hypothyroidism to that of primary hypothyroidism, or "atrophic" thyroiditis. Primary hypothyroidism is considered to be the end-stage of Hashimoto's thyroiditis. In the TSHR-immunized murine model of Graves' disease, Treg depletion (particularly CD25)-induced thyroid lymphocytic infiltrates with transient or permanent hypothyroidism [209]. Lymphocytic infiltration was associated with inter-molecular spreading of the TSHR antibody response to other self-thyroid antigens, murine thyroid peroxidase, and Tg. These data suggest a role for (regulatory T-cells) Tregs in the natural progression of hyperthyroid Graves' disease to Hashimoto's thyroiditis and hypothyroidism in humans.

9.6.6.2 Thyroid-Stimulation Blocking Antibodies (TSB-Ab)

An alternative cause of "atrophic" hypothyroidism is the development of thyroid-stimulation blocking antibodies (TSB-Ab), which, as the name implies, prevent TSH binding to TSH-R, but do not stimulate thyroid cells and cause hypothyroidism. It has been proposed that TSB-Ab bind to epitopes near the carboxyl end of the TSH-R extra-cellular domain, in contrast to thyroid-stimulating antibodies (TS-Ab), which bind to epitopes near aa 40 at the amino terminus [210]. This syndrome occurs in neonates, children, and adults. The prevalence of TSB-Ab in adult hypothyroid patients was reported back in 1990 by Okamura et al. to be 10% [211]. However, in contrast to the usual progressive and irreversible thyroid damage occurring in the usual setting, these blocking antibodies tend to follow the course of TSAb—that is, they decrease or disappear over time, and the patient may become euthyroid again [211]. A change from a predominant TSAb response to a predominant TSB-Ab response can cause patients to have sequential episodes of hyper- and hypothyroid function [212]. HLA antigens of hypothyroid patients with TSB-Ab were found to be different from patients with idiopathic myxedema or Hashimoto's thyroiditis, and rather similar to patients with Graves' disease [213].

9.6.6.3 Apoptotic Processes

Apoptosis is defined as "a type of cell death in which a series of molecular steps in a cell lead to its death." Thyroid destruction in Hashimoto's thyroiditis is mostly a consequence of the "apoptotic processes" combined with CD8+ cell-mediated cytotoxicity, changes in cell junctions, and complement activation. Apoptosis is characterized by cytoskeletal disruption, cell shrinkage, chromatin condensation, nuclear fragmentation, membrane blebbing, and DNA fragmentation [214]. In general, apoptosis enables adult healthy tissue homeostasis, while excessive cell death causes a loss of active tissue and an impaired function [214].

Two major apoptotic signal pathways have been thoroughly investigated [215]:

1. The first pathway consists of Fas receptor (Apo-1 or CD95), a type I trans-membrane protein and a member of TNF receptor superfamily, and Fas ligand (Fas-L), a type II trans-membrane protein, which binds to Fas receptor and activates apoptotic process [216]. The ligand for Fas (Fas-L) was shown to be constitutively expressed on thyrocytes and IL-1α, abundantly produced in the thyroid gland of Hashimoto's thyroiditis, induced Fas expression on thyrocytes. Thus Fas-FasL interaction on thyrocytes may induce apoptosis and thyroid cell destruction [217]. Furthermore, in relation to the Fas-Fas-L system, Dong et al. (2002) [218] reported that mutations of Fas, which induce loss of function, were found in thyroid lymphocytes in 38.1% of patients with Hashimoto's thyroiditis. These mutations are found in 65.4% of patients with lymphoma [219], which usually develops from Hashimoto's thyroiditis. These changes are possibly important for progression of Hashimoto's thyroiditis.
2. The second pathway includes tumor necrosis factor (TNF)-related apoptosis-inducing ligand (TRAIL) (Apo2L), a member of TNF receptor family, which activates apoptosis by binding to its receptors TRAIL-R1 (DR4) and TRAIL-R2 (DR5) [220, 221]. Both pathways lead to the activation of proteolytic enzymes caspases, which destroy thyroid cells. In normal conditions, the Fas pathway is inhibited, whereas in inflammation, it is activated by cytokines [222]. In vitro studies have shown that TSH inhibited Fas-mediated apoptosis, while the absence of TSH induced apoptosis [223]. A combination of IFN-γ with TNF-α or IL-1β stimulated the Fas-activated apoptosis in cultured thyroid follicular cells [224]. TRAIL receptors are also expressed in thyroid cells by cytokines [225], and TRAIL could mediate the programmed cell death under appropriate conditions [226]. Thyroid follicular cells were able to express TRAIL in the presence of IFN-γ, TNF-α, and IL-1β in vitro. Thus, such inflammatory cytokines can influence immune-mediated apoptosis [226]. Additional inductor of programmed cell death is TGF-β [227]. Its release from thyroid cells is stimulated by the epidermal growth factor (EGF) [228]. Thus, the mechanism of apoptosis in Hashimoto's thyroiditis seems to be induced by cytokines secreted from local lymphocytes [229, 230].

The main apoptotic mechanism in Hashimoto's thyroiditis represents Fas-mediated apoptosis together with down-regulation of Bcl-2, which is an inhibitor of apoptosis highly expressed in normal thyrocytes [231–234]. Immuno-histochemically, patients with Hashimoto's thyroiditis had a lower percentage of Bcl-2 stainings and a higher percentage of caspase-3 reactions than control subjects [235]. In thyroid glands with Hashimoto's thyroiditis, a strong staining for Fas and Fas-L and a high percentage of apoptosis were observed in thyroid follicles adjacent to lymphocytes when compared with healthy thyroid tissue.

9.6.6.4 CD8+ Cell-Mediated Cytotoxicity

In addition to apoptosis, CD8+ cell-mediated cytotoxicity contributes to thyroid destruction mediated by intracellular circulating adhesion molecule-1 (ICAM-1)

(CR 54), which is expressed by thyroid follicular cells and increases CD8+ cell binding [193]. Levels of ICAM-1, vascular cell adhesion molecule-1 (VCAM-1), and tissue inhibitor of metallo-proteinases 1 (TIMP-1) were significantly higher in patients with functional abnormality due to the AITD than in euthyroid subjects. Authors postulated that the autoimmune process itself may have an impact on vascular inflammation, endothelial dysfunction, and tissue remodeling [236].

9.6.6.5 Changes in Gap Junctions

Finally, changes in gap junctions consequently leading to cell-to-cell communication changes may contribute to the thyroid destruction. In Hashimoto's thyroiditis, decreased levels of connexin 43 (Cx43) were observed immuno-histochemically when compared with the normal thyroid tissue [237]. Cx43 is a part of connexons, which constitute a gap junction channel in organized tissues and in thyroid tissues. Similarly, reduced proteins Cx43, Cx32, and Cx26 were established in animal models of AITD [238]. Mitasíková et al. (2009) also showed that T3 increased the level of Cx43 [239]. Thus, the number of gap junctions may be increased in Graves' disease and decreased in Hashimoto's thyroiditis [237]. Disruption of thyroid integrity may allow TPO-Abs to bind to TPO and activate complement [193].

9.6.7 IgG4-Related Disease (IgG4-RD)

The IgG4-related disease (IgG4-RD) is a new disease entity first proposed in relation to autoimmune pancreatitis (AIP) by Hamano et al. in 2001 [208]. A high prevalence of hypothyroidism has been reported in patients with AIP [240]. In 2009, it was reported that on the basis of the immunohistochemistry (IHC) of IgG4, Hashimoto's thyroiditis can be divided into two groups, which were proposed as IgG4 thyroiditis (IgG4-positive plasma cell-rich group) and non-IgG4 thyroiditis (IgG4-positive plasma cell poor group) [241]. The IgG4 thyroiditis group shows indistinguishable histological features and may have a close relationship with IgG4-RD in other organs. In 2010, it was demonstrated that IgG4 thyroiditis is clinically associated with a lower female-to-male ratio, more rapid progress, subclinical hypothyroidism, diffuse low echogenicity, and a higher level of circulating thyroid autoantibodies than non-IgG4 thyroiditis [242].

Riedel thyroiditis is another candidate for IgG4-RD. It is a rare form of chronic thyroiditis, characterized by inflammatory proliferative fibrosis which involves the thyroid parenchyma and surrounding tissue structures. In 2010, Dahlgren and colleagues reported that IgG4-RD was the underlying condition in a part of the cases of Riedel thyroiditis [243]. When IgG4-RD occurs in a systemic pattern, the thyroid involvement may present as Riedel thyroiditis rather than Hashimoto's thyroiditis [244].

9.6.8 Summary [108]

Hashimoto's thyroiditis is one of the most prevalent autoimmune diseases provoked in genetically susceptible individuals by several triggers, including female gender, immune changes after delivery, fetal micro-chimerism, increased iodine intake, selenium deficiency, and other environmental factors. Multiple susceptibility genes may be involved in the disease development, some of which are also common for other autoimmune diseases, while others are specific for thyroid autoimmunity. It is now clear that immune-regulatory genes such as *HLA*, *CTLA-4*, and *PTPN22* play a major role in the pathogenesis of Hashimoto's thyroiditis, Graves' disease, and several other autoimmune diseases. The only thyroid-specific gene currently showing the association with Hashimoto's thyroiditis (and also Graves' disease) is the gene for Tg. The *VDR* gene is another Hashimoto's thyroiditis predisposing gene, common for other organ-specific autoimmune diseases such as type-I diabetes or Addison's disease. Furthermore, recent studies of cytokine genes such as *IFN-γ*, *IL-4*, or *TGF-β* indicate the association with the development and severity of Hashimoto's thyroiditis, presumably influencing the balance between Th1 and Th2 mechanisms.

Accordingly, it is conceivable that a complex interaction between genetic and non-genetic factors results in enhanced thyroid antigen presentation and reduced immune tolerance, leading to predominantly Th1-type autoimmunity, thyroid destruction, and clinical disease.

Despite tremendous progress made in the understanding of Hashimoto's thyroiditis during the past two decades, the exact mechanisms of its initiation and progression are yet to be clarified. A better insight into the disease pathogenesis may help us identify subjects at risk and may be even enable us to prevent the development of clinical disease.

9.7 Clinical Presentation and Course

9.7.1 Demographics and Family History

Hashimoto's disease is about seven times more common in women than in men. It can occur in teens and young women, but more commonly shows up in middle age, particularly in men. Patients with Hashimoto's thyroiditis often have family members who have thyroid or *other autoimmune diseases*, and sometimes have other autoimmune diseases themselves.

9.7.2 Clinical Course

Patients with Hashimoto's thyroiditis may present initially with features of hyperthyroidism (Hashitoxicosis), especially during the early phase of the disease, due to the release of preformed thyroxin from the destroyed thyroid follicles. The disease then progresses to subclinical (normal FT4 but elevated TSH) and overt hypothyroidism. Progression from *subclinical hypothyroidism* to *overt hypothyroidism* (low FT4 but elevated TSH) occurs in approximately 3–5% of patients each year. Finally, thyroid atrophy (failure) and *myxedema* may develop [245]. Symptoms and signs of *mild hypothyroidism* may be present in 20% of patients when first seen [246] or commonly develop over a period of several years. Thus, HT begins as a gradual, painless, homogeneous enlargement of the thyroid gland and gradual development of manifestations of hypothyroidism [247]. Furthermore, Hashimoto's thyroiditis is characterized by invasion of thyroid tissue by leukocytes, mainly T-lymphocytes. A rare, but serious complication is thyroid lymphoma, generally the B-cell type, non-Hodgkin lymphoma (NHL).

Being an autoimmune disease, the clinical course of Hashimoto's thyroiditis is one of relapsing episodes, with up to 25% of the patients showing a spontaneous recovery. The binding of autoantibodies to the thyrocytes accounts for complement and T-lymphocyte-mediated lysis of the thyrocytes and non-regulated release of T3 and T4, resulting in the transient hyperthyroidism occasionally noted. Later on, destruction of the thyroid parenchyma may lead to permanent hypothyroidism.

9.7.3 Clinical Presentation

Clinically, the patient with Hashimoto's thyroiditis can be euthyroid, hyperthyroid or hypothyroid based on the degree of thyroid destruction. There are many *symptoms* that are attributed to Hashimoto's thyroiditis or Hashimoto's disease. The most common symptoms include the following: fatigue, weight gain, pale or puffy face, feeling cold, joint and muscle pain, constipation, dry and thinning hair, heavy menstrual flow or irregular periods, depression, panic disorder, a slowed heart rate, and problems getting pregnant and maintaining pregnancy [247].

As may be seen in Table 9.2, the various clinical presentations of Hashimoto's thyroiditis include the following:

Table 9.2 Clinical presentations of Hashimoto's thyroiditis

Clinical presentation
Euthyroidism and goiter
Subclinical hypothyroidism and goiter
Primary thyroid failure
Hypothyroidism
Adolescent goiter
Painless thyroiditis or silent thyroiditis
Postpartum painless thyrotoxicosis
Alternating hypo- and hyperthyroidism

9.7.4 Goiter (Neck Swelling)

In Hashimoto's thyroiditis, the thyroid gland shows gradual, painless, homogenous enlargement; however, in some cases, the thyroid gland may become firm, large, and lobulated, rarely causing pressure symptoms such as dyspnea or dysphagia, or mild pain and tenderness. The goiter of Hashimoto's thyroiditis may remain unchanged for decades [247], but usually it gradually increases in size. Enlargement of the thyroid gland in Hashimoto's thyroiditis is due to lymphocytic infiltration and fibrosis rather than tissue hypertrophy.

9.7.5 Pain/Tenderness

Occasionally, patients with Hashimoto's thyroiditis have persistent pain, which is unresponsive to non-steroidal anti-inflammatory drugs (NSAIDs), or replacement with L-thyroxin, and recurs after therapy with steroids. In 2003, Kon and DeGroot [248] reported seven patients who finally underwent subtotal or near-total thyroidectomy, some of whom received subsequent radioactive iodide (RAI) thyroid ablation, with final relief of symptoms.

9.7.6 Hypothyroidism

Generally, the progress from euthyroidism to hypothyroidism has been considered an "irreversible process" due to thyroid cell damage and loss of thyroidal iodine stores. However, it is currently evident that up to 25% of patients who are hypothyroid may spontaneously return to normal function over the course of several years. This sequence may reflect the initial effect of high titers of thyroid-stimulation blocking antibodies, which fall with time and allow thyroid function to return [212].

At 5 years of follow-up of the natural course of euthyroid Hashimoto's thyroiditis in Italian children, more than 50% of the patients remained or became euthyroid [249]. The presence of goiter and elevated Tg-Ab at presentation, together with progressive increase in both TPO-Ab and TSH, may be predictive factors for the future development of hypothyroidism.

"Myxedema psychosis," more colloquially known as "myxedema madness," is a relatively uncommon consequence of hypothyroidism, such as in Hashimoto's thyroiditis or in patients who have had their thyroids removed surgically, and are not taking thyroxin replacement therapy. A chronically under-active thyroid can lead to slowly progressive dementia, delirium, and in extreme cases to hallucinations, coma, or psychosis, particularly in the elderly. It was first recognized by Dr. Richard Asher of London in 1949. Treatment is via the standard treatment for hypothyroidism with levothyroxine (L-T4) replacement, or in especially acute cases, liothyoxine (sodium salt of T3). Hormone replacement in these patients usually reverses the psychotic symptoms, but may not help with cognitive deficits caused by changes in metabolic activity in the central nervous system (CNS). The "myxedema" part of the name simply refers to the non-pitting edema common to hypothyroidism.

9.7.7 Associated "Unusual" Syndromes

In the past few years, several unusual syndromes believed to be associated with or part of the clinical spectrum of HT have been described; occasional patients develop "amyloid deposits" in the thyroid [250]. In 1991, Shaw et al. [251] described five patients with a relapsing steroid-responsive "encephalopathy" including episodes of stroke and seizures, high CSF protein, abnormal EEG, and normal CT scans. In the same year, Khardon et al. [252] reported a steroid-responsive lymphocytic "interstitial pneumonitis" in four patients. It remains uncertain how these illnesses relate to lymphocytic thyroiditis, which has until now been largely identified as an organ-specific disease.

When euthyroid and hypothyroid patients with orbitopathy are TRAb-negative, but associated with HT, "Hashimoto's ophthalmopathy" may be considered [253, 254]. Because patients with HT test negative for TRAb, other autoantibodies against an eye muscle antigen, such as calsequestrin, flavoprotein, or G2s, were postulated [255].

Hashimoto's thyroiditis and hypothyroidism are associated with Addison's disease, diabetes mellitus (DM), hypogonadism, hypo-parathyroidism, and pernicious anemia. Such combinations are described as the "polyglandular failure syndrome." Two forms of polyglandular autoimmunity have been recognized [256]. In the *Type I* syndrome, patients have hypoparathyroidism, muco-cutaneous candidiasis, Addison's disease, and occasionally hypothyroidism. The more frequent *Type II* often includes familial associations of diabetes mellitus, hypothyroidism, hypoadrenalism, and occasionally gonadal or pituitary failure. In these syndromes, antibodies reacting with the affected end organs are characteristically present.

Vitiligo, hives, and alopecia are associated with thyroiditis. There is also a clear association with primary and secondary Sjogren's syndrome [257]. Some patients appear to start with Hashimoto's thyroiditis, and progress with time to the picture of Riedel's thyroiditis including the frequently associated retro-peritoneal fibrosis [258].

"Musculo-skeletal" symptoms, including chest pain, fibrositis, and rheumatoid arthritis, occur in nearly 25% of patients [259], and any of the musculo-skeletal symptoms of hypothyroidism may occur. It has also been suggested that thyroiditis predisposes to vascular disease and coronary occlusion. Abnormally elevated titers of thyroid autoantibodies and the morphological changes of thyroiditis are said to occur with an increased frequency among patients with coronary artery disease.

Mild hypothyroidism associated with asymptomatic atrophic thyroiditis could predispose patients to heart disease [260]. However, other researchers have failed to find increased Tg-Ab in patients with coronary artery disease or increased coronary disease in association with thyroiditis [261].

Finally, in *children*, retarded growth, retarded bone age, decreased hydroxyproline excretion, and elevated cholesterol levels may be seen.

The autoimmune phenomena that may occur or be found in association with Hashimoto's thyroiditis are summarized in Table 9.3.

9.7.8 Neoplastic Transformation

Although chronic inflammation, leading to neoplastic transformation, is a well-established clinical phenomenon, the link between Hashimoto's thyroiditis and thyroid cancer remains controversial [262, 263]. In 2007, Larson et al. [264] reported that patients with Hashimoto's thyroiditis were three times more likely to have thyroid cancer, suggesting a strong link between chronic inflammation and development of cancer.

The association between Hashimoto's thyroiditis and papillary thyroid carcinoma (PTC) has been a subject of long and ongoing debate; Hashimoto's thyroiditis has shown a wide range of occurrence from 5% to 85% in thyroid specimens resected for PTC [265]. In addition, the clinico-pathological characteristics of PTC with concomitant Hashimoto's thyroiditis have not been definitively proposed [266, 267].

PI3K/Akt expression was increased in both Hashimoto's thyroiditis and well-differentiated thyroid cancer (WDTC), suggesting a possible molecular mechanism for thyroid carcinogenesis. Several authors reported that thyroid cancer may be associated with less aggressive disease and better outcome in patients with coexisting Hashimoto's thyroiditis [263, 268, 269].

Table 9.3 Autoimmune phenomena associated with Hashimoto's thyroiditis

Addison's disease
Alopecia (areata, totalis, and universalis)
Autoimmune gastritis (pernicious anemia)
Chronic active hepatitis (CAH)
Idiopathic hypo-parathyroidism
Poly-myalgia rheumatica and giant cell arteritis
Primary biliary cirrhosis (PBC)
Primary ovarian or testicular failure
Rheumatoid arthritis
Sjögren syndrome
Systemic lupus erythematosus (SLE)
Systemic sclerosis (scleroderma)
Type-1 diabetes mellitus (DM)
Vitiligo

9.7.9 Remission of Hashimoto's Thyroiditis: Pregnancy

Remission of Hashimoto's thyroiditis, with loss of goiter, hypothyroidism, and serum thyroid autoantibodies, has been reported during pregnancy, with relapse after delivery [270]. Antibody levels have been reported to fall during pregnancy [271]. These phenomena may reflect the immunosuppressive effects of pregnancy. However, after delivery thyroid autoantibody levels rise, and after 2–6 months, there may be sudden development of goiter and hypothyroidism [272]. The Endocrine Society Clinical Practice Guidelines were developed for the management of thyroid dysfunction during pregnancy and postpartum [273]. In such cases, management requires special considerations because pregnancy induces major changes in thyroid function, and maternal thyroid disease can have adverse effects on the pregnancy and the fetus. Avoiding maternal (and fetal) hypothyroidism is of major importance because of potential damage to fetal neural development, an increased incidence of miscarriage, and preterm delivery.

Women who have low thyroid function that has not been stabilized are at greater risk of having an infant with low birth weight, neonatal respiratory distress, hydrocephalus, hypospadias, miscarriage, and pre-term delivery. Successful pregnancy outcomes are improved when Hashimoto's thyroiditis is treated. Recommendations are to only treat pregnant women who are TPOAb-positive throughout the entirety of their pregnancies and to screen all pregnant women for thyroid levels. Close cooperation between the endocrinologist and obstetrician benefits both the woman and the infant. The Endocrine Society also recommends screening in pregnant women who are considered high-risk for thyroid autoimmune disease.

Maternal hyperthyroidism and its treatment may be accompanied by coincident problems in fetal thyroid function. Autoimmune thyroid disease is associated with both increased rates of miscarriage and postpartum thyroiditis (PPT). Fine-needle aspiration cytology (FNAC) should be performed for dominant thyroid nodules discovered in pregnancy. Radioactive isotopes must be avoided during pregnancy and lactation. Universal screening of pregnant women for thyroid disease is *not* yet supported by adequate studies, but case finding targeted to specific groups of patients who are at increased risk is strongly supported. The study by Dosiou et al. (2008) recommended screening all pregnant women for autoimmune thyroid disease in the first trimester in terms of cost-effectiveness [274].

Maternal antibodies are known to cross the placenta and, as in Graves' disease, may affect the fetus and neonate. The TPO-Ab and Tg-Ab typically appear to have no adverse effect. Some evidence suggests cytotoxic antibodies, which are thought to be different from TPO-Ab or Tg-Ab, could cause fetal hypothyroidism [275]. However, TSH-Ab can rarely produce neonatal hypothyroidism, which is self-limiting over 4–6 weeks as the maternal IgG is metabolized. Women with positive TPO antibody before assisted reproduction have a significantly increased risk for miscarriage [276].

Testing of thyroid peroxide (TPO) antibodies is recommended for women who have ever been pregnant regardless of pregnancy outcome. Previous pregnancy plays a major role in the development of autoimmune overt hypothyroidism in premenopausal women, and the number of previous pregnancies should be taken into account when evaluating the risk of hypothyroidism in young women.

9.7.10 Variants of Hashimoto's Thyroiditis

9.7.10.1 Fibrotic Hashimoto's Thyroiditis

Fibrotic HT is a fibrotic variant of HT that accounts for up to 10% of cases, mainly in elderly patients with a pre-existing goiter. It is characterized by a rapid increase in goiter size, which may lead to the suspicion of malignancy or Riedel's fibrosing thyroiditis. However, the extensive fibrotic changes and metaplasia noted on biopsies are always limited to the gland in this variant.

9.7.10.2 Atrophic Hashimoto's (Autoimmune) Thyroiditis (Primary or Idiopathic Myxedema)

The atrophic autoimmune thyroiditis is the cause of primary myxedema and should *not* be confused with end-stage fibrotic HT. Most of the patients do not show signs or symptoms of hypothyroidism till the fourth to sixth decade of life, and women are five times more affected than men [277].

9.7.10.3 Painless (Silent) and Postpartum Thyroiditis (PPT)

"Silent (painless) thyroiditis" is a syndrome that has a clinical course of thyroid dysfunction similar to subacute thyroiditis, but with no anterior neck pain and no thyroid tenderness. Initially, patients have a thyrotoxic phase, later passing through euthyroidism to hypothyroidism and, finally, return to euthyroidism. "Postpartum thyroiditis" (PPT) occurs within 6 months after delivery and runs an identical clinical course [275]. It is now considered to be identical to silent thyroiditis, and this term is used for patients who developed silent thyroiditis in the postpartum period [275].

After delivery, other forms of autoimmune thyroid dysfunction also occur, including Graves' disease, transient hypothyroidism without preceding destructive thyrotoxicosis, and persistent hypothyroidism. In recent years, the term painless thyroiditis also has been used frequently, and the same disorder has been described using different names, such as thyrotoxicosis with painless thyroiditis [278], occult subacute thyroiditis [279], hyper-thyroiditis [280], lymphocytic thyroiditis with spontaneously resolving hyperthyroidism [281], painless thyroiditis and transient hyperthyroidism without goiter [282], and transient hyperthyroidism with lymphocytic thyroiditis [283]. The thyrotoxicosis is induced by leakage of intra-thyroidal hormones into the circulation caused by damage to thyroid epithelial cells from inflammation. Thus, the thyroid radioactive iodine uptake (RAIU) is low [284].

Therefore, the early phase of thyrotoxicosis in silent thyroiditis, PPT, and subacute thyroiditis can be grouped together as "destruction-induced thyrotoxicosis" or simply as "destructive thyrotoxicosis" [285]. When the measurement of RAIU is difficult, the measurement of anti-TSH receptor antibody and/or thyroid blood flow by ultrasonography (US) may be useful to differentiate between destruction-induced thyrotoxicosis and Graves' thyrotoxicosis. The quantitative measurement by power Doppler US was more effective than that of anti-TSH receptor antibody for differential diagnosis of these two types of thyrotoxicosis and may omit the radioactive iodine uptake test [286].

During the clinical course of subclinical or very mild autoimmune thyroiditis, "aggravating factors" cause exacerbation of the destructive process. All women with subclinical autoimmune thyroiditis [287] and anti-thyroid microsomal antibodies of more than 1:5120 before pregnancy develop postpartum thyroiditis [275]. A significant percentage of patients with silent thyroiditis have personal or family history of autoimmune thyroid disease. Most patients have a complete remission, but some develop persistent hypothyroidism [288]. Some patients have had alternating episodes of typical "high-uptake" thyrotoxicosis and episodes of "transient" low-uptake thyrotoxicosis [289].

"Recurrence" of disease is common in silent thyroiditis but very rare in subacute thyroiditis. Considering all these data, it is conceivable that silent thyroiditis is caused by an exacerbation of autoimmune thyroiditis induced by aggravating factors. Thyroiditis frequently recurs, and seasonal *allergic rhinitis* is reported to be an initiation factor [290]. Physically vigorous *massage on the neck* also was reported to be a contributing factor for silent thyroiditis [291]. The prevalence of silent thyroiditis, including postpartum disease, is approximately 5% of all types of thyrotoxicosis. Spontaneous silent thyroiditis is three times more frequent than PPT.

An immune rebound mechanism has been established for the induction of PPT [275]. Postpartum thyroid destruction is associated with an increase in NK-cell counts and activity [26]. Cessation of steroid therapy has initiated silent thyroiditis in a patient with autoimmune thyroiditis and rheumatoid arthritis [292], presumably because this also allows immune rebound. In patients with Cushing's syndrome who have associated subclinical autoimmune thyroiditis, silent thyroiditis has occurred after unilateral adrenalectomy [293].

Typically, painless thyroiditis or destructive thyrotoxicosis occurs at 2–4 months postpartum. The prevalence of PPT ranges from 3 to 8% of all pregnancies (26). Possible prevention of PPT was shown in a randomized prospective controlled study where 77 TPO+ pregnant women received 200 μg seleno-methionine daily starting at the 12th week of pregnancy, and 74 TPO+ women received a placebo. The treated group had significantly lower TPO antibody levels at the end of pregnancy and during the postpartum while on treatment. The incidence of PPT was reduced from 48.6 to 28.6% in the treated group, and the incidence of permanent hypothyroidism was equivalently reduced. Thyroid hormone levels did not differ [294].

9.7.11 Hashimoto's Encephalopathy

Hashimoto's encephalopathy or encephalitis is a very rare complication of Hashimoto's thyroiditis. Neurological complications are sometimes associated with thyroid dysfunction, but patients with this encephalopathy are usually euthyroid. It is treatable, steroid-responsive, progressive, or relapsing encephalopathy associated with elevation of thyroid-specific autoantibodies [295]. This condition was first described in 1966 [296] and may present as a subacute or acute encephalopathy with seizures and stroke-like episodes, often in association with myoclonus and tremor [297]. It is associated with abnormal EEG and high CSF proteins without pleocytosis. Some patients suffer from a significant residual disability [298]. Antibody to α-enolase has been identified in some patients, but this antibody is also frequently found in other autoimmune diseases [299].

In 2002, Sawka et al. [300] reported that Hashimoto's encephalopathy is *not* caused by thyroid dysfunction or anti-thyroid antibodies but represents an "association of an uncommon autoimmune encephalopathy" with a common autoimmune thyroid disease. Identification of antibodies to brain specific antigens may disclose the real pathogenesis of this condition. Recently, autoantibodies against the amino NH2-terminal of α-enolase (referred to as NAE) were reported to be highly specific in the serum of a limited number of Hashimoto's encephalopathy patients (11%, 2/17), but in none of the controls ($n = 25$) including those with other neurological or immunological conditions involving encephalopathy [301, 302].

Steroid-reversible cerebral hypo-metabolism was recently documented by PET-scan in this condition [303]. There is a report that Hashimoto's encephalopathy is associated with elevated intra-thecal and serum IgG4 levels [304]. Additional case studies, including histological investigations as well as measurements of IgG4, are needed to elucidate the pathological role of IgG4 in Hashimoto's encephalopathy.

9.7.12 Hashimoto's Ophthalmopathy

Thyroid-associated orbitopathy (TAO) usually occurs in Graves' disease with hyperthyroidism, and sometimes in euthyroid and hypothyroid patients. Since most euthyroid and hypothyroid patients with orbitopathy are thyrotropin receptor antibody (TRAb)-positive, they are diagnosed as having euthyroid Graves' disease or hypothyroid Graves' disease. When euthyroid and hypothyroid patients with orbitopathy are TRAb-negative but associated with Hashimoto's thyroiditis, "Hashimoto's ophthalmopathy" may be considered [253, 254]. Because patients with Hashimoto's thyroiditis test negative for TRAb, other autoantibodies against an eye muscle antigen, such as calsequestrin, flavoprotein, or G2s, were postulated [255].

9.7.13 Summary of Hashimoto's Thyroiditis Presentations

Hashimoto's thyroiditis presents in the age group of 40–60 years with female predominance as painless enlargement of the thyroid gland. Cases of painful goiter in Hashimoto's thyroiditis have been reported. Clinically, the patient can be euthyroid, hyperthyroid, or hypothyroid based on the degree of thyroid destruction. Patients with Hashimoto's thyroiditis present initially with features of hyperthyroidism due to the release of preformed thyroxin from the destroyed thyroid follicles. The disease then progresses to subclinical and overt hypothyroidism and ultimately thyroid failure.

There can be local compressive effect of the goiter such as dysphagia (esophagus), dysphonia (recurrent laryngeal nerve (RLN)), and dyspnea (trachea). In the fibrous form, the thyroid gland appears lobulated with features of hypothyroidism. In the fibrous atrophy variant, the gland may not be palpable, and the patient presents with idiopathic myxedema. The IgG4-variant presents at the fifth decade with a female-to-male ratio of 3:1 and has a rapid and aggressive course. The juvenile variant presents before 18 years of age and is usually asymptomatic. The Hashitoxicosis variant has clinical features similar to Graves' hyperthyroidism initially, but finally hypothyroidism evolves. Painless (silent variant) occurs within 12 months after delivery (also known as postpartum thyroiditis). Spontaneous recovery is possible after a period of time [305].

9.8 Diagnosis

9.8.1 Clinical Evaluation

A diffuse, firm goiter with pyramidal lobe enlargement, and without signs of thyrotoxicosis, should suggest the diagnosis of Hashimoto's thyroiditis. Most often, the gland is bosselated. It is usually symmetrical, although much variation in symmetry (as well as consistency) can occur. The trachea is rarely deviated or compressed. The association of goiter with hypothyroidism is almost diagnostic of Hashimoto's disease, but is also seen in certain syndromes due to defective hormone synthesis or hormone response.

Pain and tenderness are unusual but may be present. A rapid onset is also unusual, but the goiter may rarely grow from normal to several times the normal size in a few weeks. Most commonly, the gland is 2–4 times the normal size. Satellite lymph nodes may be present, especially the Delphian node above the isthmus. Multinodular goiter (MNG) occurs in significant incidence in adult women; thus, the association of MNG and Hashimoto's thyroiditis is not rare and may provide the finding of a grossly nodular gland in a patient who is mildly hypothyroid and has positive antibody tests.

9.8.1.1 History-Taking

Common, early-presenting symptoms of hypothyroidism, such as fatigue, constipation, dry skin, and weight gain, are non-specific. Weight gain due to hypothyroidism is usually no greater than 10% of the baseline euthyroid weight and is mostly attributable to fluid accumulation in interstitial tissues.

Other symptoms of hypothyroidism include the following:

- Cold intolerance.
- Hoarseness of voice and pressure symptoms in the neck from thyroid enlargement.
- Laziness and loss of energy (chronic fatigue syndrome), and less frequently, erectile dysfunction.
- Decreased sweating.
- Mild nerve deafness.
- Peripheral neuropathy.
- Galactorrhea (may occur because of the increased prolactin levels).
- Depression, dementia, and other psychiatric disturbances. Hashimoto's when presenting as "mania" is known as "Prasad's syndrome" after *Ashok Prasad*, the psychiatrist who first described it.
- Memory loss.
- Joint pains and muscle cramps.
- Hair loss from an autoimmune process directed against the hair follicles.
- Menstrual irregularities (typically menorrhagia, infertility, and loss of libido). Increased prolactin secondary to increased thyrotropin-releasing hormone (TRH) leads to decreased luteinizing hormone (LH) and follicle-stimulating hormone (FSH) and to decreased response to gonadotropin-releasing hormone (GnRH), resulting in anovulatory cycles with menstrual irregularities
- Sleep apnea and daytime somnolence ("obstructive sleep apnea" in hypothyroidism is thought to be partly caused by hypofunction of upper airway muscles and weakness of the diaphragm).

9.8.1.2 Physical Examination

Physical findings are variable and depend on the extent of hypothyroidism and other factors such as *age* of the patient. Findings include the following:

- Puffy face and peri-orbital edema typical of hypothyroid facies.
- Cold, dry skin, which may be rough and scaly. The skin may appear yellow but does not involve the sclera, which distinguishes it from the yellowing of jaundice due to hyper-carotenemia.
- Peripheral edema of hands and feet, typically non-pitting.

- Thickened and brittle nails (may appear ridged).
- Hair loss involving the scalp, the lateral third of eyebrows, and possibly skin, genital, and facial hair.
- Bradycardia.
- Elevated blood pressure (typically diastolic hypertension); however, most often, blood pressure is normal or even low.
- Diminished deep tendon reflexes and the classic prolonged relaxation phase, most notable and initially described at the Achilles tendon (although it may be present in other deep tendon reflexes as well).
- Macroglossia.
- The thyroid gland is typically enlarged, firm, and rubbery, without any tenderness or bruit; it may be normal in size or not palpable at all.
- Hoarseness of voice.
- Slow speech.
- Impaired memory.
- Peripheral neuropathy (either mono-neuropathy as exemplified by carpal tunnel syndrome, or poly-neuropathy due to involvement of several peripheral nerves, manifesting as paresthesia).
- Cerebellar ataxia.

9.8.2 Laboratory Studies

9.8.2.1 Overview

Thyroid function tests are commonly employed to assess the hormonal status of Hashimoto's thyroiditis by assessing the levels of thyroid-stimulating hormone (TSH), tri-iodothyronine (T3), and tetra-iodothyronine (T4). Among these, TSH is the sensitive marker of hypothyroidism and diagnosis of subclinical hypothyroidism. Frequent monitoring of TSH is needed to assess the response of the treatment and disease progression.

Low levels of thyroid hormones (T4 and T3) with high TSH and circulating thyroid autoantibodies against TPO (in 70–90% of cases) and Tg (in 40–70% of cases) suggest the diagnosis of Hashimoto's thyroiditis [5]. Occasionally, the patient presents initially with hyperthyroidism associated with the presence of anti-TSH receptor antibodies [265].

9.8.2.2 Thyroxin (T4) Level

Total thyroxin (TT4) and free thyroxin (FT4) concentrations range from low to high, but are most typically in the normal or low range [306]. The radioactive iodine uptake (RAIU) (rarely required) is variable and ranges from below normal to elevated values, depending on such factors as TSH levels, the efficiency of use of iodide by the thyroid, and the nature of the components being released into the circulation.

When the serum TSH and the free T4 levels are low in the outpatient setting, the case for central hypothyroidism is strengthened. However, in the acutely ill patient, non-thyroidal illness (euthyroid sick syndrome) is the more likely possibility. The TSH level cannot be reliably used in some clinical settings to distinguish central hypothyroidism from non-thyroidal illness. Physical findings suggestive of thyroid disease, as well as the presence of obvious or subtle clinical features of hypothyroidism, become pivotal in establishing the correct diagnosis.

9.8.2.3 Tri-iodothyronine (T3) Level

A low T3 level and a high reverse T3 level may be of additional help in the diagnosis of non-thyroidal illness. Serum T3 levels are most often maintained within reference ranges (even in the very late stages of hypothyroidism), and T3 measurement has little value in the diagnosis of hypothyroidism. Furthermore, T3 levels may be low in up to 70% of hospitalized patients without hypothyroidism or any thyroid disease, as is the case with non-thyroidal illness.

9.8.2.4 Serum TSH Level

Serum TSH reflects the patient's metabolic status. However, some patients are clinically euthyroid, with normal FT4 and T3 levels, but have mildly elevated TSH. Whether this "subclinical hypothyroidism" represents partial or complete compensation is a matter of debate. In the outpatient setting, when there is no cause to suspect hypothalamic or pituitary disease and in the absence of non-thyroidal illness and of medications that suppress TSH production in the inpatient setting, a normal TSH level excludes primary hypothyroidism from any cause. Medications that suppress TSH production include steroids, dopamine, dobutamine, and octreotide.

9.8.2.5 Gamma-Globulin Level

Gamma-globulin levels may be elevated, although usually they are normal. This alteration evidently reflects the presence of high concentrations of circulating antibodies to thyroglobulin (Tg), for an antibody concentration as high as 5.2 mg/ml has been reported [307].

9.8.2.6 Thyroid Antibodies

Thyroid peroxidase antibodies (TPO-Ab), and less frequently, thyroglobulin antibodies (Tg-Ab) are found in the serum of patients with Hashimoto's thyroiditis. High levels are diagnostic of autoimmune thyroid disease. However, 10–15% of patients with Hashimoto's thyroiditis may be antibody-negative. Anti-TPO-Abs are considered as the best serological marker to establish the diagnosis of Hashimoto's thyroiditis. It is positive in about 95% of patients, whereas anti-Tg-Abs are positive in 60–80%. Young patients tend to have lower and occasionally negative levels. In this age group, even low titers signify the presence of thyroid autoimmunity [306].

9.8.3 Cytology/Histology

Hashimoto's thyroiditis is a "histological" diagnosis. Fine-needle aspiration (FNA) can be a useful diagnostic procedure, but it is infrequently required, except in patients who have a discrete "nodule" in the gland. The FNAC may frequently show

Hürthle cells, and it may be difficult to distinguish Hashimoto's thyroiditis at times from a follicular neoplasm, PTC, or low-grade MALT lymphoma. Immunohistochemistry (IHC) studies may help to reach the diagnosis.

Histologically, the thyroid gland typically shows diffuse lymphocytic and plasma cell infiltration with formation of lymphoid follicles from follicular hyperplasia and damage to the follicular basement membrane. Atrophy of the thyroid parenchyma is usually evident. It also reveals scant colloid, and a few epithelial cells, which may show Hürthle cell change. In this context, Hürthle cells do *not* represent a discrete adenoma. However, if only abundant Hürthle cells dominate the specimen, and there are few or no lymphocytes or macrophages, the biopsy must be interpreted as a possible Hürthle cell tumor. Correlation of FNA findings with the presence of anti-TPO and anti-Tg antibodies is helpful in confirming the diagnosis of Hashimoto's thyroiditis. Biopsy results are less frequently diagnostic in children [308].

9.8.4 Isotope Scanning

Thyroid isotope scan is *not* usually necessary, but can be helpful. The image is characteristically that of a diffuse or mottled uptake in an enlarged gland, in striking contrast to the focal "cold" and "hot" areas of multinodular goiter. Focal loss of isotope accumulation may occur in severely diseased portions of the thyroid. A cold thyroid nodule would indicate a higher risk for malignancy and therefore a need for fine-needle aspiration (FNA).

9.8.5 Ultrasound Imaging

Ultrasound (US) may display an enlarged thyroid gland with "normal" texture, focal or diffuse glandular enlargement with coarse, heterogenous, and hypo-echoic pattern, or a suggestion of multiple ill-defined nodules (Fig. 9.5) [199]. The

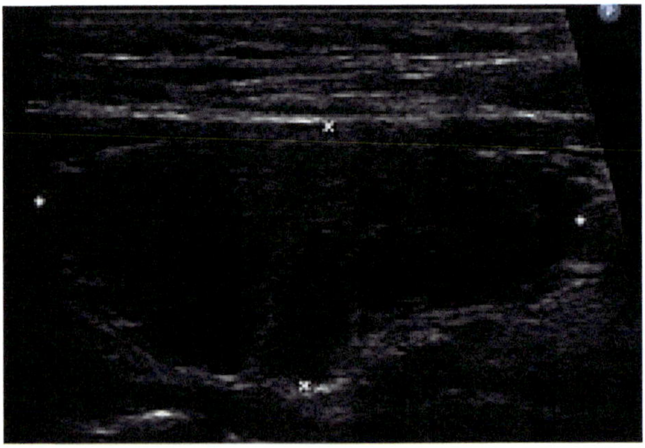

Fig. 9.5 Ultrasound imaging of the thyroid gland (right lobe longitudinal) in a patient with Hashimoto's thyroiditis

presence of discrete hypo-echoic micro-nodules (1–6 mm) is strongly suggestive of chronic thyroiditis. Fine echogenic fibrous septa may produce a pseudo-lobulated appearance. Color Doppler shows extensive hyper-vascularity.

Although features of Hashimoto's thyroiditis are usually identifiable on US, it is usually not necessary for diagnosing the condition. However, US is useful for assessing thyroid size, echo-texture, and, most importantly, whether thyroid nodules are present. Ultrasonographic study aids in confirming the presence of a thyroid nodule, in defining a nodule as solid or cystic, and in defining features suggestive of malignancy, such as irregular margins, a poorly defined halo, micro-calcification, and increased vascularity on Doppler examination. Ultrasonography is also useful in facilitating FNA of nodules in general and, in particular, small or poorly defined nodules when indicated and in patients with distorted neck anatomy. A definite diagnosis of benign versus malignant thyroid lesion can be confirmed only by cytological or histological examination of thyroid tissue.

9.8.6 Evaluating Variations in Presentation of Hashimoto's Thyroiditis

Small "atrophic gland" may be present at end stage of disease. A "nodular" form may be present in the background of diffuse thyroiditis seen on ultrasound. Benign and malignant nodules may co-exist in the background of diffuse thyroiditis. For differentiation between both, FNAC is needed.

9.8.7 Evaluating Complications of Hypothyroidism

The following tests are *not* necessary for the diagnosis of primary hypothyroidism, but may be performed to evaluate complications of hypothyroidism in some patients, when clearly indicated.

9.8.7.1 Complete Blood Count

Up to 30–40% of patients with hypothyroidism have anemia, usually from decreased erythropoiesis. In 15% of patients, it is a microcytic, hypochromic iron deficiency anemia. Although this can be a normocytic normochromic anemia, the most common morphologic abnormality is a macrocytic anemia that may be partially due to insufficient vitamin B_{12} and folate intake.

9.8.7.2 Total and Fractionated Lipid Profile

Total cholesterol, low-density lipid (LDL), and triglyceride levels may be elevated in hypothyroidism and may be responsive to levothyroxine (L-T4) replacement.

9.8.7.3 Basic Metabolic Panel

Glomerular filtration rate (GFR), renal plasma flow, and renal free water clearance are all decreased in hypothyroidism and may result in hyponatremia.

9.8.7.4 Creatine Kinase

Creatine kinase levels, predominantly the MM isoenzyme from skeletal muscle and the aldolase enzyme, are frequently elevated in severe hypothyroidism.

9.8.7.5 Prolactin

Prolactin may be elevated in primary hypothyroidism, probably due to overlap secretion due to stimulation of the lactotroph by the elevated thyrotropin-releasing hormone (TRH) level. The decreased clearance of prolactin in hypothyroidism may also play a contributory role. The elevated prolactin level leads to decreased gonadotropin secretion and decreased responsiveness to gonadotropin-releasing hormone (GnRH). The result of this is anovulatory cycles with menstrual abnormalities, galactorrhea, and infertility in some patients.

9.8.8 Additional Studies

Other studies that are usually *not* routinely necessary for diagnosis or evaluation of hypothyroid patients, but may be performed for evaluation of complications of primary hypothyroidism (when indicated), include:

- *Chest radiograph*: It may show small pleural effusions.
- *Electrocardiogram (ECG):* It may show low-voltage QRS tracing, nonspecific ST-wave changes, and premature ventricular contractions; prolongation of the QT interval, and ventricular tachycardia may be noted.
- *Echocardiogram*: It may show some pericardial effusion in severe cases of hypothyroidism.

9.9 Differential Diagnosis

In general, diseases that should be considered in the differential diagnosis of HT include subacute thyroiditis and Riedel's thyroiditis, Graves' disease, hypopituitarism, lithium-induced goiter, non-toxic goiter, thyroid neoplasm (PTC) [309, 310], lymphoma [311–314], toxic nodular goiter, and type-I and type-II poly-glandular autoimmune syndrome.

9.9.1 Thyroiditis

Hashimoto's thyroiditis should be distinguished from other forms of thyroiditis.

- *Subacute granulomatous thyroiditis:* It is a self-limiting, painful disorder of the thyroid. Clinical examination, elevated erythrocyte sedimentation rate (ESR), elevated thyroglobulin (Tg) level, and decreased radioactive iodine (RAI) uptake confirm the diagnosis.

- *Acute suppurative thyroiditis*: It is a rare infectious condition of the thyroid.
- *Riedel's thyroiditis*: It is a fibrosing disorder of thyroid characterized by hypothyroidism and hypocalcemia, and diagnosis is made by histopathology.

9.9.2 Multinodular Goiter (MNG)

Hashimoto's thyroiditis is to be also distinguished from non-toxic nodular goiter or Graves' disease. The presence of gross nodularity is strong evidence against Hashimoto's thyroiditis, but differentiation on this basis is not reliable. In multinodular goiter (MNG), thyroid function test results are usually normal, and the patient is only rarely clinically hypothyroid. Thyroid autoantibodies tend to be absent or titers are low, and the scan result is typical. Fine-needle aspiration (FNA) can resolve the question, but it is usually unnecessary. In fact, the two conditions quite commonly occur together in adult women. Whether this is a coincidence or due to the effect of thyroid growth-stimulating antibodies (or other causes) is still unknown.

Moderately and diffusely enlarged thyroid glands in teenagers are usually the result of thyroiditis, but some may be true adolescent goiters; that is, the enlargement may result from moderate hyperplasia of the thyroid gland in response to a temporarily increased demand for hormone. This condition is more often diagnosed than proved. Thyroid function test results should be normal. Antibody assays may resolve the issue. The diagnosis can be settled with certainty only by a biopsy disclosing normal or hyperplastic thyroid tissue and absence of findings of thyroiditis.

9.9.3 Colloid Goiter

The possibility of "colloid goiter" may also be entertained in the differential diagnosis of Hashimoto's thyroiditis. Colloid goiter is a definite pathological entity. Presumably, it is the resting phase after a period of thyroid hyperplasia.

9.9.4 Thyroid Neoplasm

A thyroid tumor must also be considered in the differential diagnosis of Hashimoto's disease, particularly if there is rapid growth of the gland or persistent pain. The diffuse nature of autoimmune thyroiditis, the characteristic hypothyroidism, and involvement of the pyramidal lobe are usually sufficient for differentiation. It is still uncertain whether FNA is indicated. However, it must be remembered that lymphoma or a small-cell carcinoma of the thyroid can be and has been mistaken for Hashimoto's thyroiditis.

Clusters of nodes at the upper poles strongly suggesting papillary thyroid carcinoma (PTC) may disappear when thyroid hormone replacement therapy is given.

However, a sufficient number of patients with both thyroiditis and tumor have been recorded. Thus, one diagnosis in no way excludes the other. Papillary thyroid carcinoma with Hashimoto's thyroiditis is characterized by (1) female predominance, (2) multi-focality, (3) no extra-thyroid extension, (4) no lymph node metastasis, and (5) better recurrence-free survival [309–311].

Thyroid lymphoma must always be considered if there is continued (especially asymmetric) enlargement of a Hashimoto's gland, or if pain, tenderness, hoarseness, or nodes develop. Thyroiditis is a risk factor for thyroid lymphoma, although the incidence is very low. Distinguishing thyroid lymphoma from Hashimoto's thyroiditis is sometimes quite difficult by cytology alone. Flow cytometry, immunehistochemistry (IHC), or polymerase chain reaction (PCR) should aid in diagnosis. Reverse transcription-polymerase chain reaction (RT-PCR) detecting the monoclonality of immunoglobulin heavy chain mRNA is useful for differentiation between the two [311–314].

9.9.5 Thyrotoxicosis

Occasionally, the picture of Hashimoto's thyroiditis blends rather imperceptibly into that of thyrotoxicosis, and some patients have symptoms of mild thyrotoxicosis, but then develop typical Hashimoto's thyroiditis. In fact, it is best to think of Graves' disease and Hashimoto's thyroiditis as two very closely related syndromes produced by thyroid autoimmunity. Categorization depends on associated eye findings and the metabolic level, but the pathogenesis, histological picture, and function may overlap. Some patients may have a mixture of Hashimoto's thyroiditis and subacute thyroiditis, with goiter, positive thyroid autoantibodies, and normal or low FT4 [309, 310].

9.9.6 Amyloidosis

A form of painful chronic thyroiditis with amyloid infiltration has also been described, and is probably etiologically distinct from Hashimoto's thyroiditis [315].

9.9.7 Other Autoimmune Diseases

Other autoimmune diseases like Addison's disease, diabetes mellitus (DM) type-1, rheumatoid arthritis, systemic lupus erythematosus (SLE), or vitiligo can co-exist with Hashimoto's thyroiditis.

Diseases that should be considered in the differential diagnosis of Hashimoto's thyroiditis are summarized in Table 9.4.

Table 9.4 Differential diagnosis of Hashimoto's disease

Subacute thyroiditis and Riedel's thyroiditis
Diffuse toxic goiter (Graves' disease)
Euthyroid sick syndrome
Goiter
Hypopituitarism (pan-hypopituitarism)
Lithium-induced goiter
Simple nodular (non-toxic) goiter
Thyroid lymphoma
Toxic nodular goiter
Type-I poly-glandular autoimmune syndrome
Type-II poly-glandular autoimmune syndrome

9.10 Management

9.10.1 Introduction

Hypothyroidism caused by Hashimoto's thyroiditis is treated with thyroid hormone replacement agents such as levothyroxine (L-T4), tri-iodothyronine, or desiccated thyroid extract. A tablet taken once a day generally keeps the thyroid hormone levels normal. In most cases, the treatment needs to be taken for the rest of the person's life. In the event that hypothyroidism is caused by Hashimoto's thyroiditis, it is recommended that the TSH levels be kept under 3.0.

9.10.2 No Treatment: Observation and Monitoring

Many patients with HT require no treatment, for frequently the disease is *asymptomatic* and the goiter is small. This approach is justified by the old study of Vickery and Hamlin (1961) [316] who found, on both clinical and pathological grounds, that the disease may remain static and the clinical condition unchanged over many years. Some cases of spontaneous recovery of HT have been reported [317].

9.10.3 Medical Treatment/Balanced Diet

9.10.3.1 Overview

Treatment of Hashimoto's thyroiditis is mainly medical, supplementing L-thyroxin (L-T4) for overt hypothyroidism, usually for life. L-thyroxin has proved to reduce the volume of the thyroid gland in both hypothyroidism and even euthyroid state [315]. The dosage of thyroxin should normally be that required to bring the serum TSH level to the low normal range, such as 0.3–1 μU/ml. This is typically achieved with 1 μg L-T4/lb body weight/day, ranging from 75 to 125 μg/day in women and 125 to 200 μg/day in men. The level of TSH is frequently monitored for dose adjustment till euthyroid state is attained thereafter every 6–12 months. Treatment of children and adolescents with 1.3 μg/kg/day thyroxine for 24 months was shown in a recent study to cause a significant reduction in thyroid size in patients with autoimmune thyroiditis, but *not* affect antibody levels, or significantly alter TSH or free T4 [318].

When L-T4 and seleno-methionine are given together, they reduce the release of cytokines from monocytes and lymphocytes, thus reducing the thyroid peroxidase antibody titer and autoimmune process in Hashimoto's thyroiditis [319].

The additional role of diet for the management of Hashimoto's thyroiditis is usually overlooked, and careful supplementation of possible deficiencies in Hashimoto's thyroiditis is recommended for the dietary management of these patients. There are specific nutrients that should be regularly taken to maintain a healthy and functional thyroid. The top nutrients are iodine (I_2), selenium (Se), and zinc (Zn). A diet optimizing these nutrients is vital to an overall recovery plan. Diets beneficial for patients with HT include paleo diet, gluten-free diet, and vegetarian or vegan diet. Gluten and goitrogens are the worst foods to have in the diet of patients with HT as they can have a negative impact on the thyroid.

9.10.3.2 L-Thyroxine (L-T4) Replacement Therapy

Indications

If the goiter is problematic because of local pressure symptoms or disfigurement, thyroid hormone therapy is indicated. Thyroid hormone often causes a gratifying reduction in the size of the goiter after several months of treatment [315], particularly in young patients. It seems likely that in older patients there may be more fibrosis and therefore a less tendency for the thyroid to shrink. In young patients, the response often occurs within 2–4 weeks, but in older ones, the thyroid decreases in size more gradually. In 2005, Aksoy et al. [320] reported that "prophylactic" thyroid hormone treatment is associated with a decrease in thyroid size and in thyroid antibody levels 15 months after initiation of therapy.

Thyroid hormone in a full replacement dose is, of course, indicated if hypothyroidism is present. Therapy is probably indicated if the TSH level is elevated and the FT4 is low normal (subclinical hypothyroidism), since the onset of hypothyroidism is predictable in such patients. There is no evidence that thyroid replacement actually halts the ongoing process of thyroiditis, but in some patients receiving treatment, antibody levels gradually fall over many years [321].

Dosage of Levo-thyroxine (L-T4)

The dosage of thyroxine should normally be that required to bring the serum TSH level to the low normal range, such as 0.3–1 μU/ml. This is typically achieved with 1 μg L-T4/lb body weight/day, ranging from 75 to 125 μg/day in women and 125 to 200 μg/day in men. Elderly patients and patients on androgens for various reasons usually require decreased levothyroxine replacement dosing. Patients who have undergone bowel resection and have short-bowel syndrome (or malabsorption for any reason) often require increased doses of levothyroxine to maintain the euthyroid state.

It is sensible to initiate therapy with a partial dose, since in some instances the thyroid gland may be non-suppressible even though functioning at a level below normal. Once thyroxine treatment is initiated, it is required indefinitely in most patients. However, it has been reported that up to 20% of initially hypothyroid individuals will later recover and have normal thyroid function if challenged by replacement hormone withdrawal. This may represent subsidence of cytotoxic antibodies, modulation of TSH-Ab, or some other mechanism [211]. These individuals can be identified by administration of TRH, which will induce an increase in serum T4 and T3 if the thyroid has recovered [322].

Replacement L-T4 therapy should be taken several hours before or after medications such as cholesterol-binding resins (cholestyramine), sucralfate, calcium carbonate, aluminium hydroxide, and other antacids, in addition to ferrous sulfate and iron-containing multi-vitamins, all of which can reduce absorption of L-T4 [323]. Medications that enhance the metabolism and clearance of levothyroxine may necessitate an increase in the replacement dose. These medications include phenytoin, carbamazepine, and rifampin.

Autoimmune disease usually takes an ongoing process, and Hashimoto's thyroiditis develops into hypothyroidism. Recent trial of "prophylactic" treatment with L-T4 (1.0–2.0 μg/Kg/day) for 1 year in "euthyroid" patients with Hashimoto's thyroiditis showed decrease of anti-TPO antibodies and thyroid B-lymphocytes [324] suggesting that prophylactic L-T4 therapy might be useful in stopping progression of the disease. The long-term clinical benefit should be established in the future.

Whether or not "subclinical" hypothyroidism should be treated is still under debate. Cardiac dysfunction may be associated with subclinical hypothyroidism, even when serum TSH is still in the normal range. These abnormalities are reversible with L-T4 replacement therapy [325]. In their study of 830 patients with Hashimoto's thyroiditis, Tagami et al. [82] (2009) reported that, following treatment with small doses of L-T4 in 32 of patients with subclinical hypothyroidism, significant decreases occurred in the patients' total cholesterol, low-density lipids (LDL), and non-HDL levels, as well as in their LDL/HDL ratios.

Treatment of children and adolescents with 1.3 μg/kg/day thyroxine for 24 months was shown in a recent study to cause significant reduction in thyroid size in patients with autoimmune thyroiditis, but not affect antibody levels, or significantly alter TSH or freeT4 [326].

Combination Therapy

One popular treatment, more so among patients than physicians, is the combined use of liothyronine (T3) and levothyroxine (L-T4) in an effort to mimic more closely thyroid hormone physiology. However, review of literature showed that out of nine controlled clinical trials, only one indicated that combined therapy seemed to improve the mood, quality of life, and psychometric performance of patients more than did L-T4 alone [327]. Until investigators can demonstrate a definite advantage to the administration of L-T4 plus T3, the use of levothyroxine alone should remain the treatment of choice for replacement therapy in hypothyroidism.

Replacement Therapy During Pregnancy

Pregnancy induces a state of increased need for levothyroxine. In women with hypothyroidism and in women with inadequate thyroid reserve from Hashimoto's thyroiditis or partial thyroidectomy, this is manifested by an increase in the level of TSH and a decrease in the level of free T4 (overt hypothyroidism).

The increase in L-T4 requirement is thought to be due to increased levels of thyroid hormone–binding protein, increased use by the fetus, and increased metabolism of thyroxine by the feto-placental unit. The increase usually resolves, and levothyroxine requirements return to the pre-pregnancy levels 6–8 weeks postpartum. The pregnancy-induced increased need for T4 occurs in the first trimester, usually within the first 8 weeks, and persists throughout pregnancy. Patients with hypothyroidism may require up to a 45–50% increase in L-T4 dose.

Patients who are diagnosed with Hashimoto's thyroiditis or hypothyroidism from any cause during pregnancy should be started on a levothyroxine dose close to their replacement requirement, and the TSH level should be normalized as soon as possible. Untreated hypothyroidism carries increased maternal and fetal complications. The incidence of fetal loss is increased in patients who are TPO antibody positive.

Patients with hypothyroidism are best followed up by monitoring the TSH and free T4 levels. Upon becoming pregnant, patients should have the TSH and free T4 levels checked within 4–8 weeks and then every 6–8 weeks while dose adjustments are being made. Patients who are adequately dosed and who are in a clinically and biochemically euthyroid state should have thyroid function tests (TSH and free T4) every 8 weeks. Dose adjustments should be made to keep the free T4 and TSH within reference ranges.

A transient reduction in serum TSH levels occurs toward the end of the first trimester, owing to high circulating levels of human chorionic gonadotropin (hCG); this phenomenon is often confused with hyperthyroidism.

Levothyroxine Replacement for Myxedema Coma

Myxedema coma is a state of extreme hypothyroidism with a very high mortality rate (approaching 60%). Patients with this condition usually present with an acute precipitating condition, most often in the setting of long-standing, undiagnosed hypothyroidism, discontinuation of L-T4 replacement therapy, or failure to institute T4 replacement after radioactive iodine (RAI) ablation of the thyroid in Graves' disease or after total thyroidectomy. The usual precipitating causes include infection, cardiovascular accident, pulmonary infection, congestive cardiac failure, and drugs such as narcotics, sedatives, anesthetic agents, anti-depressants, and tranquilizers (all of which depress the respiratory drive).

Myxedema coma typically manifests in winter (or during extremely cold weather) in an elderly woman who has long-standing hypothyroidism. Hospitalized patients may have a history of sedating medication use. Typical clinical findings include hypothermia, obtundation or coma, hypoventilation, bradycardia, hyponatremia, hypoglycemia, and hypotension. Those patients have an elevated TSH level and may have undetectable free T4 levels.

Therapy should be conducted in an intensive care unit (ICU), where patients may require the following:

- Ventilatory support for hypoventilation and carbon dioxide retention.
- Electrocardiographic monitoring and a Swan-Ganz catheter insertion for hemodynamic monitoring.
- Judicious re-warming to avoid excessive vasodilatation, which would increase oxygen consumption and could lead to worsening of hypotension and vascular collapse.
- Steroids, preferably hydrocortisone in stress doses.
- Treatment of infection or any other precipitating causes.
- Fluid restriction with or without hypertonic saline and Lasix to promote water diuresis.
- Levothyroxine: L-T4 is administered intravenously (IV) in a loading dose of 4 mcg/kg of lean body weight (approximately 300–600 mcg), which should be administered by rapid IV injection. The daily maintenance dose is 50–100 mcg/d, administered IV until the patient can take it orally.

9.10.3.3 Glucocorticoids

In some instances, the acute onset of Hashimoto's disease, in association with pain, has prompted therapy with glucocorticoids. This treatment alleviates the symptoms and improves the associated biochemical abnormalities, and in some studies has been shown to increase plasma T3 and T4 levels by suppression of the autoimmune process [327]. Blizzard and co-workers (1962) [328] prescribed steroids for children with Hashimoto's disease over several months in an attempt at suppressing antibody production and possibly achieving a permanent remission. The adrenocortical hormones dramatically depress clinical activity of the disease and antibody titers, but all return to pre-therapy levels when treatment is withdrawn. Steroid therapy is currently *not* recommended for Hashimoto's thyroiditis because of the undesirable side effects of the drug.

9.10.3.4 Chloroquine

Chloroquine has been reported in one study to reduce antibody titers [329]. However, because of the toxicity of this drug, its use is *not advised*.

9.10.3.5 Selenium

In a randomized prospective controlled study, 77 TPO+ pregnant women received 200 μg seleno-methionine daily starting at the 12th week of pregnancy, and 74 TPO+ women received a placebo. The treated group had significantly lower TPO antibody levels at the end of pregnancy and during the postpartum while on treatment. The incidence of postpartum thyroiditis (PPT) was reduced from 48.6 to 28.6% in the treated group, and the incidence of permanent hypothyroidism was equivalently reduced. However, thyroid hormone levels did *not* differ [330]. Confirming earlier studies, in Hashimoto's patients, 200 mμg Se in the form of L-seleno-methionine orally for 6 months caused a significant reduction of 21% in serum anti-TPO levels, but cessation caused an increase in the anti-TPO concentrations [331].

A slightly opposing study, however, reported no immunological benefit of selenium in patients with moderate disease activity (in terms of TPO-Ab and cytokine production patterns) or those with high disease activity [332]. Selenium responsiveness may be different among patients with Hashimoto's thyroiditis. A systematic review and meta-analysis revealed that selenium supplementation reduced serum TPO-Ab levels after 3, 6, and 12 months in an LT4-treated Hashimoto's population, and after 3 months in an untreated population [332]. However, no effect of selenium supplementation on thyroid-stimulating hormone, health-related quality of life, or thyroid ultrasound was found in levothyroxine substitution-untreated individuals, and sporadic evaluation of clinically relevant outcomes in levothyroxine substitution-treated patients [333].

Future well-powered randomized controlled trials (RCTs), evaluating disease progression or health-related quality of life, are warranted before determining the relevance of selenium supplementation in autoimmune thyroiditis. Further, combined treatment with *myo-inositol and selenium* was reported that the beneficial effects obtained by seleno-methionine treatment on patients affected by subclinical hypothyroidism were further improved by combination with myo-inositol [334]. Myo-inositol is an isomer of a C6 sugar alcohol and plays an important role in several cellular processes. In particular, it has been demonstrated that myo-inositol is the precursor for the synthesis of phospho-inositides, which are part of the phosphatidyl-inositol (Ptd-Ins) signal transduction pathway. In one study, the administration of myo-inositol plus selenium has been reported to be effective in decreasing TSH, TPO-Ab, and Tg-Ab levels, as well as enhancing thyroid hormones and personal wellbeing, therefore restoring euthyroidism in patients diagnosed with Hashimoto's thyroiditis [335].

9.10.3.6 Anatabine

Anatabine, an alkaloid found in "Solanaceae plants" including tobacco, has been reported to ameliorate a mouse model of Hashimoto's thyroiditis [336]. In a double-blind, randomized, placebo-controlled multi-center study for 3 months, anatabine-treated patients had a significant reduction in absolute serum Tg-Ab levels from baseline by study end relative to those on placebo [337]. Further studies are warranted to determine longer-term effects and possible actions of anatabine on the course of Hashimoto's thyroiditis.

9.10.4 Surgical Treatment

9.10.4.1 Indications

Surgery has been used as a method of therapy for Hashimoto's disease. This treatment, of course, removes the goiter, but usually results in hypothyroidism. Generally, surgery is *not* indicated unless significant pain, cosmetic problems, or pressure symptoms (e.g., dysphagia, dyspnea, and dysphonia) remain after a fair trial of thyroid therapy. Among patients with postpartum thyroid dysfunction, the most common type is destructive thyrotoxicosis, and simple symptomatic treatment, using beta-adrenergic antagonists, is usually sufficient [338]. In the case of postpartum hypothyroidism, replacement with a submaximal dose of T3 is useful to relieve symptoms more quickly and to predict spontaneous recovery which is detected by an increase of T4 level.

Some patients do not fit easily into the usual diagnostic categories; accordingly, choosing an appropriate course of therapy is more difficult. Frequently, it is impossible to differentiate Hashimoto's thyroiditis from multinodular goiter (MNG) short of performing an open biopsy. In these cases, if there is no suggestion of carcinoma, it is logical to treat the patient with hormone replacement and to observe closely. A reduction in the goiter justifies continuation of the therapy, even in the absence of a diagnosis.

In some patients, especially teenagers, the examination discloses peri-thyroidal lymph nodes or an apparent discrete nodule, in addition to the diffusely enlarged thyroid of Hashimoto's thyroiditis. Such nodules should be evaluated by fine-needle aspiration cytology (FNAC), ultrasound, and possibly scintiscan. Thyroid hormone treatment may cause regression of the nodes or the nodule. If after full evaluation uncertainty persists, if nodes remain present, or if a nodule grows, surgical exploration is indicated.

Thyroidectomy is also considered in patients with suspicion of malignancy as papillary thyroid carcinoma (PTC) is commonly associated with Hashimoto's thyroiditis [339].

Indications of thyroidectomy for patients with Hashimoto's thyroiditis are summarized in Table 9.5.

Table 9.5 Indications of surgery in Hashimoto's thyroiditis

A large goiter with obstructive symptoms (dysphagia, voice hoarseness, and stridor) (evaluation should include pulmonary function tests and a neck CT scan)
Presence of a malignant nodule as found by FNAC
Presence of a lymphoma diagnosed on FNA (thyroid lymphoma responds very well to radiotherapy—the treatment modality of choice
Cosmetic reasons—for large, unsightly goiters
Associated severe pain (painful thyroiditis)

CT computed tomography, *FNA* fine-needle aspiration cytology

9.10.4.2 Complications of Thyroidectomy

The morbidity associated with thyroid surgery is very low, but remains a matter of concern since thyroid disease often occurs in younger patients who have a long life expectancy. Most complications can be avoided by an experienced endocrine surgeon.

General complications associated with thyroidectomy include cardiac and pulmonary problems; gastrointestinal dysfunction such as nausea, vomiting, and ileus; and renal and urinary tract problems. Local complications common to all operations include post-operative bleeding, infection and keloid formation, while those specific to thyroidectomy include injury to the RLN, external branch of the superior laryngeal nerve, hypo-parathyroidism, and airway obstruction. Other local complications such as injury to the esophagus, trachea, thoracic duct, internal jugular vein (IJV), carotid artery, and spinal accessory nerve (SAN) are extremely rare [340–345].

Bleeding

The thyroid gland is extremely vascular, and bleeding can occur anywhere in the operative field. Special care must be taken with the superior thyroid vessels as these can retract and become difficult to control. Post-operative bleeding can be life-threatening by compromising the airway. Any post-operative respiratory distress can be thought of as attributable to a neck hematoma until proved otherwise. Most bleeding occurs within 4 h of operation, and virtually all occur within 24 h. Several studies have reported the successful use of bipolar vessel sealing systems [346–348] or the harmonic scalpel [349, 350] in shortening the length of thyroid surgery and reducing blood loss, while retaining good hemostasis.

Drains do *not* prevent hemorrhage and are unlikely to prevent airway compromise since they are usually blocked by clot formation. If respiratory distress occurs, the wound should be opened immediately to release and drain the hematoma. If respiratory distress is not relieved, a tracheostomy should be performed. An alternative approach is to insert an endotracheal tube to secure the airway and then return the patient to the operating theatre to gain hemostasis. Seromas also occur after thyroidectomy, and most of them are small and do not pose any respiratory problem. They resolve spontaneously, though some must be aspirated [351–353].

Respiratory Distress

Respiratory distress does not only occur due to respiratory compression and/or laryngeal edema by bleeding and hematoma formation. It can also occur with tracheal collapse from chondromalacia or kinking of a soft tortuous trachea. These problems are quite rare and usually occur with long-standing large multinodular goiters. Tracheostomy is the standard treatment in such cases, although prolonged endotracheal intubation and external splinting of the trachea by custom-made rings or Marlex mesh has been tried [354].

Recurrent Laryngeal Nerve (RLN) Injury

Patients with a *single RLN injury* may remain asymptomatic, but are more likely to have temporary or permanent hoarseness. Injury of the RLN associated with thyroidectomy has progressively decreased but still occurs in 0.1–5% of patients. If the nerve is inadvertently transected, it should be re-anastomosed immediately, if recognized intra-operatively, to avoid permanent hoarseness (more than 1 year). In such cases, a number of measures can help lessen hoarseness. These include speech therapy, Teflon injection into the vocal cord, and nerve anastomoses. "Bilateral" RLN injury will cause respiratory distress and stridor since both vocal cords will assume a midline position. Patients will require reintubation or tracheostomy to secure an airway. A vocal cord lateralization procedure can be performed if the injury has been present for over a year [355].

External Branch of Superior Laryngeal Nerve Injury

Damage to the external branch of the superior laryngeal nerve occurs in 0.3–2% of patients undergoing thyroidectomy. The nerve may be injured when taking down the superior pole of the thyroid lobe. The patient will complain of voice weakness and a subtle loss of voice pitch. In case of bilateral injury, patients can experience swallowing disorders and be susceptible to aspiration [356].

Other Nerve Injuries

Rarely the *cervical sympathetic trunk* may be injured during thyroidectomy, resulting in Horner's syndrome. This is a rare complication but can occur with very large glands, invasive tumors, or with recurrent goiters due to obliteration of normal tissue planes by scar tissue. Injury to the *spinal accessory nerve* can occur with neck dissections when combined with thyroidectomy but should not occur with thyroidectomy alone [356].

Hypoparathyroidism

"Transient asymptomatic hypocalcemia" occurs in most patients undergoing thyroidectomy, but this complication has decreased dramatically with the increased understanding of the anatomy and physiology of the parathyroid glands. "Permanent hypo-parathyroidism" has been reported in <1–2% of patients. It occurs if all the parathyroid glands are removed, injured, or rendered ischemic during thyroidectomy. Symptoms of acute post-operative hypocalcemia usually develop 1–7 days post-operatively. If untreated, carpal pedal spasm, tetany, and life-threatening cardiac arrhythmias may occur [357].

For "symptomatic" patients, intravenous (IV) calcium gluconate must be administered. Asymptomatic patients with mild hypocalcemia should be treated with oral calcium supplements. If the total serum calcium is <8 mg/dl, vitamin D replacement therapy should be initiated with one alpha-hydroxy cholecalciferol. It is important to also measure serum phosphorous in these patients. If the serum phosphorous is low, the cause of hypocalcemia may be the "bone hunger" syndrome, but if the serum phosphorous is high, the cause of hypocalcemia is hypo-parathyroidism. If hypocalcemia and hyperphosphatemia remain after a year, permanent hyperparathyroidism is present and the patient will require long-term therapy with oral calcium and vitamin D.

Permanent hypoparathyroidism can be prevented by giving special attention to identifying the parathyroid glands and preserving their blood supply during thyroidectomy by individually ligating the branches of the inferior thyroid artery. If a gland cannot be left in situ with an intact vascular pedicle, it should be removed and autotransplanted (after being confirmed by frozen-section) into the ipsilateral sternocleidomastoid (SCM) muscle or brachioradialis of the non-dominating hand.

9.10.5 Radioactive Iodine (RAI)

Radioactive iodine (RAI) treatment of Hashimoto's thyroiditis can be considered as a "last option" in elderly patients with a large goiter in whom thyroiditis is *not* responding to L-T4 and the patient is generally unfit for anesthesia and/or refusing surgery [332].

9.10.6 Long-Term Monitoring

Upon the initiation of the L-T4 replacement therapy, thyroid function tests, specifically TSH, should be checked, initially every 6–8 weeks as dose adjustments are made. After the attainment of the clinical euthyroid state and a normal TSH level, patients and TSH levels may be checked every 6–12 months.

More frequent follow-up and TSH checks may need to be performed when patients start taking medications, such as ferrous sulfate, calcium supplementation, and multivitamins, that have the potential to impair the absorption of levothyroxine and therefore affect the TSH level. Patients need to be advised to separate these medications from levothyroxine by at least 4 h.

Follow-up care should include clinical evaluation for symptoms of hypothyroidism or iatrogenic hyperthyroidism. Physical examination should routinely include weight measurement, pulse and blood pressure determinations, and thyroid examination for the presence of nodules.

9.10.7 Patient Education

Patients should know that thyroid replacement therapy in Hashimoto's thyroiditis is, except in very rare cases, lifelong. Patients must be informed about the importance of compliance with their replacement therapy and must be instructed to report any symptoms suggestive of hyperthyroidism caused by over-replacement.

Patients must also be instructed to separate—by at least 4 h—ingestion of L-T4 from ingestion of cholestyramine, ferrous sulfate, sucralfate, calcium carbonate, aluminum hydroxide (and other antacids), and iron-containing multivitamins, all of which impair the absorption of L-T4.

9.10.8 Summary of Treatment

Treatment of Hashimoto's thyroiditis is mainly medical, supplementing L-thyroxine (L-T4) for hypothyroidism. L-thyroxine has proved to reduce the volume of the thyroid gland in both hypothyroidism and even euthyroid state. The dose of L-T4 is tailored according to the patient's needs; the standard dosage is 1.6–1.8 mcg/kg/day. The level of TSH is frequently monitored for dose adjustment till euthyroid state is attained and thereafter every 6–12 months. Some cases of spontaneous recovery of Hashimoto's thyroiditis have been reported [317]. When L-T4 and selenomethionine are given together, they reduce the release of cytokines from monocytes and lymphocytes, thus reducing the thyroid peroxidase antibody titer and autoimmune process in Hashimoto's thyroiditis [319].

Surgery is generally avoided in Hashimoto's thyroiditis as it is unnecessary to induce hypothyroidism. Thyroidectomy is considered in patients with cosmetic problem, with compressive symptoms (like dysphagia, dyspnea, change of voice), and suspicion of malignancy as papillary thyroid carcinoma is commonly associated. Surgery has also a beneficial effect in cases of painful thyroiditis [332].

Radioactive iodine treatment can be considered as a *last option* in elderly patients with large goiter in whom thyroiditis is *not* responding to L-T4 and refusing surgery [339].

9.11 Prognosis

Morbidity related to Hashimoto's thyroiditis typically results from failure to reach the diagnosis of hypothyroidism or to institute L-thyroxine (L-T4) replacement therapy in adequate doses on part of the treating physician, or from failure on the part of the patient to take the replacement medication (i.e., non-compliance of the patient). With early diagnosis, timely institution of L-T4 replacement therapy, informed patient follow-up care, and attention to other attendant complications, the prognosis of Hashimoto's thyroiditis is excellent, with patients leading a normal life.

Untreated myxedema coma has a poor prognosis and a high mortality rate. The increased prevalence of "lipid disorders" in association with untreated hypothyroidism has the potential to increase morbidity from coronary artery disease.

Transient periods of thyrotoxicosis sometimes occur, and rarely the illness may progress to full hyperthyroid Graves' disease with active orbitopathy (bulging, inflamed eyes). A recent study (2016) by Kahaly et al. [339] indicated that a strong link exists between the presence of TSH receptor-stimulating antibodies (TS-Abs) in patients with Hashimoto's thyroiditis and the development of thyroid-associated orbitopathy (TAO). The study, which included 700 patients with Hashimoto's thyroiditis, found higher serum levels of TS-Abs in those with TAO than in those without this condition, while patients with active and severe TAO had higher TS-Ab levels than did patients with mild and inactive TAO. Healthy controls were negative for TS-Abs.

The risk of papillary thyroid carcinoma (PTC) is increased in patients with Hashimoto's thyroiditis, though not clearly more aggressive than other PTCs [358]. Primary thyroid B-cell lymphoma affects <1/1000 patients, and it is more likely to affect those with long-standing autoimmune thyroiditis.

Complications of over-replacement with L-T4 include accelerated bone loss, reduction in bone mineral density, osteoporosis, tachycardia, and increased cardiac wall thickness and contractility, which raise the risk of cardiac arrhythmias (especially atrial fibrillation), particularly in the elderly.

Although it is difficult to predict the severity and intractability of Hashimoto's thyroiditis, the prognosis of this disease is acknowledged to be affected by genes associated with the production or expression of immune regulatory factors. These include interleukin-1beta (1IL-1β), IL-4, IL-5, IL-6, IL-13, interferon-gamma (IFN-γ), transforming growth factor-beta (TGF-β), tumor necrosis factor-alpha (TNF-α), FoxP3, glucocorticoid-induced tumor necrosis factor receptor (GITR), and T-box 21 (TBX21) [146, 147, 149, 150, 359–362].

References

1. Fava A, Oliverio R, Giuliano S, et al. Clinical evolution of autoimmune thyroiditis in children and adolescents. Thyroid. 2009;19(4):361–7.
2. Nagar S, Angelos P. Hakaru Hashimoto. In: Surgical Endocrinopathies. New York: Springer International Publishing; 2015. p. 43–8.
3. Rose NR, Witebsky E. Studies on organ specificity. Changes in thyroid glands of rabbits following active immunization with rabbit thyroid extracts. J Immunol. 1956;76:417–9.
4. Roitt IM, Doniach D, Campbell PN, Hudson RV. Auto- antibodies in Hashimoto's thyroiditis (lymphadenoid goiter). Lancet. 1956;2:820–3.
5. Vanderpump MPJ. The epidemiology of thyroid disease. Br Med Bull. 2011;99(1):39–51.
6. Gordin A, Maatela J, Miettinen A, Helenius T, Lamberg B-A. Serum thyrotrophin and circulating thyroglobulin and thyroid microsomal antibodies in a Finnish population. Acta Endocrinol. 1979;l 90:33–39.
7. Ling SM, Kaplan SA, Weitzman JJ, Reed GB, Costin G, Landing BH. Euthyroid goiters in children. Correlation of needle biopsy with other clinical and laboratory findings in chronic lymphocytic thyroiditis and simple goiter. Pediatrics. 1969;44:695699.
8. Tunbridge WM, Evered DC, Hall R, Appleton D, Brewis M, Clark F, et al. The spectrum of thyroid disease in a community. The Whickham Survey. Clin Endocrinol. 1977;7:481–6.
9. Vanderpump MP, French JM, Appleton D. The prevalence of hyperprolactinaemia and association with markers of autoimmune thyroid disease in survivors of the Whickham Survey cohort. Clin Endocrinol. 1998;48(1):39–44.
10. Vanderpump MP, Tunbridge WM, French JM. The incidence of thyroid disorders in the community: a twenty-year follow-up of the Whickham Survey. Clin Endocrinol. 1995;43(1):55–68.
11. Staii A, Mirocha S, Todorova-Koteva K, Glinberg S, Jaume JC. Hashimoto thyroiditis is more frequent than expected when diagnosed by cytology which uncovers a pre-clinical state. Thyroid Res. 2010;3:11–6.
12. Hall R, Stanbury JB. Familial studies of autoimmune thyroiditis. Clin Exp Immunol. 1967;2:719–25.
13. Inoue M, Taketani N, Sato T, Nakajima H. High incidence of chronic lymphocytic thyroiditis in apparently healthy school children: epidemiological and clinical study. Endocrinol Jpn. 1975;22:483–7.

14. Aho K, Gordin A, Sievers K, Takala J. Thyroid autoimmunity in siblings: a population study. Acta Endocrinol Suppl (Copenh). 1983;251:11–5.
15. Phillips DI, Shields DC, Dugoujon JM, rentice L, McGuffin P, Ree Smith B. Complex segregation analysis of thyroid autoantibodies: are they inherited as an autosomal dominant trait? Hum Hered. 1993;43:141–6.
16. Desai MP, Karandikar S. Autoimmune thyroid disease in childhood: a study of children and their families. Indian Pediatr. 1999;36:659–68.
17. Segni M, Wood J, Pucarelli I, Toscano V, Toscano R, Pasquino AM. Clustering of autoimmune thyroid diseases in children and adolescents: a study of 66 families. J Pediatr Endocrinol Metab. 2001;14:1271–5.
18. Marwaha RK, Sen S, Tandon N, Sahoo M, Walia RP, Singh S, et al. Familial aggregation of autoimmune thyroiditis in first-degree relatives of patients with juvenile autoimmune thyroid disease. Thyroid. 2003;13:297–300.
19. Villanueva R, Greenberg DA, Davies TF, Tomer Y. Sibling recurrence risk in autoimmune thyroid disease. Thyroid. 2003;13:761–4.
20. Dittmar M, Libich C, Brenzel T, Kahaly GJ. Increased familial clustering of autoimmune thyroid diseases. Horm Metab Res. 2011;43:200–4.
21. Aghini-Lombardi F, Antonangeli L, Martino E, Vitti P, Maccherini D, Leoli F, et al. The spectrum of thyroid disorders in an iodine-deficient community: the Pescopagano survey. J Clin Endocrinol Metab. 1999;84:561–6.
22. Hollowell JG, Staehling NW, Flanders WD, Hannon WH, Gunter EW, Spencer CA, et al. Serum TSH, T(4), and thyroid antibodies in the United States population (1988 to 1994): National Health and Nutrition Examination Survey (NHANES III). J Clin Endocrinol Metab. 2002;87:489–99.
23. Spencer CA, Hollowell JG, Kazarosyan M, Braverman LE. National Health and Nutrition Examination Survey III thyroid-stimulating hormone (TSH)-thyroperoxidase antibody relationships demonstrate that TSH upper reference limits may be skewed by occult thyroid dysfunction. J Clin Endocrinol Metab. 2007;92:4236–40.
24. Lucas A, Julián MT, Cantón A, Castell C, Casamitjana R, Martínez-Cáceres EM, et al. Undiagnosed thyroid dysfunction, thyroid antibodies, and iodine excretion in a Mediterranean population. Endocrine. 2010;38:391–6.
25. Knudsen N, Jorgensen T, Rasmussen S, Christiansen E, Perrild H. The prevalence of thyroid dysfunction in a population with borderline iodine deficiency. Clin Endocrinol. 1999;51:361–7.
26. Pedersen IB, Knudsen N, Jørgensen T, Perrild H, Ovesen L, Laurberg P. Thyroid peroxidase and thyroglobulin autoantibodies in a large survey of populations with mild and moderate iodine deficiency. Clin Endocrinol. 2003;58:36–42.
27. Hoogendoorn EH, Hermus AR, de Vegt F, Ross HA, Verbeek AL, Kiemeney LA, et al. Thyroid function and prevalence of anti-thyroperoxidase antibodies in a population with borderline sufficient iodine intake: influences of age and sex. Clin Chem. 2006;52:104–11.
28. Simmonds MJ, Kavvoura FK, Brand OJ, Newby PR, Jackson LE, Hargreaves CE, et al. Skewed X chromosome inactivation and female preponderance in autoimmune thyroid disease: an association study and meta-analysis. J Clin Endocrinol Metab. 2014;99(1):27–31.
29. Hansen PS, Brix TH, Iachine I, Kyvik KO, Hegedüs L. The relative importance of genetic and environmental effects for the early stages of thyroid autoimmunity: a study of healthy Danish twins. Eur J Endocrinol. 2006;154:29–38.
30. Klintschar M, Schwaiger P, Mannweiler S, Regauer S, Kleiber M. Evidence of fetal microchimerism in Hashimoto's thyroiditis. J Clin Endocrinol Metab. 2001;86:2494–8.
31. Klintschar M, Immel UD, Kehlen A, Schwaiger P, Mustafa T, Mannweiler S, et al. Fetal microchimerism in Hashimoto's thyroiditis: a quantitative approach. Eur J Endocrinol. 2006;154:237–41.
32. Renné C, Ramos Lopez E, Steimle-Grauer SA, Ziolkowski P, Pani MA, Luther C, et al. Thyroid fetal male micro-chimerism in mothers with thyroid disorders: presence of Y-chromosomal immuno-fluorescence in thyroid infiltrating lymphocytes is more prevalent

in Hashimoto's thyroiditis and Graves' disease than in follicular adenomas. J Clin Endocrinol Metab. 2004;89:5810–4.
33. Totterman TH, Maenpaa J, Gordin A, Makinen T, Andersson AC. Blood and thyroid-infiltrating lymphocyte subclasses in juvenile autoimmune thyroiditis. Clin Exp Immunol. 1977;30:193–7.
34. Paolieri F, Pronzato C, Battifora M, Fiorino N, Canonica GW, Bagnasco M. Infiltrating gamma/delta T-cell receptor-positive lymphocytes in Hashimoto's thyroiditis, Graves' disease and papillary thyroid cancer. J Endocrinol Investig. 1995;18:295–8.
35. Iwatani Y, Hidaka Y, Matsuzuka F, Kuma K, Amino N. Intrathyroidal lymphocyte subsets, including unusual CD4+ CD8+ cells and CD3loTCR alpha beta lo/-CD4-CD8- cells, in autoimmune thyroid disease. Clin Exp Immunol. 1993;93:430–6.
36. Davies TF, Martin A, Concepcion ES, Graves P, Cohen L, Ben NA. Evidence of limited variability of antigen receptors on intra-thyroidal T cells in autoimmune thyroid disease. N Engl J Med. 1991;325:238–44.
37. Davies TF, Concepcion ES, Ben Nun A, Graves PN, Tarjan G. T-cell receptor V gene use in autoimmune thyroid disease: direct assessment by thyroid aspiration. J Clin Endocrinol Metab. 1993;76:660–6.
38. Heuer M, Aust G, Ode-Hakim S, Scherbaum WA. Different cytokine mRNA profiles in Graves' disease, Hashimoto's thyroiditis, and non-autoimmune thyroid disorders determined by quantitative reverse transcriptase polymerase chain reaction (RT-PCR). Thyroid. 1996;6:97–106.
39. Gunn A, Michie W, Irvine WJ. The thymus in thyroid disease. Lancet. 1964;2:776–9.
40. Michie W, Beck JS, Mahaffy RG, Honein EF, Fowler GB. Quantitative radiological and histological studies of the thymus in thyroid disease. Lancet. 1967;1:691–4.
41. Mizukami Y, Michigishi T, Hashimoto T, Tonami N, Hisada K, Matsubara F, et al. Silent thyroiditis: a histologic and immunohistochemical study. Hum Pathol. 1988;19:423–31.
42. Zaletel K, Gaberek S. Hashimoto's thyroiditis: from genes to the disease. Curr Genomics. 2011;12:576–88.
43. Hadj-Kacem H, Rebuffat S, Mnif-Feki M, Belguith-Maalej S, Ayadi H, Péraldi-Roux S. Autoimmune thyroid diseases: genetic susceptibility of thyroid-specific genes and thyroid autoantigens contributions. Int J Immunogenet. 2009;36(2):85–96.
44. Duntas LH. Environmental factors and autoimmune thyroiditis. Nat Clin Pract Endocrinol Metab. 2008;4(8):454–60.
45. Tomer Y, Huber A. The etiology of autoimmune thyroid disease: a story of genes and environment. J Autoimmun. 2009;32(3–4):231–9.
46. Jørgensen KT, Rostgaard K, Bache I, Biggar RJ, Nielsen NM, Tommerup N, et al. Autoimmune diseases in women with Turner's syndrome. Arthritis Rheum. 2010;62(3):658–66.
47. Wiebolt J, Achterbergh R, den Boer A, van der Leij S, Marsch E, Suelmann B, et al. Clustering of additional autoimmunity behaves differently in Hashimoto's patients compared with Graves' patients. Eur J Endocrinol. 2011;164(5):789–94.
48. Vestgaard M, Nielsen LR, Rasmussen AK, Damm P, Mathiesen ER. Thyroid peroxidase antibodies in pregnant women with type 1 diabetes: impact on thyroid function, metabolic control and pregnancy outcome. Acta Obstet Gynecol Scand. 2008;87(12):1336–42.
49. Ruggeri RM, Trimarchi F, Giuffrida G, Certo R, Cama E, Campennì A, et al. Autoimmune co-morbidities in Hashimoto's thyroiditis: different patterns of association in adulthood and childhood/adolescence. Eur J Endocrinol. 2017;176(2):133–41.
50. Bothra N, Shah N, Goroshi M, Jadhav S, Padalkar S, Thakkar H, et al. Hashimoto's thyroiditis: relative recurrence risk ratio and implications for screening of first degree relatives. Clin Endocrinol. 2017;87(2):201–6.
51. McCombe PA, Greer JM, Mackay IR. Sexual dimorphism in autoimmune disease. Curr Mol Med. 2009;9:1058–79.
52. Invernizzi P, Miozzo M, Selmi C, Persani L, Battezzati PM, Zuin M, et al. X chromosome monosomy: a common mechanism for autoimmune diseases. J Immunol. 2005;175:575–8.

53. Larizza D, Calcaterra V, Martinetti M. Increased prevalence of autoimmunity in Turner syndrome--influence of age. J Autoimmun. 2009;33:25–30.
54. Brix TH, Knudsen GP, Kristiansen M, Kyvik KO, Orstavik KH, Hegedüs L. High frequency of skewed X-chromosome inactivation in females with autoimmune thyroid disease: a possible explanation for the female predisposition to thyroid autoimmunity. J Clin Endocrinol Metab. 2005;90:5949–53.
55. Ozcelik T, Uz E, Akyerli CB, Bagislar S, Mustafa CA, Gursoy A, et al. Evidence from autoimmune thyroiditis of skewed X-chromosome inactivation in female predisposition to autoimmunity. Eur J Hum Genet. 2006;14:791–7.
56. Yin X, Latif R, Tomer Y, Davies TF. Thyroid epigenetics: X chromosome inactivation in patients with autoimmune thyroid disease. Ann N Y Acad Sci. 2007;1110:193–200.
57. Chabchoub G, Uz E, Maalej A, Mustafa CA, Rebai A, Mnif M, et al. Analysis of skewed X-chromosome inactivation in females with rheumatoid arthritis and autoimmune thyroid diseases. Arthritis Res Ther. 2009;11:R106.
58. Brix TH, Hansen PS, Kyvik KO, Hegedüs L. Preliminary evidence of a noncausal association between the X-chromosome inactivation pattern and thyroid autoimmunity: a twin study. Eur J Hum Genet. 2010;18:254–7.
59. Guerin LR, Prins JR, Robertson SA. Regulatory T-cells and immune tolerance in pregnancy: a new target for infertility treatment? Hum Reprod Update. 2009;15:517–35.
60. Weetman AP. Immunity, thyroid function and pregnancy: molecular mechanisms. Nat Rev Endocrinol. 2010;6:311–8.
61. Kämpe O, Jansson R, Karlsson FA. Effects of L-thyroxine and iodide on the development of autoimmune postpartum thyroiditis. J Clin Endocrinol Metab. 1990;70:1014–8.
62. Kuijpens JL, Pop VJ, Vader HL, Drexhage HA, Wiersinga WM. Prediction of post partum thyroid dysfunction: can it be improved? Eur J Endocrinol. 1998;139:36–43.
63. Smyth PP, Wijeyaratne CN, Kaluarachi WN, Smith DF, Premawardhana LD, Parkes AB, et al. Sequential studies on thyroid antibodies during pregnancy. Thyroid. 2005;15:474–7.
64. Lazarus JH. The continuing saga of postpartum thyroiditis. J Clin Endocrino Metab. 2011;96:614–6.
65. Kokandi AA, Parkes AB, Premawardhana LD, John R, Lazarus JH. Association of postpartum thyroid dysfunction with antepartum hormonal and immunological changes. J Clin Endocrinol Metab. 2003;88:1126–32.
66. Bianchi DW, Zickwolf GK, Weil GJ, Sylvester S, DeMaria MA. Male fetal progenitor cells persist in maternal blood for as long as 27 years postpartum. Proc Natl Acad Sci USA. 1996;93:705–8.
67. Evans PC, Lambert N, Maloney S, Furst DE, Moore JM, Nelson JL. Long-term fetal microchimerism in peripheral blood mononuclear cell subsets in healthy women and women with scleroderma. Blood. 1999;93:2033–7.
68. Koopmans M, Kremer Hovinga IC, Baelde HJ, Harvey MS, de Heer E, Bruijn JA, et al. Chimerism occurs in thyroid, lung, skin and lymph nodes of women with sons. J Reprod Immunol. 2008;78:68–75.
69. Srivatsa B, Srivatsa S, Johnson KL, Samura O, Lee SL, Bianchi DW. Microchimerism of presumed fetal origin in thyroid specimens from women: a case-control study. Lancet. 2001;358:2034–8.
70. Renne C, Ramos Lopez E, Steimle-Grauer SA, Ziolkowski P, Pani MA, Luther C, et al. Thyroid fetal male microchimerisms in mothers with thyroid disorders: presence of Y-chromosomal immunofluorescence in thyroid-infiltrating lymphocytes is more prevalent in Hashimoto's thyroiditis and Graves' disease than in follicular adenomas. J Clin Endocrinol Metab. 2004;89:5810–4.
71. Brix TH, Hansen PS, Kyvik KO, Hegedüs L. Aggregation of thyroid autoantibodies in twins from opposite-sex pairs suggests that microchimerism may play a role in the early stages of thyroid autoimmunity. J Clin Endocrinol Metab. 2009;94:4439–43.

72. Strieder TG, Prummel MF, Tijssen JG, Endert E, Wiersinga WM. Risk factors for and prevalence of thyroid disorders in a cross-sectional study among healthy female relatives of patients with autoimmune thyroid disease. Clin Endocrinol. 2003;59:396–401.
73. Walsh JP, Bremner AP, Bulsara MK, O'Leary P, Leedman PJ, Feddema P, et al. Parity and the risk of autoimmune thyroid disease: a community-based study. J Clin Endocrinol Metab. 2005;90:5309–12.
74. Bülow Pedersen I, Laurberg P, Knudsen N, Jørgensen T, Perrild H, Ovesen L, et al. Lack of association between thyroid autoantibodies and parity in a population study argues against microchimerism as a trigger of thyroid autoimmunity. Eur J Endocrinol. 2006;154:39–45.
75. Friedrich N, Schwarz S, Thonack J, John U, Wallaschofski H, Völzke H. Association between parity and autoimmune thyroiditis in a general female population. Autoimmunity. 2008;41:174–80.
76. Sgarbi JA, Kasamatsu TS, Matsumura LK, Maciel RM. Parity is not related to autoimmune thyroid disease in a population-based study of Japanese-Brazilians. Thyroid. 2010;20:1151–6.
77. Gordin A, Saarinen P, Pelkonen A, Lamberg B-A. Serum thyroglobulin and the response to thyrotropin releasing hormone in symptomless autoimmune thyroiditis and in borderline and overt hypothyroidism. Acta Endocrinol. 1974;75:274–7.
78. Tunbridge WMG, Brewis M, French JM, Appleton D, Bird T, Clark F, et al. Natural history of autoimmune thyroiditis. Br Med J. 1981;282:258–63.
79. Marwaha RK, Tandon N, Karak AK, Gupta N, Verma K, Kochupillai N. Hashimoto's thyroiditis: countrywide screening of Goitrous healthy young girls in post-iodization phase in India. New Delhi: All India Institute of Medical Sciences; 2000.
80. Mazokopakis EE, Papadomanolaki MG, Tsekouras KC, Evangelopoulos AD, Kotsiris DA, Tzortzinis AA. Is vitamin D related to pathogenesis and treatment of Hashimoto's thyroiditis? Hell J Nucl Med. 2015;18(3):222–7.
81. Blum S. The immune system recovery plan. New York: Scribner; 2013.
82. Tagami T, Tamanaha T, Shimazu S, Honda K, Nanba K, Nomura H, et al. Lipid profiles in the untreated patients with Hashimoto thyroiditis and the effects of thyroxine treatment on subclinical hypothyroidism with Hashimoto thyroiditis. Endocr J. 2010;57(3):253–8.
83. Zeitlin AA, Heward JM, Newby PR, Carr-Smith JD, Franklyn JA, Gough SC, et al. Analysis of HLA class II genes in Hashimoto's thyroiditis reveals differences compared to Graves' disease. Genes Immun. 2008;9(4):358–63.
84. Brix TH, Kyvik KO, Hegedus L. A population-based study of chronic autoimmune hypothyroidism in Danish twins. J Clin Endocr Metab. 2000;85:536–9.
85. Jacobson EM, Huber A, Tomer Y. The HLA gene complex in thyroid autoimmunity: from epidemiology to etiology. J Autoimmun. 2008;30:58–62.
86. Hunt PJ, Marshall SE, Weetman AP, Bunce M, Bell JI, Wass JA, et al. Histocompatibility leucocyte antigens and closely linked immunomodulatory genes in autoimmune thyroid disease. Clin Endocrinol. 2001;55:491–9.
87. Badenhoop K, Schwartz G, Walfish PG, Drummond V, Usadel KH, Bottazzo GF. Susceptibility to thyroid autoimmune disease: molecular analysis of HLA-D region genes identifies new markers for goitrous Hashimoto's thyroiditis. J Clin Endocrinol Metab. 1990;71:1131–7.
88. Petrone A, Giorgi G, Mesturino CA, Capizzi M, Cascino I, Nistico L, et al. Association of DRB1*04-DQB1*0301 haplotype and lack of association of two polymorphic sites at CTLA-4 gene with Hashimoto's thyroiditis in an Italian population. Thyroid. 2001;11:171–5.
89. Wan XL, Kimura A, Dong RP, Honda K, Tamai H, Sasazuki T. HLA-A and -DRB4 genes in controlling the susceptibility to Hashimoto's thyroiditis. Hum Immunol. 1995;42:131–6.
90. Honda K, Tamai H, Morita T, Kuma K, Nishimura Y, Sasazuki T. Hashimoto's thyroiditis and HLA in Japanese. J Clin Endocrinol Metab. 1989;69:1268–73.
91. Hawkins BR, Lam KSL, Ma JTC, Wang C, Yeung RTT. Strong association between HLA-DRw9 and Hashimoto's thyroiditis in Southern Chinese. Acta Endocrinol. 1987;114:543–6.
92. Jacobson EM, Tomer Y. The CD40, CTLA-4, thyroglobulin, TSH receptor, and PTPN22 gene quintet and its contribution to thyroid autoimmunity: back to the future. J Autoimmun. 2007;28:85–98.

93. Kotsa K, Watson PF, Weetman AP. A CTLA-4 gene polymorphism is associated with both Graves' disease and autoimmune hypothyroidism. Clin Endocrinol. 1997;46:551–4.
94. Akamizu T, Sale MM, Rich SS, Hiratani H, Noh JY, Kanamoto N, et al. Association of autoimmune thyroid disease with microsatellite markers for the thyrotropin receptor gene and CTLA-4 in Japanese patients. Thyroid. 2000;10:851–8.
95. Donner H, Braun J, Seidl C, Rau H, Finke R, Ventz M, et al. Codon 17 polymorphism of the cytotoxic T lymphocyte antigen 4 gene in Hashimoto's thyroiditis and Addison's disease. J Clin Endocrinol Metab. 1997;82:4130–2.
96. Nithiyananthan R, Heward JM, Allahabadia A, Franklyn JA, Gough SC. Polymorphism of the CTLA-4 gene is associated with autoimmune hypothyroidism in the United Kingdom. Thyroid. 2002;12:3–6.
97. Terauchi M, Yanagawa T, Ishikawa N, Ito K, Fukazawa T, Maruyama H, et al. Interactions of HLA-DRB4 and CTLA-4 genes influence thyroid function in Hashimoto's thyroiditis in Japanese population. J Endocrinol Investig. 2003;26:1208–12.
98. Park YJ, Chung HK, Park DJ, Kim WB, Kim SW, Koh JJ, et al. Polymorphism in the promoter and exon 1 of the cytotoxic T lymphocyte antigen-4 gene associated with autoimmune thyroid disease in Koreans. Thyroid. 2000;10:453–9.
99. Sahin M, Gursoy A, Erdogan MF. Cytotoxic T lymphocyte-associated molecule-4 polymorphism in Turkish patients with Hashimoto thyroiditis. Int J Immunogenet. 2009;36:103–6.
100. Bicek A, Zaletel K, Gaberscek S, Pirnat E, Krhin B, Stopar TG, et al. 49A/G and CT60 polymorphisms of the cytotoxic T-lymphocyte-associated antigen 4 gene associated with autoimmune thyroid disease. Hum Immunol. 2009;70:820–4.
101. Kavvoura FK, Akamizu T, Awata T, Ban Y, Chistiakov DA, Frydecka I, et al. Cytotoxic T-lymphocyte associated antigen 4 gene polymorphisms and autoimmune thyroid disease: a meta-analysis. J Clin Endocrinol Metab. 2007;92:3162–70.
102. Ueda H, Howson JM, Esposito L, Heward J, Snook H, Chamberlain G, et al. Association of the T-cell regulatory gene CTLA4 with susceptibility to autoimmune disease. Nature. 2003;423:506–11.
103. Ban Y, Tozaki T, Taniyama M, Tomita M, Ban Y. Association of a CTLA-4 3′ untranslated region (CT60) single nucleotide polymorphism with autoimmune thyroid disease in the Japanese population. Autoimmunity. 2005;38:151–3.
104. Ikegami H, Awata T, Kawasaki E, Kobayashi T, Maruyama T, Nakanishi K, et al. The association of CTLA4 polymorphism with type 1 diabetes is concentrated in patients complicated with autoimmune thyroid disease: a multicenter collaborative study in Japan. J Clin Endocrinol Metab. 2006;91:1087–92.
105. Tomer Y, Greenberg DA, Barbesino G, Concepcion E, Davies TF. CTLA-4 and not CD28 is a susceptibility gene for thyroid autoantibody production. J Clin Endocrinol Metab. 2001;86:1687–93.
106. Ban Y, Davies TF, Greenberg DA, Kissin A, Marder B, Murphy B, et al. Analysis of the CTLA-4, CD28, and inducible costimulator (ICOS) genes in autoimmune thyroid disease. Genes Immun. 2003;4:586–93.
107. Ban Y, Greenberg DA, Davies TF, Jacobson E, Concepcion E, Tomer Y. Linkage analysis of thyroid antibody production: evidence for shared susceptibility to clinical autoimmune thyroid disease. J Clin Endocrinol Metab. 2008;93:3589–96.
108. Zaletel K, Gaberscek S. Hashimoto's thyroiditis: from genes to the disease. Curr Genomics. 2011;12(8):576–88.
109. Zaletel K, Krhin B, Gaberscek S, Hojker S. Thyroid autoantibody production is influenced by exon 1 and promoter CTLA-4 polymorphisms in patients with Hashimoto's thyroiditis. Int J Immunogenet. 2006;33:87–91.
110. Zaletel K, Krhin B, Gaberscek S, Bicek A, Pajic T, Hojker S. Association of CT60 cytotoxic T lymphocyte antigen-4 gene polymorphism with thyroid autoantibody production in patients with Hashimoto's and postpartum thyroiditis. Clin Exp Immunol. 2010;161:41–7.

111. Begovich AB, Carlton VE, Honigberg LA, Schrodi SJ, Chokkalingam AP, Alexander HC, et al. A missense single-nucleotide polymorphism in a gene encoding a protein tyrosine phosphatase (PTPN22) is associated with rheumatoid arthritis. Am J Hum Genet. 2004;75:330–7.
112. Bottini N, Musumeci L, Alonso A, Rahmouni S, Nika K, Rostamkhani M, et al. A functional variant of lymphoid tyrosine phosphatase is associated with type I diabetes. Nat Genet. 2004;36:337–8.
113. Criswell LA, Pfeiffer KA, Lum RF, Gonzales B, Novitzke J, Kern M, et al. Analysis of families in the multiple autoimmune disease genetics consortium (MADGC) collection: the PTPN22 620W allele associates with multiple autoimmune phenotypes. Am J Hum Genet. 2005;76:561–71.
114. Kyogoku C, Langefeld CD, Ortmann WA, Lee A, Selby S, Carlton VE, et al. Genetic association of the R620W polymorphism of protein tyrosine phosphatase PTPN22 with human SLE. Am J Hum Genet. 2004;75:504–7.
115. Smyth D, Cooper JD, Collins JE, Heward JM, Franklyn JA, Howson JM, et al. Replication of an association between the lymphoid tyrosine phosphatase locus (LYP/PTPN22) with type 1 diabetes, and evidence for its role as a general autoimmunity locus. Diabetes. 2004;53:3020–3.
116. Velaga MR, Wilson V, Jennings CE, Owen CJ, Herington S, Donaldson PT, et al. The codon 620 tryptophan allele of the lymphoid tyrosine phosphatase (LYP) gene is a major determinant of Graves' disease. J Clin Endocrinol Metab. 2004;89:5862–5.
117. Burn GL, Svensson L, Sanchez-Blanco C, Saini M, Cope AP. Why is PTPN22 a good candidate susceptibility gene for autoimmune disease? FEBS Lett. 2011;585:3689.
118. Kahles H, Ramos-Lopez E, Lange B, Zwermann O, Reincke M, Badenhoop K. Sex-specific association of PTPN22 1858T with type 1 diabetes but not with Hashimoto's thyroiditis or Addison's disease in the German population. Eur J Endocrinol. 2005;153:895–9.
119. Chabchoub G, Teixiera EP, Maalej A, Ben Hamad M, Bahloul Z, Cornelis F, et al. The R620W polymorphism of the protein tyrosine phosphatase 22 gene in autoimmune thyroid diseases and rheumatoid arthritis in the Tunisian population. Ann Hum Biol. 2009;36:342–9.
120. Ban Y, Tozaki T, Taniyama M, Tomita M, Ban Y. The codon 620 single nucleotide polymorphism of the protein tyrosine phosphatase-22 gene does not contribute to autoimmune thyroid disease susceptibility in the Japanese. Thyroid. 2005;15:1115–8.
121. Dultz G, Matheis N, Dittmar M, Röhrig B, Bender K, Kahaly GJ. The protein tyrosine phosphatase non-receptor type 22 C1858T polymorphism is a joint susceptibility locus for immunthyroiditis and autoimmune diabetes. Thyroid. 2009;19:14–148.
122. Kordonouri O, Hartmann R, Badenhoop K, Kahles H, Ilonen J. PTPN22 1858T allele is associated with younger age at onset of type 1 diabetes and is not related to subsequent thyroid autoimmunity. Hum Immunol. 2010;71:731–2.
123. Ban Y, Tozaki T, Taniyama M, Nakano Y, Ban Y, Ban Y, et al. Association of the protein tyrosine phosphatase nonreceptor 22 haplotypes with autoimmune thyroid disease in the Japanese population. Thyroid. 2010;20:893–9.
124. Sakai K, Shirasawa S, Ishikawa N, Ito K, Tamai H, Kuma K, et al. Identification of susceptibility loci for autoimmune thyroid disease to 5q31-q33 and Hashimoto's thyroiditis to 8q23-q24 by multipoint affected sib-pair linkage analysis in Japanese. Hum Mol Genet. 2001;10:1379–86.
125. Tomer Y, Ban Y, Concepcion E, Barbesino G, Villanueva R, Greenberg DA, et al. Common and unique susceptibility loci in Graves and Hashimoto diseases: results of whole-genome screening in a data set of 102 multiplex families. Am J Hum Genet. 2003;73:736–47.
126. Tomer Y, Greenberg DA, Concepcion E, Ban Y, Davies TF. Thyroglobulin is a thyroid specific gene for the familial autoimmune thyroid diseases. J Clin Endocrinol Metab. 2002;87:404–7.
127. Ban Y, Tozaki T, Taniyama M, Tomita M, Ban Y. Association of a thyroglobulin gene polymorphism with Hashimoto's thyroiditis in the Japanese population. Clin Endocrinol. 2004;61:263–8.

128. Collins J, Heward JM, Carr-Smith J, Daykin J, Franklyn JA, Gough SC. Association of a rare thyroglobulin gene microsatellite variant with autoimmune thyroid disease. J Clin Endocrinol Metab. 2003;88:5039–42.
129. Ban Y, Greenberg DA, Concepcion E, Skrabanek L, Villanueva R, Tomer Y. Amino acid substitutions in the thyroglobulin gene are associated with susceptibility to human and murine autoimmune thyroid disease. Proc Natl Acad Sci USA. 2003;100:15119–24.
130. Collins JE, Heward JM, Howson JM, Foxall H, Carr-Smith J, Franklyn JA, Gough SC. Common allelic variants of exons 10, 12, and 33 of the thyroglobulin gene are not associated with autoimmune thyroid disease in the United Kingdom. J Clin Endocrinol Metab. 2004;89:6336–9.
131. Maierhaba M, Zhang JA, Yu ZY, Wang Y, Xiao WX, Quan Y, et al. Association of the thyroglobulin gene polymorphism with autoimmune thyroid disease in Chinese population. Endocrine. 2008;33:294–9.
132. Toubi E, Shoenfeld Y. The role of vitamin D in regulating immune responses. Isr Med Assoc J. 2010;12:174–5.
133. Ban Y, Taniyama M, Ban Y. Vitamin D receptor gene polymorphisms in Hashimoto's thyroiditis. Thyroid. 2001;11:607–8.
134. Lin WY, Wan L, Tsai CH, Chen RH, Lee CC, Tsai FJ. Vitamin D receptor gene polymorphisms are associated with risk of Hashimoto's thyroiditis in Chinese patients in Taiwan. J Clin Lab Anal. 2006;20:109–12.
135. Stefani M, Papi S, Suver M, Glavas-Obrovac L, Karner I. Association of vitamin D receptor gene 3′-variants with Hashimoto's thyroiditis in the Croatian population. Int J Immunogenet. 2008;35:125–31.
136. Zaletel K, Gaberšček S. Hashimoto's thyroiditis: from genes to the disease. Curr Genomics. 2011;12(8):576–88.
137. Kochi Y, Myouzen K, Yamada R, Suzuki A, Kurosaki T, Nakamura Y, et al. FCRL3, an autoimmune susceptibility gene, has inhibitory potential on B-cell receptor-mediated signaling. J Immunol. 2009;183:5502–10.
138. Gibson AW, Li FJ, Wu J, Edberg JC, Su K, Cafardi J, et al. The FCRL3–169CT promoter single-nucleotide polymorphism, which is associated with systemic lupus erythematosus in a Japanese population, predicts expression of receptor protein on CD19+B cells. Arthritis Rheum. 2009;60:3510–2.
139. Duchatelet S, Caillat-Zucman S, Dubois-Laforgue D, Blanc H, Timsit J, Julier C. FCRL3–169CT functional polymorphism in type 1 diabetes and autoimmunity traits. Biomed Pharmacother. 2008;62:153–7.
140. Ikari K, Momohara S, Nakamura T, Hara M, Yamanaka H, Tomatsu T, et al. Supportive evidence for a genetic association of the FCRL3 promoter polymorphism with rheumatoid arthritis. Ann Rheum Dis. 2006;65:671–3.
141. Mao C, Pan H, Chen Q, Wang X, Ye D, Qiu L. Association between Fc receptor-like 3 C169T polymorphism and risk of systemic lupus erythematosus: a meta-analysis. Mol Biol Rep. 2010;37:191–6.
142. Matesanz F, Fernandez O, Milne RL, Fedetz M, Leyva L, Guerrero M, et al. The high producer variant of the Fc-receptor like-3 (FCRL3) gene is involved in protection against multiple sclerosis. J Neuroimmunol. 2008;195:146–50.
143. Koyanagi M, Nakabayashi K, Fujimoto T, Gu N, Baba I, Takashima Y, et al. ZFAT expression in B and T lymphocytes and identification of ZFAT-regulated genes. Genomics. 2008;91:451–7.
144. Fujimoto T, Doi K, Koyanagi M, Tsunoda T, Takashima Y, Yoshida Y, et al. ZFAT is an antiapoptotic molecule and critical for cell survival in MOLT-4 cells. FEBS Lett. 2009;583:568-572.
145. Shirasawa S, Harada H, Furugaki K, Akamizu T, Ishikawa N, Ito K, et al. SNPs in the promoter of a B cell-specific antisense transcript, SAS-ZFAT, determine susceptibility to autoimmune thyroid disease. Hum Mol Genet. 2004;13:2221–31.

146. Ito C, Watanabe M, Okuda N, Watanabe C, Iwatani Y. Association between the severity of Hashimoto's disease and the functional +874A/T polymorphism in the interferon-gamma gene. Endocr J. 2006;53:473–8.
147. Nanba T, Watanabe M, Akamizu T, Iwatani Y. The -590CC genotype in the IL4 gene as a strong predictive factor for the development of hypothyroidism in Hashimoto disease. Clin Chem. 2008;54:621–3.
148. Yamada H, Watanabe M, Nanba T, Akamizu T, Iwatani Y. The +869T/C polymorphism in the transforming growth factor-beta1 gene is associated with the severity and intractability of autoimmune thyroid disease. Clin Exp Immunol. 2008;151:379–82.
149. Inoue N, Watanabe M, Morita M, Tomizawa R, Akamizu T, Tatsumi K, et al. Association of functional polymorphisms related to the transcriptional level of FOXP3 with prognosis of autoimmune thyroid diseases. Clin Exp Immunol. 2010;162:402–6.
150. Inoue N, Watanabe M, Nanba T, Wada M, Akamizu T, Iwatani Y. Involvement of functional polymorphisms in the TNFA gene in the pathogenesis of autoimmune thyroid diseases and production of anti-thyrotropin receptor antibody. Clin Exp Immunol. 2009;156:199–204.
151. Tomer Y. Genetic susceptibility to autoimmune thyroid disease: past, present, and future. Thyroid. 2010;20:715–25.
152. Simmonds MJ. GWAS in autoimmune thyroid disease: redefining our understanding of pathogenesis. Nat Rev Endocrinol. 2013;9(5):277–87.
153. Cai T, Li J, An X, Yan N, Li D, Jiang Y, et al. Polymorphisms in MIR499A and MIR125A gene are associated with autoimmune thyroid diseases. Mol Cell Endocrinol. 2017;15:106–15.
154. Xiao C, Rajewsky K. MicroRNA control in the immune system: basic principles. Cell. 2009;136:26–36.
155. Zhu J, Zhang Y, Zhang W, Zhang W, Fan L, Wang L, et al. MicroRNA-142-5p contributes to Hashimoto's thyroiditis by targeting CLDN1. J Transl Med. 2016;14(1):166–8.
156. Duntas LH. Environmental factors and autoimmune thyroiditis. Nat Clin Pract Endocrinol Metab. 2010;4:454–60.
157. Pacini F, Vorontsova T, Molinaro E, Kuchinskaya E, Agate L, Shavrova E, et al. Prevalence of thyroid autoantibodies in children and adolescents from Belarus exposed to the Chernobyl radioactive fallout. Lancet. 1998;352(9130):763–7666.
158. Kasagi K, Takahashi N, Inoue G, Honda T, Kawachi Y, Izumi Y. Thyroid function in Japanese adults as assessed by a general health checkup system in relation with thyroid-related antibodies and other clinical parameters. Thyroid. 2009;19:937–44.
159. Heydarian P, Ordookhani A, Azizi F. Goiter rate, serum thyrotropin, thyroid autoantibodies and urinary iodine concentration in Tehranian adults before and after national salt iodization. J Endocrinol Investig. 2007;30:404–10.
160. Gokowski F, Buziak-Bereza M, Trofimiuk M, Badys-Waligórska A, Szybiski Z, Huszno B. Increased prevalence of hyperthyroidism as an early and transient side-effect of implementing iodine prophylaxis. Public Health Nutr. 2007;10:799–802.
161. Fountoulakis S, Philippou G, Tsatsoulis A. The role of iodine in the evolution of thyroid disease in Greece: from endemic goiter to thyroid autoimmunity. Hormones (Athens). 2007;6:25–35.
162. Kahaly GJ, Dienes HP, Beyer J, Hommel G. Iodide induces thyroid autoimmunity in patients with endemic goitre: a randomised, double-blind, placebo-controlled trial. Eur J Endocrinol. 1998;139:290–7.
163. Rose NR, Bonita R, Burek CL. Iodine: an environmental trigger of thyroiditis. Autoimmun Rev. 2002;1:97–103.
164. Burek CL, Talor MV. Environmental triggers of autoimmune thyroiditis. J Autoimmun. 2009;33:183–9.
165. Yu X, Li L, Li Q, Zang X, Liu Z. TRAIL and DR5 promote thyroid follicular cell apoptosis in iodine excess-induced experimental autoimmune thyroiditis in NOD mice. Biol Trace Elem Res. 2011;143(2):1064–76.
166. Xu J, Yang X-F, Guo H-L, Hou X-H, Liu L-G, Sun X-F. Selenium supplement alleviated the toxic effects of excessive iodine in mice. Biol Trace Elem Res. 2006;111:229–38.

167. Thomson CD, Campbell JM, Miller J, Skeaff SA. Minimal impact of excess iodate intake on thyroid hormones and selenium status in older New Zealanders. Eur J Endocrinol. 2011;165(5):745–52.
168. Tomer Y. Hepatitis C and interferon induced thyroiditis. J Autoimmun. 2010;34:322–6.
169. Barbesino G. Drugs affecting thyroid function. Thyroid. 2010;20:763–70.
170. Baethge C, Blumentritt H, Berghöfer A, Bschor T, Glenn T, Adli M, et al. Long-term lithium treatment and thyroid antibodies: a controlled study. J Psychiatry Neurosci. 2005;30:423–7.
171. Martino E, Bartalena L, Bogazzi F, Braverman LE. The effects of amiodarone on the thyroid. Endocr Rev. 2001;22:240–54.
172. Desailloud R, Hober D. Viruses and thyroiditis: an update. Virol J. 2009;6:5.
173. Wasserman EE, Nelson K, Rose NR, Rhode C, Pillion JP, Seaberg E, et al. Infection and thyroid autoimmunity: a seroepidemiologic study of TPOa-Ab. Autoimmunity. 2009;42:439–46.
174. de Freitas CU, Grimaldi Campos RA, Rodrigues Silva MA, Panachão MR, de Moraes JC, Waissmann W, et al. Can living in the surroundings of a petrochemical complex be a risk factor for autoimmune thyroid disease? Environ Res. 2010;110:112–7.
175. Langer P, Tajtáková M, Kocan A, Petrík J, Koska J, Ksinantová L, et al. Thyroid ultrasound volume, structure and function after long-term high exposure of large population to polychlorinated biphenyls, pesticides and dioxin. Chemosphere. 2007;69:118–217.
176. Agate L, Mariotti S, Elisei R, Mossa P, Pacini F, Molinaro E, et al. Thyroid autoantibodies and thyroid function in subjects exposed to Chernobyl fallout during childhood: evidence for a transient radiation-induced elevation of serum thyroid antibodies without an increase in thyroid autoimmune disease. J Clin Endocrinol Metab. 2008;93(7):2729–36.
177. Elfström P, Montgomery SM, Kämpe O, Ekbom A, Ludvigsson JF. Risk of thyroid disease in individuals with celiac disease. J Clin Endocrinol Metab. 2008;93(10):3915–21.
178. Shevach EM. From vanilla to 28 flavours: multiple varieties of T regulatory cells. Immunity. 2006;25:195–201.
179. Sakaguchi S, Yamaguchi T, Nomura T, Ono M. Regulatory T cells and immune tolerance. Cell. 2008;133:775–87.
180. Baecher-Allan C, Wolf E, Hafler DA. Functional analysis of highly defined, FACS-isolated populations of human regulatory CD4+CD25+T cells. Clin Immunol. 2005;115:10–8.
181. Kong YM, Morris GP, Brown NK, Yan Y, Flynn JC, David CS. Autoimmune thyroiditis: a model uniquely suited to probe regulatory T cell function. J Autoimmun. 2009;33:239–46.
182. Watanabe M, Yamamoto N, Marouka H, Tamai H, Matsuzuka F, Miyauchi A, et al. Independent involvement of CD8+CD25+ cells and thyroid autoantibodies in disease severity of Hashimoto's disease. Thyroid. 2002;12:801–8.
183. Nakano A, Watanabe M, Iida T, Kuroda S, Matsuzuka F, Miyauchi A, et al. Apoptosis-induced decrease of intrathyroidal CD4(+)CD25(+) regulatory T cells in autoimmune thyroid diseases. Thyroid. 2007;17:25–31.
184. Baecher-Allan C, Wolf E, Hafler DA. Class II expression identifies functionally distinct human regulatory T cells. J Immunol. 2006;176:4622–31.
185. Fountoulakis S, Vartholomatos G, Kolaitis N, Frillingos S, Philippou G, Tsatsoulis A. Differential expression of Fas system apoptotic molecules in peripheral lymphocytes from patients with Graves' disease and Hashimoto's thyroiditis. Eur J Endocrinol. 2008;158:853–9.
186. Toda S, Nishimura T, Yamada S, Koike N, Yonemitsu N, Watanabe K, et al. Immunohistochemical expression of growth factors in subacute thyroiditis and their effects on thyroid folliculogenesis and angiogenesis in collagen gel matrix culture. J Pathol. 1999;188:415–22.
187. Betteli E, Korn T, Kuchroo VK. Th17: the third member of the effector T cell trilogy. Curr Opin Immunol. 2007;19:652–7.
188. Akinci B, Comlekci A, Yener S, Bayraktar F, Demir T, Ali Ozcan M, et al. Hashimoto's thyroiditis, but not treatment of hypothyroidism, is associated with altered TGF-β1 levels. Arch Med Res. 2008;39:397–401.
189. Guimaraes VC, Quintans J, Fisfalen ME, Straus FH, Fields PE, Medeiros-Neto DeGroot LJ. Immunosupression of thyroiditis. Endocrinology. 1996;137:2199–207.

190. Chen K, Wei Y, Sharp GC, Braley-Mullen H. Mechanism of spontaneous resolution versus fibrosis in granulomatous experimental autoimmune thyroiditis. J Immunol. 2003;171:6236–43.
191. Ajjan RA, Watson PF, Weetman AP. Cytokines and thyroid function. Adv Neuroimmunol. 1996;6:359–86.
192. Battifora M, Pesce G, Paolieri F, Fiorino N, Giordano C, Riccio AM, et al. B7.1 costimulatory molecule is expressed on thyroid follicular cells in Hashimoto's thyroiditis, but not in Graves' disease. J Clin Endocrinol Metab. 1998;83:4130–9.
193. Weetman AP. Cellular immune responses in autoimmune thyroid disease. Clin Endocrinol. 2004;61:405–13.
194. Ajjan RA, Watson PF, Mcintosh RS, Weetman AP. Intrathyroidal cytokine gene expression in Hashimoto's thyroiditis. Clin Exp Immunol. 1996;105:523–8.
195. Nielsen CH, Hegedüs L, Rieneck K, Moeller AC, Leslie RGQ, Bendtzen K. Production of interleukin (IL)-5 and IL-10 accompanies T helper cell type 1 (Th2) cytokine responses to a major thyroid self-antigen, thyroglobulin, in health and autoimmune thyroid disease. Clin Exp Immunol. 2006;147:287–95.
196. Nanba T, Watanabe M, Inoue N, Iwatani Y. Increases of the Th1/Th2 cell ratio in severe Hashimoto's disease and in the proportion of Th17 cells in intractable Graves' disease. Thyroid. 2009;19:495–501.
197. Karanikas G, Shuetz M, Wahl K, Paul M, Kontur S, Pietschmann P, et al. Relation of anti-TPO autoantibody titer and T lymphocyte cytokine production patterns in Hashimoto's thyroiditis. Clin Endocrinol. 2005;63:191–6.
198. Nielsen CH, Brix TH, Leslie RG, Hegedüs L. A role for autoantibodies in enhancement of proinflammatory cytokine responses to a self-antigen, thyroid perioxidise. Clin Immunol. 2009;133:118–27.
199. Kawakami Y, Fisfalen M-E, DeGroot LJ. Proliferative responses of peripheral blood mononuclear cells from patients with autoimmune thyroid disease to synthetic peptide epitopes of human thyroid peroxidase. Autoimmunity. 1992;13:17–26.
200. Ng HP, Kung AW. Induction of autoimmune thyroiditis and hypothyroidism by immunization of immunoactive T cell epitope of thyroid peroxidase. Endocrinology. 2006;147(6):3085–92.
201. Hidaka Y, Amino N, Iwatani Y, Kaneda T, Nasu M, Mitsuda N, et al. Increase in peripheral natural killer cell activity in patients with autoimmune thyroid disease. Autoimmunity. 1992;11:239–43.
202. Muixí L, Carrascal M, Alvarez I, Daura X, Martí M, Armengol MP, et al. Thyroglobulin peptides associate in vivo to HLA-DR in autoimmune thyroid glands. J Immunol. 2008;181(1):795–807.
203. Itoh M, Takahashi T, Sakaguchi N, Kuniyasu Y, Shimizu J, Otsuka F, et al. Thymus and autoimmunity: production of CD25+CD4+ naturally anergic and suppressive T cells as a key function of the thymus in maintaining immunologic self-tolerance. J Immunol. 1999;162:5317–26.
204. McLachlan SM, Nagayama Y, Pichurin PN, Mizutori Y, Chen CR, Misharin A, et al. The link between Graves' disease and Hashimoto's thyroiditis: a role for regulatory T cells. Endocrinology. 2007;148(12):5724–33.
205. Figueroa-Vega N, Alfonso-Pérez M, Benedicto I, Sánchez-Madrid F, González-Amaro R, Marazuela M. Increased circulating pro-inflammatory cytokines and Th17 lymphocytes in Hashimoto's thyroiditis. J Clin Endocrinol Metab. 2010;95:953–62.
206. Shi Y, Wang H, Su Z, Chen J, Xue Y, Wang S, et al. Differentiation imbalance of Th1/Th17 in peripheral blood mononuclear cells might contribute to pathogenesis of Hashimoto's thyroiditis. Scand J Immunol. 2010;72:250–5.
207. Li C, Yuan J, Zhu YF, Yang XJ, Wang Q, Xu J, et al. Imbalance of Th17/Treg in different subtypes of autoimmune thyroid diseases. Cell Physiol Biochem. 2016;40(1–2):245–52.
208. Hamano H, Kawa S, Horiuchi A, Unno H, Furuya N, Akamatsu T, et al. High serum IgG4 concentrations in patients with sclerosing pancreatitis. N Engl J Med. 2001;344(10):737–328.

209. Kosugi S, Ban T, Akamizu T, Kohn LD. Identification of separate determinants on the thyrotropin receptor reactive with Graves' thyroid-stimulating antibodies and with thyroid-stimulating blocking antibodies in idiopathic myxedema: these determinants have no homologous sequence on gonadotropin receptors. Molecul Endocrinol. 1992;6:168–80.
210. Tamaki H, Amino N, Kimura M, Hidaka Y, Takeoka K, Miyai K. Low prevalence of thyrotropin receptor antibody in primary hypothyroidism in Japan. J Clin Endocrinol Metab. 1990;71:1382–7.
211. Okamura K, Sato K, Yoshinari M, Ikenoue H, Kuroda T, Nakagawa M, et al. Recovery of the thyroid function in patients with atrophic hypothyroidism and blocking type TSH binding inhibitor immunoglobulin. Acta Endocrinol. 1990;122:107–14.
212. Takasu N, Yamada T, Takasu M, Komiya I, Nagasawa Y, Asawa T, et al. Disappearance of thyrotropin-blocking antibodies and spontaneous recovery from hypothyroidism in autoimmune thyroiditis. N Engl J Med. 1992;326:513–8.
213. Mori T, Akamizu T, Kosugi S, Sugawa H, Inoue D, Okuda J, et al. Recent progress in TSH receptor studies with a new concept of "Autoimmune TSH receptor disease". Endocr J. 1994;41:1–11.
214. Thompson CB. Apoptosis in the pathogenesis and treatment of disease. Science. 1995,267.1456–62.
215. Mitsiades N, Poulaki V, Mitsiades CS, Koutras DA, Chrousos GP. Apoptosis induced by FasL and TRAIL/Apo2L in the pathogenesis of thyroid diseases. Trends Endocrinol Metab. 2001;12:384–90.
216. Nagata S, Golstein P. The Fas death factor. Science. 1995;267:1449–56.
217. Giordano C, Stassi G, Maria R, Todaro M, Richiusa P, Papoff G, et al. Potential involvement of Fas and its ligand in the pathogenesis of Hashimoto's thyroidiitis. Science. 1997;275:960–5.
218. Dong Z, Takakuwa T, Takayama H, Luo WJ, Takano T, Amino N, et al. Fas and Fas ligand gene mutations in Hashimoto's thyroiditis. Lab Investig. 2002;82:1611–6.
219. Takakuwa T, Dong Z, Takayama H, Matsuzuka F, Nagata S, Aozasa K. Frequent mutations of Fas gene. Cancer Res. 2001;61(4):1382–5.
220. Pan G, Ni J, Wei YF, Yu G, Gentz R, Dixit VM. An antagonist decoy receptor and a death domain-containing receptor for TRAIL. Science. 1997;277:815–8.
221. Pan G, O'Rourke K, Chinnaiyan AM, Gentz R, Ebner R, Ni JK, et al. The receptor for the cytotoxic ligand TRAIL. Science. 1997;276:111–3.
222. Wang SH, Bretz JD, Phelps E, Mezosi E, Arscott PL, Utsugi S, et al. A unique combination of inflammatory cytokines enhances apoptosis of thyroid follicular cells and transforms nondestructive to destructive thyroiditis in experimental autoimmune thyroiditis. J Immunol. 2002;168:2470–4.
223. Kawakami A, Eguchi K, Matsouka N, Tsuboi M, Kawabe Y, Ishikawa N, et al. Thyroid-stimulating hormons inhibits Fas antigen-mediated apoptosis of human thyrocytes *in vitro*. Endocrinology. 1996;137:3163–9.
224. Bretz JD, Rymaszewski M, Arscott PL, Myc A, Ain KB, Thompson NW, et al. TRAIL death pathway expression and induction in thyroid follicular cells. J Biol Chem. 1999;274:23627–32.
225. Bretz JD, Baker JR. Apoptosis and autoimmune thyroid disease: following a TRAIL to thyroid destruction? Clin Endocrinol. 2001;55:1–11.
226. Bretz JD, Arscott PL, Myc A, Baker JR. Inflammatory cytokine regulation of Fas-mediated apoptosis in thyroid follicular cells. J Biol Chem. 1999;274:25433–8.
227. Bursch W, Oberhammer F, Jirtle RL, Askari M, Sedivy R, Grasl-Kraupp B, et al. Transforming growth factor-beta 1 as a signal for induction of cell death by apoptosis. Br J Cancer. 1993;67:531–6.
228. Gartner R, Schopohl D, Schaefer S, Dugrillon A, Erdmann A, Toda S, et al. Regulation of transforming growth factor beta-1 messenger ribonucleic acid expression in porcine thyroid follicles *in vitro* by growth factors, iodine, or delta-iodolactone. Thyroid. 1997;7:633–40.
229. Bechtner G, Fröschl H, Sachse A, Schopohl D, Gärtner R. Induction of apoptosis in porcine thyroid follicles by transforming growth factor β1 and epidermal growth factor. Biochimie. 1999;81:315–20.

230. Giordano C, Stassi G, De Maria R, Todaro M, Richiusa P, Papoff G, et al. Potential involvement of Fas and its ligand in the pathogenesis of Hashimoto's thyroiditis. Science. 1997;275:960–3.
231. Arscott PL, Baker JR. Short analytical review. Apoptosis and thyroiditis. Clin Immunol Immunopathol. 1998;87:207–17.
232. Mitsiades N, Poulaki V, Kotoula V, Astorakos G, Tseleni-Balafouta S, Koutras DA, et al. Fas/Fas ligand up-regulation and Bcl-2 down-regulation may be significant in the patogenesis of Hashimoto's thyroiditis. J Clin Endocrinol Metab. 1998;83:2199–203.
233. Fountoulakis S, Vartholomatos G, Kolaitis N, Frillingos S, Philippou G, Tsatsoulis A. HLA-DR expressing peripheral T regulatory cells in newly diagnosed patients with different forms of autoimmune thyroid disease. Thyroid. 2008;18:1195–200.
234. Wang SH, Van Antwerp M, Kuick R, Gauger PG, Doherty GM, Fan YY, et al. Microarray analysis of cytokine activation of apoptosis pathways in the thyroid. Endocrinology. 2007;148:4844–52.
235. Kaczmarek E, Lacka K, Jarmolowska-Jurczyszyn D, Sidor A, Majewski P. Changes of B and T lymphocytes and selected apopotosis markers in Hashimoto's thyroiditis. J Clin Pathol. 2011;64(7):626–30.
236. Jublanc C, Beaudeux JL, Aubart F, Raphael M, Chadarevian R, Chapman MJ, et al. Serum levels of adhesion molecules ICAM-1 and VCAM-1 and tissue inhibitor of metallo-proteinases, TIMP-1, are elevated in patients with autoimmune thyroid disorders: relevance to vascular inflammation. Nutr Metab Cardiovasc Dis. 2010;10:817–22.
237. Jiang X, Feng X, Li G, Zhao Q, Yin H. Differential expression of connexin 43 in human autoimmune thyroid disease. Acta Histochem. 2010;112:278–83.
238. Green LM, Lazarus JP, LaBue M, Shah MM. Reduced cell-cell communication in a spontaneous murine model of autoimmune thyroid disease. Endocrinology. 1995;136:3611–8.
239. Mitasíková M, Lin H, Soukup T, Imanaga I, Tribulová N. Diabetes and thyroid hormones affect connexin-43 and PKC-epsilon expression in rat heart atria. Physiol Res. 2009;58:211–7.
240. Komatsu K, Hamano H, Ochi Y, Takayama M, Muraki T, Yoshizawa K, et al. High prevalence of hypothyroidism in patients with autoimmune pancreatitis. Dig Dis Sci. 2005;50(6):1052–7.
241. Li Y, Bai Y, Liu Z, Ozaki T, Taniguchi E, Mori I, et al. Immunohistochemistry of IgG4 can help subclassify Hashimoto's autoimmune thyroiditis. Pathol Int. 2009;59(9):636–41.
242. Dahlgren M, Khosroshahi A, Nielsen GP, Deshpande V, Stone JH. Riedel's thyroiditis and multifocal fibrosclerosis are part of the IgG4-related systemic disease spectrum. Arthritis Care Res (Hoboken). 2010;62:1312–8.
243. Kakudo K, Li Y, Taniguchi E, Mori I, Ozaki T, Nishihara E, Miyauchi A, et al. IgG4-related disease of the thyroid glands [Review]. Endocr J. 2012;59(4):273–81.
244. Nystrom E, Bengtsson C, Lapidus L, Petersen K, Lindstedt G. Smoking--A risk factor for hypothyroidism. J Endocrinol Investig. 1993;16:129–31.
245. Buchanan WW, Harden RM. Primary hypothyroidism and Hashimoto's thyroiditis. Arch Intern Med. 1965;115:411–5.
246. Gordin A, Saarinen P, Pelkonen A, Lamberg B-A. Serum thyroglobulin and the response to thyrotropin releasing hormone in symptomless autoimmune thyroiditis and in borderline and overt hypothyroidism. Acta Endocrinol. 1974;75:274–9.
247. Tunbridge WMG, Evered DC, Hall R, Appleton D, Brewis M, Clark F, et al. The spectrum of thyroid disease in a community. The Whickham Survey. Clin Endocrinol. 1977;7:481–5.
248. Kon YC, Degroot LJ. Painful Hashimoto's thyroiditis as an indication for thyroidectomy: clinical characteristics and outcome in seven patients. J Clin Endocrinol Metab. 2003;88:2667–72.
249. Radetti G, Gottardi E, Bona G, Corrias A, Salardi S, Loche S. Study Group for Thyroid Diseases of the Italian Society for Pediatric Endocrinology and Diabetes (SIEDP/ISPED).The natural history of euthyroid Hashimoto's thyroiditis in children. J Pediatr. 2006;149:827–32.
250. Moriuchi A, Yokoyama S, Kashima K, Andoh T, Nakayama I, Noguchi S. Localized primary anyloid tumor of the thyroid developing in the course of Hashimoto's thyroiditis. Acta Pathol Jpn. 1992;42:210–6.

251. Shaw PJ, Walls TJ, Newman PK, Cleland PG, Cartlidge NE. Hashimoto's encephalopathy: a steroid-responsive disorder associated with high antithyroid antibody titers -- report of five cases. Neurology. 1991;41:228–33.
252. Khardori R, Eagleton LE, Soler NG, McConnachie PR. Lymphocytic interstitial pneumonitis in autoimmune thyroid disease. Am J Med. 1991;90:649–52.
253. Tateno F, Sakakibara R, Kishi M, Ogawa E. Hashimoto's ophthalmopathy. Am J Med Sci. 2011;342(1):83–5.
254. Yoshihara A, Yoshimura Noh J, Nakachi A, Ohye H, Sato S, Sekiya K, et al. Severe thyroid-associated orbitopathy in Hashimoto's thyroiditis. Report of two cases. Endocr J. 2011;58(5):343–8.
255. Skillern PG, Crile G Jr, McCullaugh EP, Hazard JB, Lewis LA, Brown H. Struma lymphomatosa: primary thyroid failure with compensatory thyroid enlargement. J Clin Endocrinol Metab. 1956;16:35–9.
256. Eisenbart GS, Wilson PW, Ward F, Buckley C, Lebovitz H. The polyglandular failure syndrome. Disease inheritance, HLA type, and immune function. Ann Intern Med. 1979;91:528.
257. Loviselli A, Mathieu A, Pala R, Mariotti S, Cau S, Marongiu C, et al. Development of thyroid disease in patients with primary and secondary Sjogren's syndrome. J Endocrinol Investig. 1988,11.653–7.
258. Best TB, Munro RE, Burwell S, Volpe R. Riedel's thyroiditis associated with Hashimoto's thyroiditis, hypoparathyroidism, and retroperitoneal fibrosis. J Endocrinol Investig. 1991;14:767–72.
259. Becker KL, Ferguson RH, McConahey WM. The connective-tissue diseases and symptoms associated with Hashimoto's thyroiditis. N Engl J Med. 1963;268:277–81.
260. Bastenie PA, Vanhaelst L, Golstein J, Smets P, Keys MJ, Karvonen MJ, et al. Asymptomatic autoimmune thyroiditis and coronary heart-disease. Lancet. 1977;1:155–9.
261. Heinonen OP, Aho K, Pyorala K, Gordin A, Punsar S, Puro K. Symptomless autoimmune thyroiditis in coronary heart disease. Lancet. 1972;1:785–9.
262. Jankovic B, Le KT, Hershman JM. Clinical review: Hashimoto's thyroiditis and papillary thyroid carcinoma: is there a correlation? J Clin Endocrinol Metab. 2013;98(2):474–82.
263. Lee JH, Kim Y, Choi JW, Kim YS. The association between papillary thyroid carcinoma and histologically proven Hashimoto's thyroiditis: a meta-analysis. Eur J Endocrinol. 2013;168(3):343–9.
264. Larson SD, Jackson LN, Riall TS, Uchida T, Thomas RP, Qiu S, et al. Increased incidence of well-differentiated thyroid cancer associated with Hashimoto thyroiditis and the role of the PI3k/Akt pathway. J Am Coll Surg. 2007;204(5):764–673.
265. Fava A, Oliverio R, Giuliano S, Parlato G, Michniewicz A, Indrieri A, et al. Clinical evolution of autoimmune thyroiditis in children and adolescents. Thyroid. 2009;19(4):361–7.
266. Muzza M, Degl'Innocenti D, Colombo C, Perrino M, Ravasi E, Rossi S, Cirello V, Beck-Peccoz P, Borrello MG, Fugazzola L. The tight relationship between papillary thyroid cancer, autoimmunity and inflammation: clinical and molecular studies. Clin Endocrinol. 2010;72:702–8.
267. Kim HS, Choi YJ, Yun JS. Features of papillary thyroid microcarcinoma in the presence and absence of lymphocytic thyroiditis. Endoc Pathol. 2010;21:149–53.
268. Dvorkin S, Robenshtok E, Hirsch D, Strenov Y, Shimon I, Benbassat CA. Differentiated thyroid cancer is associated with less aggressive disease and better outcome in patients with coexisting Hashimotos thyroiditis. J Clin Endocrinol Metab. 2013;98(6):2409–14.
269. Marotta V, Guerra A, Zatelli MC, Uberti ED, Di Stasi V, Faggiano A, et al. BRAF mutation positive papillary thyroid carcinoma is less advanced when Hashimoto's thyroiditis lymphocytic infiltration is present. Clin Endocrinol. 2013;79(5):733–8.
270. Amino N, Miyai K, Onishi T, Hashimoto T, Arai K, Ishibashi K, Kumahara Y. Transient hypothyroidism after delivery in autoimmune thyroiditis. J Clin Endocrinol Metab. 1976;42:296–301.

271. Amino N, Kuro R, Tanizawa O, Tanaka F, Hayashi C, Kotani K, et al. Changes of serum antithyroid antibodies during and after pregnancy in autoimmune thyroid diseases. Clin Exp Immunol. 1978;31:30–5.
272. Amino N, Miyai K, Kuro R, Tanizawa O, Azukizawa M, Takai S, et al. Transient postpartum hypothyroidism. Fourteen cases with autoimmune thyroiditis. Ann Intern Med. 1977;87:155–9.
273. Abalovich M, Amino N, Barbour LA, Cobin RH, De Groot LJ, Glinoer D, et al. Management of thyroid dysfunction during pregnancy and postpartum: an Endocrine Society clinical practice guideline. J Clin Endocrinol Metab. 2007;92(8 Suppl):S1–47.
274. Dosiou C, Sanders GD, Araki SS, Crapo LM. Screening pregnant women for autoimmune thyroid disease: a cost-effectiveness analysis. Eur J Endocrinol. 2008;158(6):841–51.
275. Amino N, Tada H, Hidaka Y. Postpartum autoimmune thyroid syndrome: a model of aggravation of autoimmune disease. Thyroid. 1999;9:705–13.
276. Poppe K, Glinoer D, Tournaye H, Devroey P, van Steirteghem A, Kaufman L, et al. Assisted reproduction and thyroid autoimmunity: an unfortunate combination? J Clin Endocrinol Metab. 2003;88:4129–52.
277. Pankow BG, Michalak J, McGee MK. Adult human thyroid weight. Health Phys. 1985;49:1097–103.
278. Woolf PD, Daly R. Thyrotoxicosis with painless thyroiditis. Am J Med. 1976;60:73–9.
279. Hamburger JI. Occult subacute thyroiditis: diagnostic challenge. Mich Med. 1976;70:1125–9.
280. Woolf PD. Transient painless thyroiditis with hyperthyroidism. A variant of lymphocytic thyroiditis. Endocr Rev. 1980;1:411–6.
281. Nikolai TF, Brosseau J, Kettrick MA, Roberts R, Beltaos E. Lymphocytic thyroiditis with spontaneously resolving hyperthyroidism (silent thyroiditis). Arch Intern Med. 1980;140:478–82.
282. Dorfman SG, Copperman MT, Nelson RL, Depuy H, Peake RL, Young RL. Painless thyroiditis and transient hyperthyroidism without goiter. Ann Intern Med. 1977;86:24–8.
283. Gorman CA, Duick DS, Woolner LB, Wahner HW. Transient hyperthyroidism in patients with lymphocytic thyroiditis. Mayo Clin Proc. 1978;53:359–65.
284. Gluck FB, Nusynowitz ML, Plymate S. Chronic lymphocytic thyroiditis, thyrotoxicosis, and low radioactive iodine uptake: reports of four cases. N Engl J Med. 1975;292:624–8.
285. Amino N, Yabu Y, Miyai K, Fujie T, Azukizawa M, Onishi T, et al. Differentiation of thyrotoxicosis induced by thyroid destruction from Graves' disease. Lancet. 1978;2:344–6.
286. Ota H, Amino N, Morita S, Kobayashi K, Kubota S, Fukata S, et al. Quantitative measurement of thyroid blood flow for differentiation of painless thyroiditis from Graves' disease. Clin Endocrinol. 2007;67:41–5.
287. Yoshida H, Amino N, Yagawa K, Uemura K, Satoh M, Miyai K, et al. Association of serum antithyroid antibodies with lymphocytic infiltration of the thyroid gland: studies of seventy autopsied cases. J Clin Endocrinol Metab. 1978;46:859–63.
288. Amino N, Tada H, Hidaka Y. Autoimmune thyroid disease and pregnancy. J Endocrinol Investig. 1996;19:59–64.
289. Taylor HC, Sheeler LR. Recurrence and heterogeneity in painless thyrotoxic lymphocytic thyroiditis. Report of five cases. J Am Med Assn. 1982;248:1085–8.
290. Yamamoto M, Shibuya N, Chen LC, Ogata E. Seasonal recurrence of transient hypothyroidism in a patient with autoimmune thyroiditis. Endocr J. 1988;35:135–42.
291. Tachi J, Amino N, Miyai K. Massage therapy on neck: a contributing factor for destructive thyrotoxicosis? Thyroidology. 1990;2:25–7.
292. Maruyama H, Kato M, Mizuno O, Kataoka K, Matusi S. Transient thyrotoxicosis occurred after cessation of steroid therapy in a patient with autoimmune thyroiditis and rheumatoid arthritis. Endocr J. 1982;29:583–8.
293. Takasu N, Komiya I, Nagasawa Y, Asawa T, Yamada T. Exacerbation of autoimmune thyroid dysfunction after unilateral adrenalectomy in patients with Cushing's syndrome due to an adrenocortical adenoma. N Engl J Med. 1990;322:1708–12.

294. Negro R, Greco G, Mangieri T, Pezzarossa A, Dazzi D, Hassan H. The influence of Selenium supplementation on postpartum thyroid status in pregnant women in thyroid peroxidase autoantibodies. J Clin Endocrinol Metab. 2007;92(4):1263–8.
295. Peschen-rosin R, Schabet M, Dichgans J. Manifestation of Hashimoto's encephalopathy years before onset of thyroid disease. Eur Neurol. 1999;41:79–84.
296. Brain L, Jellinek EH, Ball K. Hashimoto's disease and encephalopathy. Lancet. 1966;2:512–4.
297. Pozo-Rosich P, Villoslada P, Canton A, Simo R, Rovira A, Montalban X. Reversible white matter alterations in encephalopathy associated with autoimmune thyroid disease. J Neurol. 2002;249:1063–5.
298. Canton A, de Fabregas O, Tintore M, Mesa J, Codina A, Simo R. Encephalopathy associated to autoimmune thyroid disease: a more appropriate term for an underestimated condition? J Neurol Sci. 2000;176:65–9.
299. Ochi H, Horiuchi I, Araki N, Toda T, Araki T, Sato K, et al. Proteomic analysis of human brain identifies У-enolase as a nobel autoantigen in Hashimoto's encephalopathy. FEBS Lett. 2002;528:197–202.
300. Sawka AM, Fatourechi V, Boeve BF, Mokri B. Rarity of encephalopathy associated with autoimmune thyroiditis: a case series from Mayo Clinic from 1950 to 1996. Thyroid. 2002;12:393–8.
301. Fujii A, Yoneda M, Ito T, Yamamura O, Satomi S, Higa H, et al. Autoantibodies against the amino terminal of alpha-enolase are a useful diagnostic marker of Hashimoto's encephalopathy. J Neuroimmunol. 2005;162:130–6.
302. Yoneda M, Fujii A, Ito A, Yokoyama H, Nakagawa H, Kuriyama M. High prevalence of serum autoantibodies against the amino terminal of α-enolase in Hashimoto's encephalopathy. J Neuroimmunol. 2007;185:195–200.
303. Seo SW, Lee BI, Lee JD, Park SA, Kim KS, Kim SH, et al. Thyrotoxic autoimmune encephalopathy: a repeat positron emission tomography study. J Neurol Neurosurg Psychiatry. 2003;74(4):504–6.
304. Hosoi Y, Kono S, Terada T, Konishi T, Miyajima H. Hashimoto's encephalopathy associated with an elevated intrathecal IgG4 level. J Neurol. 2013;260(4):1174–6.
305. Caturegli P, De Remigis A, Rose NR. Hashimoto thyroiditis: clinical and diagnostic criteria. Autoimmunity Rev. 2014;13:391–7.
306. McConahey WM, Keating FR, Butt HR, Owen CA. Comparison of certain laboratory tests in the diagnosis of Hashimoto's thyroiditis. J Clin Endocrinol Metab. 1961;21:879–83.
307. Glynne A, Thomson JA. Serum immunoglobulin levels in thyroid disease. Clin Exp Immunol. 1972;12:71–7.
308. Monteleone JA, Davis RK, Tung KSK, Ramos CV, Peden VH. Differentiation of chronic lymphocytic thyroiditis and simple goiter in pediatrics. J Pediatr. 1973;83:381–5.
309. Zhang L, Li H, Ji QH, Zhu YX, Wang ZY, Wang Y, et al. Clinical features of papillary thyroid cancer in ht patients from an area wih a high prevalence of Hashimoto's disease. BMC Cancer. 2012;12:610–5.
310. Fiore E, Rago T, Latrofa F, Provenzale MA, Piaggi P, Delitala A, et al. Hashimoto's thyroiditis is associated with papillary thyroid carcinoma: role of TSH and treatment with L-thyroxine. Endocrine Related Cancer. 2011;18:429–37.
311. Krysiak R, Okopien B. The effect of levothyroxine and Selenomethionine on lymphocyte and monocyte cytokine release in women with Hashimoto's thyroiditis. J Clin Endocrinol Metab. 2011;96:2206–15.
312. Wozniak R, Beckwith L, Ratech H, Surks MI. Maltoma of the thyroid in a man with Hashimoto's thyroiditis. J Clin Endocrinol Metab. 1999;4:84–8.
313. Miller BS, Paul G. Image in endocrinology: thyroid lymphoma arising from Hashimoto's thyroiditis. J Clin Endocrinol Metab. 1991;10:3711–2.
314. Takano T, Miyauchi A, Matsuzuka F, Yoshida H, Kuma K, Amino N. Diagnosis of thyroid malignant lymphoma by reverse transcription-polymerase chain reaction detecting the monoclonality of immunoglobulin heavy chain messenger ribonucleic acid. J Clin Endocr Metab. 2000;85:671–5.

315. McConahey WM, Woolner LB, Black BM, Keating FR Jr. Effect of desiccated thyroid in lymphocytic (Hashimoto's) thyroiditis. J Clin Endocrinol Metab. 1959;19:45–9.
316. Vickery AL, Hamlin E Jr. Struma lymphomatosa (Hasimoto's thyroiditis): observations on repeated biopsies in 16 patients. N Engl J Med. 1961;264:226–9.
317. Bozkurt NC, Karbek B, Ucan B, Sahin M, Cakal E, Ozbek M, et al. The association between severity of vitamin D deficiency and Hashimoto's thyroiditis. Endocr Pract. 2013;21:1–14.
318. Karges B, Muche R, Knerr I, Ertelt W, Wiesel T, Hub R, et al. Levothyroxine in euthyroid autoimmune thyroiditis and type 1 diabetes: a randomized, controlled trial. J Clin Endocrinol Metab. 2007;92(5):1647–52.
319. Caturegli P, De Remigis A, Rose NR. Hashimoto thyroiditis: clinical and diagnostic criteria. Autoimmun Rev. 2014;4-5:391–7.
320. Aksoy DY, Kerimoglu U, Okur H, Canpinar H, Karaagaoglu E, Yetgin S, et al. Effects of prophylactic thyroid hormone replacement in euthyroid Hashimoto's thyroiditis. Endocr J. 2005;52(3):337–43.
321. Papapetrou PD, MacSween RNM, Lazarus JH, McG HR. Long-term treatment of Hashimoto's thyroiditis with thyroxine. Lancet. 1972;2:7786–9.
322. Takasu N, Komiya I, Asawa T, Nagasawa Y, Yamada T. Test for recovery from hypothyroidism during thyroxine therapy in Hashimoto's thyroiditis. Lancet. 1990;336:1084–6.
323. Campbell NR, Hasinoff BB, Stalts H, Rao B, Wong NC. Ferrous sulfate reduces thyroxine efficacy in patients with hypothyroidism. Ann Intern Med. 1992;117(12):1010–3.
324. Padberg S, Heller K, Usadel KH, Schumm-Draeger PM. One-year prophylactic treatment of euthyroid Hashimoto's thyroiditis patients with levothyroxine: is there a benefit? Thyroid. 2001;11:249–55.
325. Mariotti S, Zoncu S, Pigliaru F, Putzu C, Cambuli VM, Vargiu S, et al. Cardiac effects of l-thyroxine administration in borderline hypothyroidism. Int J Cardiol. 2008;126(2):190–5.
326. Escobar-Morreale HF, Botella-Carretero JI, Escobar del Rey F, et al. Review: treatment of hypothyroidism with combinations of levothyroxine plus liothyronine. J Clin Endocrinol Metab. 2005;90(8):4946–54.
327. Yamada T, Ikejiri K, Kotani M, Kusakabe T. An increase of plasma triiodothyronine and thyroxine after administration of dexamethasone to hypothyroid patients with Hashimoto's thyroiditis. J Clin Endocrinol Metab. 1981;46:784–9.
328. Blizzard RM, Hung M, Chandler RW, Aceto T Jr, Kyle M, Winship T, Hashimoto's thyroiditis. Clinical and laboratory response to prolonged cortisone therapy. N Engl J Med. 1962;267:1015–9.
329. Ito S, Tamura T, Nishikawa M. Effects of desiccated thyroid, prednisolone and chloroquine on goiter and antibody titer in chronic thyroiditis. Metabolism. 1968;17:317–22.
330. Negro R, Greco G, Mangieri T, Pezzarossa A, Dazzi D, Hassan H. The influence of selenium supplementation on postpartum thyroid status in pregnant women with thyroid peroxidase autoantibodies. J Clin Endocrinol Metab. 2007;92:1263–8.
331. Mazokopakis EE, Papadakis JA, Papadomanolaki MG, Batistakis AG, Giannakopoulos TG, Protopapadakis EE, Ganotakis ES. Effects of 12 months treatment with l-Selenomethionine on serum anti-TPO levels in patients with Hashimoto's thyroiditis. Thyroid. 2007;17(7):609–12.
332. Wichman J, Winther KH, Bonnema SJ, Hegedüs L. Selenium supplementation significantly reduces thyroid autoantibody levels in patients with chronic autoimmune thyroiditis: a systematic review and meta-analysis. Thyroid. 2016;26(12):1681–92.
333. Winther KH, Wichman JE, Bonnema SJ, Hegedüs L. Insufficient documentation for clinical efficacy of selenium supplementation in chronic autoimmune thyroiditis, based on a systematic review and meta-analysis. Endocrine. 2017;55(2):376–85.
334. Nordio M, Pajalich R. Combined treatment with Myo-inositol and selenium ensures euthyroidism in subclinical hypothyroidism patients with autoimmune thyroiditis. J Thyroid Res. 2013;13:4241–63.
335. Nordio M, Basciani S. Treatment with Myo-Inositol and selenium ensures Euthyroidism in patients with autoimmune thyroiditis. Int J Endocrinol. 2017:2549491.https://doi.org/10.1155/2017/2549491.

336. Caturegli P, De Remigis A, Ferlito M, Landek-Salgado MA, Iwama S, Tzou SC, Ladenson PW. Anatabine ameliorates experimental autoimmune thyroiditis. Endocrinology. 2012;153(9):4580–7.
337. Schmeltz LR, Blevins TC, Aronoff SL, Ozer K, Leffert JD, Goldberg MA, et al. Anatabine supplementation decreases thyroglobulin antibodies in patients with chronic lymphocytic autoimmune (Hashimoto's) thyroiditis: a randomized controlled clinical trial. J Clin Endocrinol Metab. 2014;99(1):E137–42.
338. Amino N, Tada H, Hidaka Y. The spectrum of postpartum thyroid dysfunction: diagnosis, management, and long-term prognosis. Endocr Pract. 1996;2:406–12.
339. Kahaly GJ, Diana T, Glang J, Kanitz M, Pitz S, König J. Thyroid stimulating antibodies are highly prevalent in Hashimoto's thyroiditis and associated Orbitopathy. J Clin Endocrinol Metab. 2016;101(5):1998–2004.
340. Harness J, Heerden J, Lennquist S, Rothmund M, Barraclough BH, Goode AW, Rosen IB, et al. Future of thyroid surgery and training surgeons to meet the expectations of 2000 and beyond. World J Surg. 2000;24:976–82.
341. Luft HS, Bunker JP, Enthoven AC. Should operations be regionalized? The empirical relation between surgical volume and mortality. N Engl J. 1979;301:1364–9.
342. Hannan EL, O'Donnell JF, Kilburn H, Bernard HR, Yazıcı A. Investigation of the relationship between volume and mortality for surgical procedures performed in New York State hospitals. JAMA. 1989;262:503–10.
343. Begg CB, Cramer LD, Hoskins WJ. Impact of hospital volume on operative mortality for major cancer surgery. JAMA. 1998;280:1747–51.
344. Birkmeyer JD, Siewers AE, Finlayson EV. Hospital volume and surgical mortality in the United States. N Engl J. 2002;346:1128–37.
345. Birkmeyer JD, Finlayson EV, Birkmeyer BS. Volume standards for high-risk surgical procedures: potential benefits of the Leapfrog initiative. Surgery. 2001;130:415–22.
346. Manouras A, Markogiannakis H, Koutras AS, Antonakis PT, Drimousis P, Lagoudianakis EE, et al. Thyroid surgery: comparison between the electrothermal bipolar vessel sealing system, harmonic scalpel, and classic suture ligation. Am J Surg. 2008;195(1):48–52.
347. Franko J, Kish KJ, Pezzi CM, Pak H, Kukora JS. Safely increasing the efficiency of thyroidectomy using a new bipolar electro-sealing device (LigaSure) versus conventional clamp-and tie technique. Am Surg. 2006;72(2):132–6.
348. Shen WT, Baumbusch MA, Kebebew E, Duh QY. Use of the electro-thermal vessel sealing system versus standard vessel ligation in thyroidectomy. Asian J Surg. 2005;28(2):86–9.
349. Cordon C, Fajardo R, Ramirez J, Herrera MF. A randomized, prospective, parallel group study comparing the harmonic scalpel to electrocautery in thyroidectomy. Surgery. 2005;137(3):337–41.
350. Kilic M, Keskek M, Ertan T, Yoldas O, Bilgin A, Koc M. A prospective randomized trial comparing the harmonic scalpel with conventional knot tying in thyroidectomy. Adv Ther. 2007;24(3):632–8.
351. Kaplan EL. Thyroid and parathyroid. In: Schwartz SI, Shires CT, Spencer FO, Storer EU, editors. Principles of surgery. 9th ed. New York: McGraw-Hill; 2009. p. 1545.
352. Kukora SS, Hardy SD. Complications of thyroid and parathyroid surgery. In: Hardy JD, editor. Complications in surgery and their management. 4th ed. Philadelphia: WB Saunders Co; 1981. p. 295–312.
353. Dudley HAF. Thyroid. In: Williamson RC, editor. Waxman BP: An aid to clinical surgery. 6th ed. London, UK: Churchill Livingstone; 1998. p. 107–20.
354. Harness JK, Fung L, Thompson NW, Burney RE, McLeod MK. Total thyroidectomy: complications and technique. World J Surg. 1986;10:781–6.
355. Roy van Zuidewijn DB, Songun I, Kievit J, van de Velde CJ. Complications of thyroid surgery. Ann Surg Oncol. 1995;2:56–60.
356. Songun I, Kievit J, van de Velde CJH. Complications of thyroid surgery. In: Clark OH, Duh Q-Y, editors. Textbook of endocrine surgery. 1st ed. Philadelphia: WB Saunders; 1997. p. 167–74.

357. Olson JA Jr, DeBenedetti MK, Baumann DS, Wells SA Jr. Parathyroid autotransplantation during thyroidectomy. Results of long-term follow-up. Ann Surg. 1996;223:472–8.
358. Kim KW, Park YJ, Kim EH, Park SY, Park DJ, Ahn SH, et al. Elevated risk of papillary thyroid cancer in Korean patients with Hashimoto's thyroiditis. Head Neck. 2011;33(5):691–5.
359. Hayashi F, Watanabe M, Nanba T, Inoue N, Akamizu T, Iwatani Y. Association of the -31C/T functional polymorphism in the interleukin-1beta gene with the intractability of Graves' disease and the proportion of T helper type 17 cells. Clin Exp Immunol. 2009;158:281–6.
360. Inoue N, Watanabe M, Morita M, Tatusmi K, Hidaka Y, Akamizu T, et al. Association of functional polymorphisms in promoter regions of IL5, IL6 and IL13 genes with development and prognosis of autoimmune thyroid diseases. Clin Exp Immunol. 2011;163:318–23.
361. Morita M, Watanabe M, Inoue N, Inaoka C, Akamizu T, Tatsumi K, et al. Functional polymorphisms in *TBX21* and *HLX* are associated with development and prognosis of Graves' disease. Autoimmunity. 2012;45(2):129–36.
362. Tomizawa R, Watanabe M, Inoue N, Takemura K, Hidaka Y, Akamizu T, et al. Association of functional GITR gene polymorphisms related to expression of glucocorticoid-induced tumour necrosis factor-receptor (GITR) molecules with prognosis of autoimmune thyroid disease. Clin Exp Immunol. 2011;165:141–67.

Chronic Thyroiditis: Hashimoto's Dietary Management

10

10.1 Introduction

Hashimoto's thyroiditis is part of the spectrum of chronic autoimmune thyroid diseases (AITD) and is associated with thyroid hypofunction, lymphocytic infiltration, and production of thyroid autoantibodies such as thyroid peroxidase antibodies (TPO-Ab) and thyroglobulin antibodies (Tg-Ab) [1–5]. Although the exact mechanism of progressive thyroid tissue destruction is not clear, Hashimoto's thyroiditis is considered a disorder of T cell-mediated immunity, caused by an interaction between susceptibility genes and environmental factors, the research of which is still inconclusive [5]. In the majority of patients with Hashimoto's thyroiditis, lifelong levothyroxine (LT4) substitution to achieve normal circulating thyrotropin (TSH) levels is required [4, 6, 7]. The additional role of diet for the management of Hashimoto's thyroiditis is usually overlooked, and careful supplementation of possible deficiencies in Hashimoto's thyroiditis is recommended for the dietary management of these patients.

In addition, the co-existence of Hashimoto's thyroiditis with other organ-specific diseases (e.g., pernicious anemia, vitiligo, celiac disease, type 1 diabetes mellitus, autoimmune liver disease, primary biliary cirrhosis, myasthenia gravis, alopecia areata, sclerosis multiplex, Addison's disease), and non-specific non-endocrine autoimmune diseases (e.g., rheumatoid arthritis, systemic lupus erythematosus, Sjögren syndrome, systemic sclerosis, mixed connective tissue disease), should be evaluated [8, 9].

10.2 The Best Diet for Hashimoto's Thyroiditis

There are specific nutrients that should be regularly taken to maintain a healthy and functional thyroid. The top nutrients are iodine (I_2), selenium (Se), and zinc (Zn). A diet optimizing these nutrients is vital to an overall recovery plan. The best way to get the daily requirement of these minerals and nutrients is to eat a balanced diet,

M. Sakr, *Thyroiditis*, https://doi.org/10.1007/978-3-032-19513-5_10

but if this is not possible, supplements are available. Diets beneficial for patients with Hashimoto's disease include paleo diet, gluten-free diet, and vegetarian or vegan diet.

10.2.1 Iodine (I_2)

Iodine is an essential micronutrient of the diet necessary for thyroid function and synthesis of thyroid hormones [10]. The recommended adult daily iodine intake is 150 g, reaching up to 250 g during pregnancy and lactation [11]. Main diet iodine sources are seafood (e.g., seaweed, scallops, cod, sardines, shrimps, salmon, and tuna), animal products (dairy products and eggs), fruits (prunes, cranberries, and strawberries), and iodinated table salt. It is important to be conscious of the iodine in diet. Too little iodine can cause goiter in some people, while too much iodine can make hypothyroidism worse.

Iodine deficiency manifests with a wide clinical range, from goiter to cretinism [12], but this problem was solved in many countries worldwide with iodized salt (IS) programs, and nowadays about two-thirds of the world's population (71%) uses IS [13]. On the other hand, most persons with thyroid disorders in iodine-replete areas have autoimmune thyroid disease (AITD), ranging from primary atrophic hypothyroidism, Hashimoto's thyroiditis to thyrotoxicosis (Graves' disease) [14].

Other studies revealed the influence of dietary iodine intake on the epidemiology of thyroid dysfunction [14]. Autoimmune hypothyroidism and thyroid antibodies are more common in iodine replete areas than in iodine deficient areas [15]. Hypothyroidism induced by iodine in AITD may be due to a persistent inhibitory effect of iodine on thyroid hormone synthesis and secretion (Wol-Chaiko effect) [6, 16]. Patients with Hashimoto's thyroiditis may have inadequate thyroid hormone synthesis, may be unable to escape from the acute Wolff-Chaikoff effect, and can develop iodine-induced hypothyroidism. Several studies reported that moderate or even mild iodine excess (median urinary iodine 220 μg/24 h) is associated with a more frequent occurrence of hypothyroidism, especially in elderly subjects, the exact mechanism of which has not been clarified [17, 18]. Furthermore, a cross-sectional study from south China showed that high iodine intake was likely to lead to the occurrence of thyroid diseases, such as Hashimoto's thyroiditis, nodular goiter, and hyperthyroidism, through a long-term process [19]. Pedersen et al. (2011) [20] reported an increased prevalence of thyroid antibodies, 4–5 years after a cautious salt iodization program, supporting the view that even a small increase in iodine supplementation may be associated with increased thyroid autoimmunity [12]. The underlying mechanism for this association is yet to be elucidated.

A recent study (2016) by Xu et al. [21] suggested that the apoptosis of thyroid follicular cells seen in Hashimoto's thyroiditis is probably caused by suppression of autophagy activity, which is induced by iodine excess. This process is mediated through transforming growth factor-1 down-regulation, activation of the Akt/mTOR signaling pathway, and enhanced reactive oxygen species (ROS) production. Another potential mechanism could be that iodine excess increases intra-thyroid infiltrating Th17-cells and inhibits T-regulatory (TREG) cells development, while it triggers an abnormal expression of tumor necrosis factor (TNF)-related apoptosis-inducing ligand (TRAIL) in thyrocytes, thus inducing apoptosis and parenchymal destruction [22]. The fact that excessive iodine plays a significant role in inducing thyroid autoimmunity is also strongly supported in genetically predisposed animals by increasing the immunogenicity of thyroglobulin (Tg) [23]. This phenomenon may be explained by the fact that Tg is the only self-antigen that undergoes post-translational modification as a consequence of the environmental supply of iodine, with the exposure of previously hidden epitopes [24–28]. Thus, high iodine supplementation in Hashimoto's thyroiditis should be discouraged and should be considered as "not beneficial" and "possibly harmful." Discouraging iodine over-supplementation must not preclude its appropriate supplementation in pregnancy to a total intake of 250 g/day [6].

10.2.2 Selenium (Se)

Selenium (Se) is an essential micronutrient of diet with many pleiotropic effects ranging from antioxidant and anti-inflammatory to increasing active thyroid hormone production [29–33]. The thyroid has the highest Se content per gram of tissue in the entire body.

Among at least 30 selenoproteins, the seleno-enzymes such as glutathione peroxidases (GPX), thioredoxin reductases (TR), iodothyronine deiodinases, and seleno-protein P seem to play a unique role in thyroid function and thyroid hormone homeostasis [2, 29, 30]. Selenium supplementation in patients with AITD, including Hashimoto's thyroiditis, seems to modify the inflammatory and immune responses, probably by enhancing plasma GPX and TR activity and by decreasing toxic concentrations of hydrogen peroxide and lipid hydroperoxides, resulting from thyroid hormone synthesis [2, 30, 31]. When Se intake is adequate, the intra-cellular GPX and TR systems protect thyrocytes from these peroxides, as oxidative stress induces TR1 and GPX [4]. The current recommended dietary intake of Se in adults, in order to achieve the maximal activity of GPX in plasma or in erythrocytes, ranges from 55 to 75 g/day [32–36]. Foods rich in Se are Brazil nuts [36], oysters, tuna, whole-wheat bread, sunflower seeds, meat (pork, beef, lamb, turkey, chicken), mushrooms, and rye. Studies have shown different results regarding the efficacy of Se supplementation in Hashimoto's thyroiditis patients [37–39].

Three meta-analysis studies confirmed that patients with Hashimoto's thyroiditis who receive selenium supplements have shown a decrease in the serum levels of antibodies (TPO-Ab and Tg-Ab) attacking the thyroid gland [37–39]. The recently published systematic review and meta-analysis of Wichman et al. (2016) [39] in particular showed that Se supplementation effectively reduces serum TPO-Ab levels at 3, 6, and 12 months and serum Tg-Ab at 12 months in LT4-treated populations, but not in non-treated ones. This meta-analysis also showed a significant decrease in serum TPO-Ab levels in patients receiving 200 g seleno-methionine, but not in those receiving 200 g sodium selenite. The difference might be related to absorption of selenite which is approximately two-thirds of the absorption of seleno-methionine [3, 39]. However, another meta-analysis in the Cochrane library concluded that the evidence to support or refute the efficacy of Se supplementation in patients with Hashimoto's thyroiditis is insufficient [40]. A most recent study from Italy showed that supplementation with L-seleno-methionine for 6 months had no effect on TPO-Ab [41], but other studies have shown that Se supplementation for 12 months decreased TPO-Ab [2, 42].

A recent population-based study in China by Wu et [43] (2015) reported that the prevalence of thyroid diseases (except Graves' and nodular disease) was higher in a region of low Se intake (serum Se < 69 g/L) compared to a region of adequate Se intake (serum Se 69 g/L or more).

However, long-term intake of large amounts of Se may have adverse effects on human health [44–49]. Consumption of approximately 330 g of Se/day could be toxic not only for growth hormones and insulin-like growth factor 1 metabolism but also in the synthesis of thyroid hormones [44, 45]. Possible major side effects include nail and hair loss, anorexia, diarrhea, depression, hemorrhage, liver and kidney necrosis, blindness, ataxia, and respiratory disturbances [45, 46]. There have also been reported cases of dermatitis and CNS disorders in an area with high Se content in Enshi, China [47]. These signs and symptoms of Se toxicity are known as selenosis. A Se intake of 50–400 g/day is considered a safe range for adults, while 850–900 g could be allowed as minimum for Se toxicity [50].

In order to predict whether a patient with Hashimoto's thyroiditis would benefit from Se supplementation, the clinician should first investigate the patient's iodine status by determining the urinary iodine excretion test in a 24-h urine sample [44]. It should be noted that excessive iodine may indicate dietary excess intake [51], recent imaging contrast media exposure or use of drugs containing iodine (e.g., amiodarone). The effect of iodine-containing antiseptic solutions appears to be negligible [52, 53]. Selenium supplementation in the form of seleno-methionine would be beneficial in Hashimoto's thyroiditis patients with Se deficiency and adequate iodine intake.

10.2.3 Zinc (Zn)

Zinc (Zn) is an essential nutrient for thyroid health that assists in the conversion of T4 to T3. The hypothalamus requires zinc to accurately gauge thyroid hormone levels to increase production when levels are low. For these reasons, zinc deficiency is linked with decreased thyroid production and hypothyroidism. A 2010 study showed that taking zinc supplements increased thyroid hormone levels in patients with goiter. Furthermore, zinc supplementation improves thymic and immune functions in children with Down syndrome [54]. Zinc deficits, like iodine, are extremely uncommon in the developed world. However, if more zinc is required to be added to diet, the following foods are excellent sources: oysters and shellfish, beef, chicken, legumes such as lentils and beans, as well as cow's milk.

10.2.4 Vitamin D

Vitamin D is now considered as both a fat-soluble vitamin and a steroid hormone that plays a central role in the regulation of calcium/phosphate homeostasis and bone intensity [55]. It is synthesized within the body via skin exposure to sunlight and through dietary intake [5]. The natural sources that provide humans with large amounts of vitamin D3 are fish (cod liver oil, wild fresh salmon, and sardines) and dairy products [5]. Its serum normal ranges between 30 and 80 ng/mL.

Several studies showed the correlation between vitamin D deficiency and thyroid autoimmunity [5, 56–60] by demonstrating that cholecalciferol supplements are effective in reducing TPO-Ab among Hashimoto's thyroiditis patients with vitamin D deficiency [60, 61], owing to its anti-inflammatory and immuno-modulatory functions [5].

The Endocrine Society of USA guidelines indicated that daily vitamin D intakes of 1500–2000 IU are needed to raise the blood level of 25(OH) D constantly above 30 ng/mL [62], while the Institute of Medicine of USA reported that the tolerable upper intake level, defined as the maximum daily intake above which the potential for adverse health effects may increase after chronic use, is 4000 IU/day [63]. Levels of 25(OH) D between 30 and 40 ng/mL that are adequate for avoiding metabolic and autoimmune disorders [64], in more than 97% of the population, can be achieved by an optimal dosage of approximately 2000 IU cholecalciferol daily, regardless of increased exposure to ultraviolet rays [65]. The main *side effects* of vitamin D over-treatment are hypercalcemia (calcium serum levels above 11 mg/dL) and nephrolithiasis. To avoid coronary artery calcification, which is an important predictor of cardiovascular disease, concomitant use of cholecalciferol with vitamin K2 (menaquinones) may be necessary [66]. Patients with renal disease cannot convert 25[OH]D to active 1,25[OH]D2 and need to receive calcitriol instead of cholecalciferol. In addition, one must consider the potential interactions of some drugs with vitamin D supplements [5, 67].

Apart from cholecalciferol or calcitriol, a regular exposure to sunlight could contribute to the prevention and management of vitamin D deficiency in Hashimoto's thyroiditis patients. It is obvious that excessive sun exposure and sunburn should be avoided because of the high risk of skin cancer (particularly melanoma) [68]. Taking into consideration the low cost and the minimal side effects of vitamin D supplementation, screening for vitamin D deficiency and careful vitamin D supplementation with monthly monitoring of calcium and 25[OH]D levels, when required, may be recommended for patients with Hashimoto's thyroiditis [5, 55].

10.2.5 Vitamin B_{12}

Vitamin B_{12} deficiency is observed in over 30% of people with autoimmune thyroid disease including Hashimoto's thyroiditis. Food sources of B_{12} include mollusks, sardines, salmon, and organ meats such as liver, muscle meat, and dairy products.

The primary sources of vitamin B_{12} in vegan diets include fortified cereals and nutritional yeast [69].

10.2.6 Gluten-Free Diet

While foods containing gluten are not the cause of Hashimoto's disease, for some people, those foods can trigger an autoimmune response [70]. This results in inflammation and tissue destruction. Gluten is part of every wheat flour product and can hide in many different foods, which thus should be avoided by patients with Hashimoto's thyroiditis, such as wheat, barley, cookies, cakes, pizza, and bread. Gluten-free alternatives for common flour-based foods are available, though they can be expensive.

Whereas it is not yet clear whether a gluten-free diet can prevent autoimmune diseases, it is worth mentioning that Hashimoto's thyroiditis patients (with or without celiac disease) benefit from a diet low in gluten as far as the progression and the potential disease complications are concerned [71]. Still, a lifelong gluten-free diet is not easy to maintain, it could be very costly, and the subject's quality of life may deteriorate [72].

10.2.7 Paleo Diet

The paleo diet (also known as caveman diet) focuses on eating what humans during the Paleolithic period of evolution ate. The focus is on "hunter-and-gatherer" style food. Because it eliminates foods that can trigger an autoimmune reaction (such as grains, dairy, and highly processed foods), the paleo diet is a highly effective diet for Hashimoto's disease. The anti-inflammatory benefits of the paleo diet can be achieved by eating the following foods: lean meat, fish, seafood, fruit, vegetables, nuts, and seeds. Starches such as potatoes should be avoided [73].

10.2.8 Vegetarian and Vegan Diets

Vegetarians do not eat meat, and vegans do not eat any animal products, including milk, butter, and eggs. These diets are said to help improve the autoimmune response involved in Hashimoto's disease. They also reduce inflammation and promote gut health. However, B-vegetarian and vegan diets are deficient in important vitamins and minerals such as iron and vitamin D. Supplements should help balance the nutritional deficiencies found in this type of diet. The following whole, plant-based foods may improve thyroid and gut health: fruits, vegetables, nuts, seeds, vegetable oils, legumes like lentils and beans, and vegetable proteins like tofu and tempeh [73].

10.3 The Worst Diet for Hashimoto's Thyroiditis

In addition to foods that help the thyroid, there are specific foods in certain amounts that can have a negative impact on the thyroid. Gluten and goitrogens are the worst foods to have in the diet of patients with Hashimoto's disease.

10.3.1 Gluten

Celiac disease is an immune-mediated disease characterized by chronic inflammation and destruction of the villous structure of the small intestine [74, 75]. It is triggered by the ingestion of gluten, a protein complex, found in wheat and related grains, such as barley, rye, and oat. Celiac disease is now considered a multi-organ disorder, often presenting with diarrhea, malabsorption syndrome, and weight loss, and has been linked to many diseases including autoimmune disorders [74–77]. According to the International Medical Bibliography, AITD and celiac disease are clearly associated [9, 77–79]. This might be explained partly by the increased immuno-sensitivity of celiac disease patients, as part of an autoimmune polyglandular syndrome, by the deficiency of key elements such as Se and iodine due to malabsorption [80, 81] or due to antibodies that affect both target tissues [82].

Some authors reported that between 3.2% [83] and 4.8% [84] of patients with autoimmune thyroid disorder tested positive for celiac disease. Valentino et al. (2002) [85] reported that 43% of Hashimoto's thyroiditis patients proved to have potential celiac disease. A study in 2003 examined 400 patients with either Grave's or Hashimoto's thyroiditis and found that 5.5% tested positive for IgA, indicating gluten sensitivity [86]. More recently, another study published in 2015 reported that 29% of patients with positive gluten sensitivity developed autoimmune disorders, most commonly Hashimoto's thyroiditis, over the course of the 10-year study [87]. These findings all suggest that gluten plays a huge rule in autoimmune disorders, specifically related to Hashimoto's thyroiditis.

Patients with Hashimoto's thyroiditis must therefore undergo celiac serological tests [serum IgA and IgG gliadin antibodies (AGA-IgA, AGA-IgG), IgA transglutaminase antibodies (TGA), and serum IgA endomysium antibodies (EMA)] [88]. If any of the celiac serological tests are positive, the patients must be investigated with gastro-duodenoscopy and duodenal biopsy [88].

Some authors suggested that gluten intolerance can be largely attributed to all autoimmune disorders. If symptoms of patients with Hashimoto's thyroiditis do not improve with lifestyle change and medication, patients may try to avoid foods that include wheat, (common in breads, cookies, and crackers), barley (common in soups and stews), and rye (common in bread and whiskey). In conclusion, any patient suffering from Hashimoto's thyroiditis should most certainly eliminate gluten from their diet.

10.3.2 Goitrogens

Goitrogens are compounds that impair the function of thyroid gland and interfere with the production of thyroxin hormones. Pro-goitrin is a biochemical from the glucosinolate family that is found in some foods. It is inactive but after ingestion is converted to goitrin, which interferes with iodine utilization in the synthesis of thyroid hormones. This has been reported to be of concern only when associated with an iodine deficiency [89]. Pro-goitrin has been isolated in cabbage, cauliflower, pricoli, spinach, kale, peanuts, mustard, and rapeseed oil. These foods do not pose much of a threat if eaten in small amounts. Moreover, heating cruciferous vegetables alters the potential goitrogenic effect.

While people with goiters should be especially wary of goitrogens, most patients with Hashimoto's disease will not negatively impact their symptoms unless they consume a large amount of these foods every day.

Soy, which comes from soybeans, is another potential goitrogen, and the isoflavone and genistein in soy inhibited the synthesis of thyroxin which could result in goiter. Nonetheless, multiple studies revealed that hypothyroidism is not associated with soy intake in people with adequate amounts of iodine [90, 91].

10.3.3 Alcohol

Alcohol feeds negative bacteria, and can allow them to get into the bloodstream through tiny holes in the epithelial cells and create an autoimmune response even in very small amounts. For this reason, alcohol is best avoided. Cooking with alcohol is also best to avoid at least initially and may be considered again after some healing has occurred [92].

10.3.4 Other Food Additives, Supplements, and Chemicals

Gums such as guar and xanthan gum, lecithin, and carrageenan act as emulsifiers and thickeners in recipes and are hidden in a lot of prepared and canned foods. They are complex sugar molecules that are very hard to digest, and therefore, anyone suffering from leaky gut should avoid them [92].

Coffee and fiber supplements lower the absorption of thyroid medication (L-thyroxine) suggesting a 1-h gap between the both with thyroid medication [93, 94]. In addition, flavonoids in fruits and vegetables exhibit a potential cardiovascular benefit; however, high dosages of flavonoid supplements attenuate thyroid function [95].

References

1. Caturegli P, De Remigis A, Rose NR. Hashimoto thyroiditis: clinical and diagnostic criteria. Autoimmun Rev. 2014;13:391–7.
2. Mazokopakis E, Papadakis JA, Papadomanolaki MG, Batistakis AG, Giannakopoulos TG, Protopapadakis EE, et al. Effects of 12 months treatment with L-selenomethionine on serum anti-TPO levels in patients with Hashimoto's thyroiditis. Thyroid. 2007;17:609–12.
3. Mazokopakis EE, Tzortzinis AA, Dalieraki-Ott EI, Tsartsalis AN, Syros PK, Karefilakis CM, et al. Coexistence of Hashimoto's thyroiditis with papillary thyroid carcinoma. A retrospective study. Hormones (Athens). 2010;9:312–7.
4. Mazokopakis EE, Chatzipavlidou V. Hashimoto's thyroiditis and the role of selenium. Current concepts. Hell J Nucl Med. 2007;10:6–8.
5. Mazokopakis EE, Kotsiris DA. Hashimoto's autoimmune thyroiditis and vitamin D deficiency. Current aspects. Hell J Nucl Med. 2014;17:37–40.
6. Topliss DJ. Clinical update in aspects of the management of autoimmune thyroid diseases. Endocrinol Metab (Seoul). 2016;31:493–9.
7. Pearce SH, Brabant G, Duntas LH, Monzani F, Peeters RP, Razvi S, et al. 2013 ETA guideline: management of subclinical hypothyroidism. Eur Thyroid J. 2013;2:215–28.
8. Dilas LT, Icin T, Paro JN, Bajkin I. Autoimmune thyroid disease and other non-endocrine autoimmune diseases. Med Pregl. 2011;64:183–7.
9. Boelaert K, Newby PR, Simmonds MJ, Holder RL, Carr-Smith JD, Heward JM, et al. Prevalence and relative risk of other autoimmune diseases in subjects with autoimmune thyroid disease. Am J Med. 2010;123:183.e1–9.
10. Rohner F, Zimmermann M, Jooste P, Pandav C, Caldwell K, Raghavan R, et al. Biomarkers of nutrition for development-iodine review. J Nutr. 2014;144:1322S–42S.
11. Zimmermann MB, Boelaert K. Iodine deficiency and thyroid disorders. Lancet Diabetes Endocrinol. 2015;3:286–95.
12. Pearce EN, Andersson M, Zimmermann MB. Global iodine nutrition: where do we stand in 2013? Thyroid. 2013;23:523–8.
13. Zimmermann MB. Iodine deficiency. Endocr Rev. 2009;30:376–408.
14. Vanderpump MPJ. The epidemiology of thyroid diseases. Br Med Bull. 2011;99:39–51.
15. Laurberg P, Pedersen KM, Hreidarsson A, Sigfusson N, Iversen E, Knudsen PR. Iodine intake and the pattern of thyroid disorders: a comparative epidemiological study of thyroid abnormalities in the elderly in Iceland and in Jutland, Denmark. J Clin Endocrinol Metab. 1998;83:765–9.
16. Markou K, Georgopoulos N, Kyriazopoulou V, Vagenakis AG. Iodine-induced hypothyroidism. Thyroid. 2001;11:501–10.
17. Laurberg P, Bulow Pedersen I, Knudsen N, Ovesen L, Andersen S. Environmental iodine intake affects the type of nonmalignant thyroid disease. Thyroid. 2001;11:457–69.
18. Bjergved L, Jorgensen T, Perrild H, Carlé A, Cerqueira C, Krejbjerg A, et al. Predictors of change in serum TSH after iodine fortification: an 11-year follow-up to the DanThyr study. J Clin Endocrinol Metab. 2012;97:4022–9.
19. Zhao H, Tian Y, Liu Z, Li X, Feng M, Huang T. Correlation between iodine intake and thyroid disorders: a cross-sectional study from the South of China. Biol Trace Elem Res. 2014;162:87–94.
20. Pedersen IB, Knudsen N, Carle A, Vejbjerg P, Jørgensen T, Perrild H, et al. A cautious iodization program bringing iodine intake to a low recommended level is associated with an increase in the prevalence of thyroid autoantibodies in the population. Clin Endocrinol. 2011;75:120–6.
21. Xu C, Wu F, Mao C, Wang X, Zheng T, Bu L, et al. Excess iodine promotes apoptosis of thyroid follicular epithelial cells by inducing autophagy suppression and is associated with Hashimoto thyroiditis disease. J Autoimmun. 2016;75:50–7.
22. Duntas LH. The role of iodine and selenium in autoimmune thyroiditis. Horm Metab Res. 2015;47:721–6.

23. Carayanniotis G. Recognition of thyroglobulin by T cells: the role of iodine. Thyroid. 2007;17:963–73.
24. Dai YD, Rao VP, Carayanniotis G. Enhanced iodination of thyroglobulin facilitates processing and presentation of a cryptic pathogenic peptide. J Immunol. 2002;168:5907–11.
25. Li HS, Jiang HY, Carayanniotis G. Modifying effects of iodine on the immunogenicity of thyroglobulin peptides. J Autoimmun. 2007;28:171–6.
26. Jiang HY, Li HS, Carayanniotis K, Carayanniotis G. Variable influences of iodine on the T-cell recognition of a single thyroglobulin epitope. Immunology. 2007;121:370–6.
27. Shi L, Bi M, Yang R, Zhou J, Zhao S, Fan C, et al. Defective expression of regulatory B cells in iodine-induced autoimmune thyroiditis in non-obese diabetic H2 (h4) mice. J Endocrinol Investig. 2014;37:43–50.
28. Fiore E, Latrofa F, Vitti P. Iodine, thyroid autoimmunity and cancer. Eur Thyroid J. 2015;4:26–35.
29. Brown KM, Arthur JR. Selenium, selenoproteins and human health: a review. Public Health Nutr. 2001;4:593–9.
30. Beckett GJ, Arthur JR. Selenium and endocrine systems. J Endocrinol. 2005;184:455–65.
31. Duntas LH. The role of selenium in thyroid autoimmunity and cancer. Thyroid. 2006;16:455–60.
32. Schomburg L. Dietary selenium and human health. Nutrients. 2016;9:E22.
33. Rayman MP. Selenium and human health. Lancet. 2012;379:1256–68.
34. Rayman MP. The importance of selenium to human health. Lancet. 2000;356:233–41.
35. Institute of Medicine. Dietary reference intakes for vitamin C, vitamin E, selenium, and carotenoids. Washington, DC: National Academic Press (US); 2000. p. 284–319.
36. Mazokopakis EE, Protopapadakis EE. Recommended dietary selenium intakes and selenium concentrations in nuts. Hell J Nucl Med. 2007;10:34.
37. Toulis KA, Anastasilakis AD, Tzellos TG, Goulis DG, Kouvelas D. Selenium supplementation in the treatment of Hashimoto's thyroiditis: a systematic review and a meta-analysis. Thyroid. 2010;20:1163–73.
38. Fan Y, Xu S, Zhang H, Cao W, Wang K, Chen G, et al. Selenium supplementation for autoimmune thyroiditis: a systematic review and meta-analysis. Int J Endocrinol. 2014;2014:904573.
39. Wichman J, Winther KH, Bonnema SJ, Hegedüs L. Selenium supplementation significantly reduces thyroid autoantibody levels in patients with chronic autoimmune thyroiditis: a systematic review and meta-analysis. Thyroid. 2016;26:1681–92.
40. van Zuuren EJ, Albusta AY, Fedorowicz Z, Carter B, Pijl H. Selenium supplementation for Hashimoto's thyroiditis: summary of a Cochrane systematic review. Eur Thyroid J. 2014;3:25–31.
41. Esposito D, Rotondi M, Accardo G, Vallone G, Conzo G, Docimo G, et al. Influence of short term selenium supplementation on the natural course of Hashimoto's thyroiditis: clinical results of a blinded placebo-controlled randomized prospective trial. J Endocrinol Investig. 2017;40:83–9.
42. Nacamulli D, Mian C, Petricca D, Lazzarotto F, Barollo S, Pozza D, et al. Influence of physiological dietary selenium supplementation on the natural course of autoimmune thyroiditis. Clin Endocrinol. 2010;73:535–9.
43. Wu Q, Rayman MP, Lv H, Schomburg L, Cui B, Gao C, et al. Low population selenium status is associated with increased prevalence of thyroid disease. J Clin Endocrinol Metab. 2015;100:4037–47.
44. Kaprara A, Krassas GE. Selenium and thyroidal function; the role of immunoassays. Hell J Nucl Med. 2006;9:195–203.
45. Vinceti M, Wei ET, Malagoli C, Bergomi M, Vivoli G. Adverse health effects of selenium. Rev Environ Health. 2001;16:233–51.
46. Fan AM, Kizer KW. Selenium. Nutritional, toxicologic and clinical aspects. West J Med. 1990;153:160–7.
47. Yang GQ, Wang SZ, Zhou RH, Sun SZ. Endemic selenium intoxication of humans in China. Am J Clin Nutr. 1983;37:872–81.

48. Vinceti M, Bonvicini F, Bergomi M, Malagoli C. Possible involvement of overexposure to environmental selenium in the etiology of amyotrophic lateral sclerosis: a short review. Ann Ist Super Sanita. 2010;46:279–83.
49. Aldosary BM, Sutter ME, Schwartz M, Morgan BW. Case series of selenium toxicity from a nutritional supplement. Clin Toxicol (Phila). 2012;50:57–64.
50. Parekh PP, Khan AR, Torres MA, Kitto ME. Concentrations of selenium, barium, and radium in Brazil nuts. J Food Compost Anal. 2008;21:332–5.
51. Katagiri R, Asakura K, Uechi K, Masayasu S, Sasaki S. Iodine excretion in 24-hour urine collection and its dietary determinants in healthy Japanese adults. J Epidemiol. 2016;26:613–21.
52. Michalaki M, Pylioti A, Loutas V, Mamali I, Markou KB. Absence of differences in urinary iodine excretion and thyroid function tests in operating room staff members using or not using iodine-containing antiseptic solutions. Thyroid. 2013;23:1659–60.
53. Markou KB, Koukkou EG. The Greek population is iodine sufficient and not at risk of iodine-induced hyperthyroidism. J Nutr. 2012;142:1611–2.
54. Ertek S, Cicero A, Caglar O, Erdogan G. Relationship between serum zinc levels, thyroid hormones and thyroid volume following successful iodine supplementation. Hormones. 2010;9(3):263–8.
55. Caprio M, Infante M, Calanchini M, Mammi C, Fabbri A. Vitamin D: not just the bone. Evidence for beneficial pleiotropic extraskeletal effects. Eat Weight Disord. 2017;22(1):27–41.
56. Kivity S, Agmon-Levin N, Zisappl M, Shapira Y, Nagy EV, Dankó K, et al. Vitamin D and autoimmune thyroid diseases. Cell Mol Immunol. 2011;8:243–7.
57. Sönmezgöz E, Ozer S, Yilmaz R, Önder Y, Bütün I, Bilge S. Hypovitaminosis D in children with Hashimoto thyroiditis. Rev Med Chile. 2016;144:611–6.
58. Muscogiuri G, Mari D, Prolo S, Fatti LM, Cantone MC, Garagnani P, et al. 25 Hydroxyvitamin D deficiency and its relationship to autoimmune thyroid disease in the elderly. Int J Environ Res Public Health. 2016;13:850.
59. Bozkurt NC, Karbek B, Ucan B, Sahin M, Cakal E, Ozbek M, et al. The association between severity of vitamin D deficiency and Hashimoto's thyroiditis. Endocr Pract. 2013;19:479–84.
60. Mazokopakis EE, Papadomanolaki MG, Tsekouras KC, Evangelopoulos AD, Kotsiris DA, Tzortzinis AA. Is vitamin D related to pathogenesis and treatment of Hashimoto's thyroiditis? Hell J Nucl Med. 2015;18:222–7.
61. Chaudhary S, Dutta D, Kumar M, Saha S, Mondal SA, Kumar A, et al. Vitamin D supplementation reduces thyroid peroxidase antibody levels in patients with autoimmune thyroid disease: an open-labeled randomized controlled trial. Indian J Endocrinol Metab. 2016;20:391–8.
62. Holick MF, Binkley NC, Bischo-Ferrari HA, Gordon CM, Hanley DA, Heaney RP, et al. Evaluation, treatment, and prevention of vitamin D deficiency: an Endocrine Society clinical practice guideline. J Clin Endocrinol Metab. 2011;96:1911–30.
63. Institute of Medicine. Dietary reference intakes for calcium and vitamin D. Editors: A. Catharine Ross, Christine L. Taylor, Ann L. Yaktine, and Heather B. Del Valle. Washington, DC: National Academic Press (US); 2011.
64. Holick MF. Vitamin D deficiency. N Engl J Med. 2007;357:266–81.
65. Heaney RP. The case for improving vitamin D status. J Steroid Biochem Mol Biol. 2007;103:635–41.
66. Beulens JW, Booth SL, van den Heuvel EG, Stoecklin E, Baka A, Vermeer C. The role of menaquinones (vitamin K) in human health. Br J Nutr. 2013;110:1357–68.
67. Robien K, Oppeneer SJ, Kelly JA, Hamilton-Reeves JM. Drug-vitamin D interactions: a systematic review of the literature. Nutr Clin Pract. 2013;28:194–208.
68. van der Rhee HJ, de Vries E, Coebergh JW. Regular sun exposure benefits health. Med Hypotheses. 2016;97:34–7.
69. Sworczak K, Wisniewski P. The role of vitamins in the prevention and treatment of thyroid disorders. Endokrynol Pol. 2011;62:340–4.
70. Volta U, De Franceschi L, Molinaro N, Tetta C, Bianchi FB. Organ-specific autoantibodies in coeliac disease: do they represent an epiphenomenon or the expression of associated autoimmune disorders? Ital J Gastroenterol Hepatol. 1997;29:18–21.

71. Lundin KE, Wijmenga C. Coeliac disease and autoimmune disease-genetic overlap and screening. Nat Rev Gastroenterol Hepatol. 2015;12:507–15.
72. Collin P. Should adults be screened for celiac disease? What are the benefits and harms of screening? Gastroenterology. 2005;128:S104–8.
73. Liontiris MI, Mazokopakis EE. A concise review of Hashimoto thyroiditis (HT) and the importance of iodine, selenium, vitamin D and gluten on the autoimmunity and dietary management of HT patients; points that need more investigation. Hell J Nucl Med. 2017;20(1):51–6.
74. Green PH, Cellier C. Celiac disease. N Engl J Med. 2007;357:1731–43.
75. Tonutti E, Bizzaro N. Diagnosis and classification of celiac disease and gluten sensitivity. Autoimmun Rev. 2014;13:472–6.
76. Kaukinen K, Collin P, Mykkanen AH, Partanen J, Mäki M, Salmi J. Celiac disease and autoimmune endocrinologic disorders. Dig Dis Sci. 1999;44:1428–33.
77. Freeman HJ. Endocrine manifestations in celiac disease. World J Gastroenterol. 2016;22:8472–9.
78. Hadithi M, de Boer H, Meijer JW, Willekens F, Kerckhaert JA, Heijmans R, et al. Coeliac disease in Dutch patients with Hashimoto's thyroiditis and vice versa. World J Gastroenterol. 2007;13:1715–22.
79. Tuhan H, Ik S, Abac A, Şimşek E, Anık A, Anal Ö, et al. Celiac disease in children and adolescents with Hashimoto thyroiditis. Turk Pediatri Ars. 2016;51:100–5.
80. Stazi AV, Trinti B. Selenium deficiency in celiac disease: risk of autoimmune thyroid diseases. Minerva Med. 2008;99:643–53.
81. Stazi AV, Trinti B. Selenium status and over-expression of interleukin 15 in celiac disease and autoimmune thyroid diseases. Ann Ist Super Sanita. 2010;46:389–99.
82. Naiyer AJ, Shah J, Hernandez L, Kim SY, Ciaccio EJ, Cheng J, et al. Tissue trans-glutaminase antibodies in individuals with celiac disease bind to thyroid follicles and extracellular matrix and may contribute to thyroid dysfunction. Thyroid. 2008;18:1171–8.
83. Lieberman S. The gluten connection. New York: Rodale Books; 2007.
84. Collin P, Salmi J, Hallstrom O, Reunala T, Pasternack A. Autoimmune thyroid disorders and coeliac disease. Eur J Endocrinol. 1994;130(2):137–40.
85. Valentino R, Savastano S, Maglio M, Paparo F, Ferrara F, Dorato M, et al. Markers of potential coeliac disease in patients with Hashimoto's thyroiditis. Eur J Endocrinol. 2002;146(4):479–83.
86. Akcay M, Akcay G. The presence of the antigliadin antibodies in autoimmune thyroid diseases. Hepatogastroenterology. 2003;50(Suppl):2.
87. Carroccio A, D'Alcamo A, Cavataio F, Soresi M, Seidita A, Sciume C, et al. High proportions of people with non-celiac what sensitivity have autoimmune disease of anti-nuclear antibodies. Gastroenterology. 2015;149(3):596–603.e1. https://doi.org/10.1053/j.gastro.2015.05.040.
88. Roy A, Laszkowska M, Sundström J, Lebwohl B, Green PH, Kämpe O, et al. Prevalence of celiac disease in patients with autoimmune thyroid disease: a meta-analysis. Thyroid. 2016;26:880–90.
89. Felker P, Bunch R, Leung AM. Concentrations of thiocyanate and goitrin in human plasma, their precursor concentrations in brassica vegetable and associated potential for hypothyroidism. Nutr Rev. 2016;74:248–58.
90. Divia RL, Changa HC, Doerge DR. Anti-thyroid isoflavones from soy bean: isolation, characterization and mechanisms of action. Biochem Pharmacol. 1997;54:1087–96.
91. Messina M, Redmond G. Effects of soy protein and soy bean isoflavones on thyroid function in healthy adults and hypothyroid patients: a review of the relevant literature. Thyroid. 2006;16:249–58.
92. Bethesda. Hypothyroidism: National endocrine and metabolic diseases information service. Department of Health and Human Services, NIH Publication No. 13-6180; 2013. p. 61–80.
93. Mazokopakis EE, Giannakopoulos TG, Starakis K. Interaction between levothyroxine and calcium carbonate. Can Fam Physician. 2008;54:39.

94. Benvenga S, Bartolone L, Pappalardo MA, Lapa RA, Trimarchi F, et al. Altered intestinal absorption of L-thyroxine cause by coffee. Thyroid. 2008;18:293–301.
95. Egert S, Rimbach G. Which sources of flavonoids: complex diets or dietary supplements? Adv Nutr. 2011;2:8–14.

Chronic Thyroiditis: Hashimoto's Encephalopathy

11

11.1 Introduction

Hashimoto's encephalopathy is an uncommon neurological condition associated with Hashimoto's thyroiditis and is characterized by encephalopathy, altered mental status, hallucinations, delusions, and sometimes seizures, in association with high serum anti-thyroid antibody concentration (thyroid autoimmunity) that is usually responsive to glucocorticoid therapy [1]. It is sometimes referred to as a "neuro-endocrine disorder," although the condition's relationship to the endocrine system is widely disputed. It is recognized as a rare disease by the National Institute of Health (NIH) Genetic and Rare Diseases Information Center [2].

Originally described in 1966, Hashimoto's encephalopathy remains a somewhat controversial disorder. It most often presents with a subacute onset of confusion with altered level of consciousness, seizures, and myoclonus. In contrast to the cognitive dysfunction associated with hypothyroidism or hyperthyroidism, Hashimoto's encephalopathy is believed to be an immune-mediated disorder rather than representing the direct effect of an altered thyroid state on the central nervous system [3]. Diagnosis requires exclusion of other identifiable causes of encephalopathy [4, 5]. Brain magnetic resonance imaging (MRI) and cerebrospinal fluid (CSF) studies are either normal or non-specific. Currently, an aggressive form of Hashimoto's thyroiditis accompanied by elevated serum IgG4 levels has been described (IgG4-related thyroiditis). In relation to Hashimoto's encephalopathy, it is possible that the IgG4 fraction may be responsible for the CNS involvement causing encephalopathy [6–8]. Negative thyroid peroxidase antibodies (anti-TPOs) may represent a valuable parameter in ruling out Hashimoto's encephalopathy. Nonetheless, this result cannot be used to confirm the diagnosis. Furthermore, the proposed anti-NH2-terminal-α-enolase (anti-NAE) is non-specific for Hashimoto's encephalopathy. The effectiveness of glucocorticoid therapy is 60.94%, although relapse occurs in 31.67% of patients following the treatment. The etiology, pathogenesis, as well as treatment of Hashimoto's encephalopathy still need to be clearly defined [9].

M. Sakr, *Thyroiditis*, https://doi.org/10.1007/978-3-032-19513-5_11

Up to the year 2005, there were almost 200 published case reports of Hashimoto's encephalopathy. From 1990 to 2000, 43 cases were published. Since that time, research has expanded, and numerous cases are being reported by scientists around the world, suggesting that this rare condition is likely to have been significantly undiagnosed in the past. Over 100 scientific articles on Hashimoto's encephalopathy were published between 2000 and 2013 [10]. So far, over 300 cases of Hashimoto's encephalopathy have been described, with approximately 30 occurring in children [11].

11.2 Definition/Synonyms

11.2.1 Definition

Hashimoto's encephalopathy is a "relapsing encephalopathy occurring in association with Hashimoto's thyroiditis with high titers of anti-thyroid antibodies." Clinically, the condition may present one or more symptoms. Onset is often gradual and may go unnoticed by the patients and their close associates. Symptoms sometimes resolve themselves within days to weeks, leaving a patient undiagnosed. For many other patients, the condition may result in ongoing problems with a variety of manifestations, often confusing clinicians due to the diffuse nature of symptoms.

11.2.2 Synonyms

Since there is no direct pathophysiological link between anti-thyroid antibodies, Hashimoto's thyroiditis, and the cerebral syndrome, the nomenclature Hashimoto's encephalopathy could be misleading. The response to steroids led to a re-naming to "steroid responsive encephalopathy associated with autoimmune thyroiditis" (SREAT), though some cases do *not* respond to steroids including Lord Brain's original patient. Another nomenclature is "non-vasculitic autoimmune inflammatory meningo-encephalitis" (NAIM), but it probably does *not* reflect the neuropathology with accuracy [12]. Hashimoto's encephalopathy has also been known as "encephalopathy associated with autoimmune thyroid disease" (EAATD).

11.3 Historical Review

The first case of Hashimoto's encephalopathy was described by Lord Brain et al. in 1966 [13]. The patient was a 49-year-old man previously diagnosed with hypothyroidism due to Hashimoto's thyroiditis, confirmed by elevated anti-thyroid antibodies. He developed a neurological illness consisting of altered mood and consciousness, along with stroke-like episodes causing transient aphasia, hemiparesis, hemisensory symptoms, hemianopia, and monocular blindness. These were followed by episodes of hallucinations, confusion, and involuntary movements (tremor and athetosis).

The patient CSF studies showed raised protein content with mild pleocytosis. Carotid angiography was normal, EEG showed generalized slowing. He was treated with prednisone and anticoagulant therapy with inconsistent response and ultimately resolved while taking only levothyroxine [13]. Since 1966, many cases of Hashimoto's encephalopathy have been reported with varied presentations—fulminant, acute, subacute, or chronic patterns of altered mental status—occurring across all ages [14].

11.4 Epidemiology

11.4.1 Prevalence

The syndrome of Hashimoto's encephalopathy is relatively rare with an estimated prevalence of 2.1/100,000 in the adult population [15].

11.4.2 Gender

Hashimoto's encephalopathy occurs much more frequently in women than in men (4:1), which may result from the higher incidence of Hashimoto's disease in the female population [1, 15].

11.4.3 Age

Although Hashimoto's encephalopathy has been described in all age groups (including children), it is most common in individuals between 40 and 60 years of age. The mean age of onset is 44 years, ranging from 41 to 48 years [11, 16], with approximately 20% of patients presenting before the age of 18 years [11, 17, 18].

11.4.4 Co-morbidities

In addition, Hashimoto's encephalopathy co-occurs with other autoimmune diseases (such as Sjögren's syndrome, type I diabetes mellitus, and systemic lupus erythematosus) in approximately 30% of patients [5]. Notably, it is also highly likely that Hashimoto's encephalopathy remains underdiagnosed [19, 20].

11.5 Pathogenesis

The pathogenesis of Hashimoto's encephalopathy is uncertain and remains unclear [1, 9, 20]. Although overt hypothyroidism can cause cerebral dysfunction, there is no evidence that thyroid hormone dysregulation (hypothyroidism or hyperthyroidism) has any role in the pathogenesis of Hashimoto's encephalopathy, as majority of the patients are euthyroid at the time of presentation [5]. Because of the uncertainty regarding its etiopathogenesis, Hashimoto's encephalopathy has remained a controversial entity. Thus, it would be relevant to address the issue of what induces and affects the development of Hashimoto's encephalopathy. Essentially, three major mechanisms have emerged [8, 18, 21–29].

11.5.1 Vasculitis

The first proposed mechanism for the development of Hashimoto's encephalopathy is related to "vasculitis." The concept assumes that the brain micro-vasculature is altered and that this condition leads to edema, or that vasculitis is a result of endothelial inflammation [22]. Histopathological and morphological examinations in patients with Hashimoto's encephalopathy revealed the presence of chronic, limited inflammatory lesions of the cortex and meninges, which have been referred to as NAIM (non-vasculitis autoimmune inflammatory meningo-encephalitis) [23]. A research published by Nolte et al. (2000). described an association between Hashimoto's encephalopathy and lymphocytic infiltration around small arterioles or venules or inflammatory lesions of the brainstem and gray matter due to vasculitis [24].

The pathogenetic process is probably associated with immune complex deposition, possibly disrupting the cerebral micro-vasculature. Consistent with this hypothesis, auto-antibodies to α-enolase have been found to be associated with Hashimoto's encephalopathy [30]. Since enolase is the penultimate step in glycolysis, if it were inhibited (e.g., by being bound by auto-antibodies), one would expect decreased energy production by each cell, leading to atrophy of the affected organ. This would occur most likely through each cell shrinking in size in response to the energy deficit (and/or in extreme situations from some cells dying via either apoptosis or necrosis, depending on location). This may occur due to lack of ATP to maintain cellular functions: notably failure of the Na/K ATPase, resulting in a loss of the gradient to drive the Na/Ca anti-porter, which normally keeps Ca+2 out of cells so that it does not build to toxic levels that will rupture cell lysosomes leading to apoptosis. An additional feature of a low-energy state is failure to maintain axonal transport via Dynein/Kinesin ATPases, which in many diseases results in neuronal injury to both the brain and/or periphery [30].

11.5.2 Anti-thyroid Antibodies (Autoimmunity)

The second hypothesis for the development of Hashimoto's encephalopathy is based on the presence of anti-thyroid antibodies. The bulk of available evidence points to an "autoimmune" disorder similar to Hashimoto's thyroiditis, as its name suggests (autoimmune vasculitis), or other inflammatory process [1, 20]. As in most autoimmune conditions, the disease is more common in women. In more than one-third of patients, there is co-morbidity with other systemic or organ-specific autoimmune diseases such as systemic lupus erythematosus (SLE), Sjögren's syndrome, pernicious anemia, sarcoidosis, and myasthenia gravis [15]. Most patients with Hashimoto's encephalopathy respond to steroids or other immunosuppressive therapies.

Elevated anti-thyroid antibodies are consistent with an autoimmune process, though it is unlikely that these antibodies have a direct pathogenic role. The thyroid antibodies are thus considered as diagnostic markers rather than etiological agents. Moreover, no correlation has been found between thyroid antibody concentration, the severity of the disease, and the constellation of symptoms [18, 21, 26, 31]. Despite high levels of anti-thyroid antibodies in the serum and cerebrospinal fluid (CSF), they have *not* been observed in the central nervous system (CNS) structures in autopsy studies [1, 19]. A review by Chong et al. (2003) entitled "Hashimoto encephalopathy—syndrome or myth?" concluded that "the combination of encephalopathy, high serum anti-thyroid antibody concentrations, and responsiveness to glucocorticoid therapy seems unlikely to be due to chance. However, there is no evidence of a pathogenic role for the antibodies, which are probably markers of some other autoimmune disorder affecting the brain" [19].

In recent years, an aggressive form of Hashimoto's thyroiditis accompanied by elevated serum IgG4 levels has been described (IgG4-related thyroiditis). Characteristic features include a higher incidence in men than in women (5:1), onset at a younger age, more intense thyroid inflammation, and higher anti-thyroid antibody titers [27, 32]. Such subjects have excessive production of IgG4 + plasmocytes, which infiltrate various organs leading to fibrosis and sclerosis, and even inflammatory tumors [7]. It has been observed that IgG4 antibodies are present in 70% of patients with hypothyroidism but only 14% in euthyroid patients [29]. Other members of the family of IgG4-related disorders include autoimmune pancreatitis, sclerosing cholangitis, interstitial nephritis, Sjögren syndrome, Riedel's goiter, and hypertrophic pachymeningitis. In relation to Hashimoto's encephalopathy, it is possible that the IgG4 fraction may be responsible for the CNS involvement causing encephalopathy [6–8].

In 2013, Hosoi et al. described a 60-year-old patient with severe Hashimoto's encephalopathy and elevated IgG4 concentrations in serum and CSF. The patient's IgG4 index was lower than that of IgG, indicating passive transport of IgG4 across the blood–brain barrier. Moreover, after corticosteroid treatment, serum IgG4 levels decreased, but were indeterminate in the cerebrospinal fluid. The described case may highlight the suspected influence of the IgG4 fraction on the development of neurological abnormalities, including Hashimoto's encephalopathy [8].

Most reports of Hashimoto's encephalopathy appeared before the spectrum of autoimmune encephalitis was recognized and so tests for other auto-antibodies were not done or done in a limited way. Thus, it is possible that some of the cases reported were actually autoimmune encephalitis patients, who are also responsive to steroids and immunosuppressive therapy, and the raised TPO antibody titer was just an incidental finding. In a recent review (2020), Mattozzi et al. [33] studied 24 patients meeting the accepted diagnostic criteria of Hashimoto's encephalopathy and lacking co-existing serum or CSF anti-glial or anti-neuronal antibodies. The patients had four clinical subtypes including rapidly progressive psychiatric syndrome in 29%, encephalopathy/cognitive impairment in 29%, new-onset refractory status epilepticus in 25%, and limbic encephalitis in 17%. There were no patients with stroke-like episodes. Surprisingly, only 32% responded to steroids. These patients were otherwise similar to those who did *not* respond, and it was not possible to distinguish them before treatment. TPO antibody levels were studied in two other groups: 74 patients with possible autoimmune encephalitis without neuronal antibodies and 205 with different neuro-immunological diseases. The frequency of Hashimoto's encephalopathy was approximately 8% in both groups, suggesting it is a non-specific finding, and of limited use in picking up possible Hashimoto's encephalopathy cases in a group of patients with encephalopathy of unknown origin with negative neuronal antibodies [33].

11.5.3 Increased Thyrotropin-Releasing Hormone (TRH)

A third hypothesis that stems from the toxic effects of increased thyrotropin-releasing hormone (TRH) on the CNS has been proposed, as some patients appear to improve with thyroid supplementation despite being euthyroid. However, these cases appear to be the exception rather than the rule. Only one study has been conducted which demonstrated that TRH triggered myoclonus and tremor similar to the symptoms that patients experience during exacerbation of Hashimoto's encephalopathy symptoms [25]. The hypothesis of a direct toxic effect of TRH on nerve cells causing inflammatory lesions of the brain and medulla, in the course of demyelination, was also considered as a causative factor when a patient developed myoclonus and tremor after an intravenous TRH infusion [25].

11.6 Pathology

Very little is known about the pathology of Hashimoto's encephalopathy. Post-mortem studies of some individuals have shown lymphocytic vasculitis of venules and veins in the brain stem and a diffuse gliosis involving gray matter more than white matter. Auto-antibodies to alpha-enolase associated with Hashimoto's encephalopathy have thus far been the most hypothesized mechanism of injury.

Autopsy and histopathological examinations have not shown the presence of antibodies in the structures of the nervous system, but only in the tissues of the thyroid gland, even if these antibodies could be detected in high concentrations in the serum and sometimes in the CSF [34]. Thyroid gland fibrosis evidenced by ultrasonography (US) is more common in patients with anti-TPO antibody than with the anti-TG antibody [14]. This prompted some workers to question the value of anti-Tg antibodies in the diagnosis of Hashimoto's encephalopathy. Furthermore, no significant decrease in the levels of such antibodies could be detected in some patients after treatment with corticosteroids [35]. This is in contrast to our observations in two of the three patients reported recently by Chaudhuri and colleagues in 2023 [14].

11.7 Clinical Presentation

11.7.1 History-Taking

Pempera et al. (2024) [36] reported that out of 48 interviewed patients, 18 (38%) reported a history of autoimmune disease in their family or personal history. Hence, Hashimoto's encephalopathy appears highly likely to co-occur with other autoimmune diseases. However, no clear data are available with regard to the most common co-morbidities. The existence of an autoimmune disease in the family or in the patient should indicate the need to monitor the disease in order to limit its development and to start treatment as early as possible.

11.7.2 Clinical Features

The onset of symptoms in Hashimoto's encephalopathy tends to be fairly gradual and to occur over 1–7 days. The clinical course is generally *not* specific; however, cognitive dysfunction has been described as the initial manifestation in over 80% of patients, and behavioral and personality disorders in over 90–100% [5, 15]. The clinical disorders observed in the course of Hashimoto's encephalopathy vary. Some patients develop tremors, myoclonus, ataxia, stupor, or coma [37, 38]. Patients less frequently report persistent headaches, gait disturbances, isolated nystagmus, opsoclonus-myoclonus syndrome, Parkinsonian syndromes, fatigue syndrome, sleep disturbances, or hallucinations [1, 15].

Seizures are common, occurring in approximately two-thirds of the patients [19, 39]. Diagnosis of Hashimoto's encephalopathy should be considered in unexplained episodes of focal or generalized seizures, refractory to common anti-epileptic drugs, with cognitive impairment and neuropsychiatric symptoms. New onset status epilepticus (SE), including epilepsia partialis continua (EPC), and non-convulsive SE (NCSE) have been reported by several authors [39–42]. A limbic encephalitis-like presentation with subacute onset memory deficits, decreased level of consciousness, seizures, and behavioral change can also occur [43]. Autoimmune encephalitis, including Anti-IgLON5 disease [44], needs to be excluded in such cases with appropriate tests for neuronal surface antibodies. Anti-IgLON5 disease is a recently defined autoimmune disorder of the nervous system associated with autoantibodies against IgLON5. It is a progressive disorder which combines autoimmunization with neuro-degeneration and may have a very heterogenous manifestations, the clinical features of which consist of a sleep disorder with non-rapid eye movement (REM) sleep parasomnia, REM behavior disorder, obstructive sleep apnea syndrome, stridor bulbar symptoms, gait abnormalities, extrapyramidal features, autonomic disturbances, and cognitive dysfunction [44].

Hashimoto's encephalopathy can cause progressive cognitive deterioration with dementia, neuro-psychiatric symptoms, and impaired consciousness [45, 46]. This is seen more in older patients, and Hashimoto's encephalopathy should be considered in the differential diagnosis of rapidly progressive dementia, especially Creutzfeldt–Jakob disease (CJD), which is an incurable, always fatal neurodegenerative disease belonging to the transmissible spongiform encephalopathy (TSE) group. Even in patients with apparent degenerative dementias like Alzheimer's disease, Lewy body dementia, fronto-temporal dementia, and cortico-basal degeneration, Hashimoto's encephalopathy needs consideration if the course is too rapid or atypical.

According to the six studies analyzed by Pempera et al. [36] and reported recently in 2024, Tang et al. (2012) [47] reported that out of 13 patients with Hashimoto's encephalopathy, memory disorders were found in 7 patients (53.8%), psychiatric symptoms in 5 (38.5%), sleep disturbance and seizures in 4 patients each (30.8%), and involuntary movement in only 1 (7.7%). Mamoudjy et al. (2013) [48], in turn, observed that out of eight patients, disorders of consciousness were present in seven (87.5%), seizures and behavioral changes in four each (50%). According to Sharma et al. (2015) [49] who studied 13 patients with Hashimoto's encephalopathy, memory disturbance and behavioral changes was recorded in 10 patients each (76.9%), sleep disturbance in 9 (69.2%), seizures in 6 (46.2%), psychiatric symptoms in 5 (38.5%), and involuntary movement in 4 (30.8%). Kishitani et al. (2017) [14] reported that out of 14 patients, disorders of consciousness were encountered in 10 patients (71.4%), memory dysfunction in 9 (64.3%), psychiatric symptoms in 7 (50%), seizures in 6 (42.9%), involuntary movement in 2 (14.3%), and respiratory impairment in only 1 (7.1%). Recently, Mattozzi et al. (2020) [33], who analyzed 24 patients with Hashimoto's encephalopathy, reported seizures in 12 patients (50%), psychiatric symptoms and disorders of consciousness in 6 patients each (25%), as well as memory impairment, behavioral changes, and involuntary movement in 4 patients each (16.7%). In another more recent study, Dumrikarnlert et al. (2023) [50] found that out of 13 studied patients, disorders of consciousness and psychiatric symptoms occurred in 6 patients each (46.2%), sleep disorders and seizures in 5 patients each (38.5%), behavioral changes in 4 patients (30.8%), and involuntary movement in 3 (23.1%). These clinical features are summarized in Table 11.1.

In general, symptoms of Hashimoto's encephalopathy can be summarized as follows [43]:

- Personality changes
- Aggression
- Delusional behavior
- Concentration and memory problems
- Decreased level of consciousness—coma
- Disorientation
- Headaches
- Jerks in the muscles (myoclonus)
- Lack of coordination (ataxia)

Table 11.1 Clinical features of Hashimoto's encephalitis reported recently in the literature [21, 33, 47–50]

Clinical features	Tang et al. $N = 13$ [47] 2012	Mamoudjy et al. $N = 8$ [48] 2013	Sharma et al. $N = 13$ [49] 2015	Kishitani et al. $N = 14$ [21] 2017	Mattozzi et al. $N = 24$ [33] 2020	Dumrikarnlert et al. $N = 13$ [50] 2023
Memory disorders	7 (53.8%)	–	10 (76.9%)	9 (64.3%)	4 (16.7%)	–
Psychiatric symptoms	5 (38.5%)	–	5 (38.5%)	7 (50%)	6 (25%)	6 (46.2%)
Sleep disorders	4 (30.8%)	–	9 (69.2%)	–	–	5 (38.5%)
Seizures	4 (30.8%)	4 (50%)	6 (46.2%)	6 (42.9%)	12 (50%)	5 (38.5%)
Involuntary movement	1 (7.7%)	–	4 (30.8%)	2 (14.3%)	4 (16.7%)	3 (23.1%)
Disorders of consciousness	–	7 (87.5%)	–	10 (71.4%),	6 (25%)	6 (46.2%)
Behavioral changes	–	4 (50%)	10 (76.9%)	–	4 (16.7%)	4 (30.8%)
Respiratory impairment	–	–	–	1 (7.1%)	–	–

- Partial paralysis on the right side
- Psychosis
- Seizures
- Status epilepticus
- Sleep abnormalities
- Speech problems (transient aphasia)
- Tremors

11.7.3 Clinical Types (Patterns) of Hashimoto's Encephalopathy

According to symptoms, two types (patterns) of Hashimoto's encephalopathy have been described in the literature. In the first, recurrent incidents appear which suggests that the underlying cause is vascular (stroke-like incidents and focal symptoms, corresponding to transient cerebral ischemia), with frequent disorders of cognitive function, although without seizures. It occurs more rarely and is milder, and thus the prognosis indicates higher chances of recovery. The other pattern or type is progressive in nature, with epileptic seizures, disturbances of consciousness, psychiatric symptoms such as mania, depression, or psychosis, and increasing dementia syndrome. It is more common, usually has acute onset and rapid course, and usually progresses without relapses. The manifestations of the second type seem to be more intense, and hence the prognosis usually remains poorer [1, 8, 11]. Myoclonus and tremors have been reported to occur in both types [51].

11.8 Investigations/Diagnosis

11.8.1 General Laboratory Findings

In general, laboratory studies may show increased liver enzyme levels in approximately 55% of patients, elevated anti-nuclear antibodies (ANA) in 31.2%, positive rheumatoid factor in 11.5%, increased thyroid-stimulating hormone (TSH) levels in about 50%, increased erythrocyte sedimentation rate (ESR) in nearly 25%, and increased C-reactive protein (CRP) in 13% [43]. Moreover, Kishitani et al. (2017) [21] reported that hyponatremia was present in 6 of 14 studied patients (42.9%). It is of note that the above-mentioned parameters do not indicate the presence of characteristic Hashimoto's encephalopathy changes. In fact, they suggest that Hashimoto's encephalopathy is a diverse disease, which differs in various patients.

11.8.2 Cerebrospinal Fluid (CSF) Findings

The CSF studies show abnormalities, usually mild, in approximately 80% of patients. The most common abnormality is raised protein content in around 75% of patients. Protein levels more than 100 mg/dl are uncommon, occurring in only 20%. A mild lymphocytic pleocytosis is present in 10–25% [52]. The CSF is characteristically negative for 14–3–3 protein in Hashimoto's encephalopathy [53] but contains anti-thyroid antibodies in the majority of patients [52].

11.8.3 Thyroid Hormone Abnormalities

Thyroid status varies from overt hypothyroidism to overt hyperthyroidism. However, most patients with Hashimoto's encephalopathy are either euthyroid or have subclinical hypothyroidism. The following thyroid hormone abnormalities may be found in more than 80% of patients with Hashimoto's encephalopathy [43]:

- Subclinical hypothyroidism (35% of cases)
- Overt hypothyroidism (20% of cases)
- Hyperthyroidism (5% of cases)
- Euthyroid on levothyroxine (10% of cases)
- Euthyroid not on levothyroxine (20% of cases)

11.8.4 Thyroid Antibodies

11.8.4.1 Anti-thyroid Peroxidase (Anti-TPO) Antibodies

In Hashimoto's encephalopathy, anti-thyroid peroxidase (anti-TPO) antibodies, anti-thyroid microsomal (anti-M) antibodies, and anti-thyroglobulin (anti-Tg) antibodies are elevated in majority of cases, and are required for diagnosis, but their levels do not correlate with the severity or disease activity. In a review of 105 patients with Hashimoto's encephalopathy, anti-TPO antibodies were elevated in 100% of patients, and anti-Tg antibodies in 48% [31, 54]. However, the presence of thyroid antibodies is not specific, as about 10% of the general population has raised serum anti-TPO [55, 56].

In the recent systematic and critical review of Pempera et al. (2024), it was reported that in six studies [21, 33, 47–50], anti-TPO antibody was measured in 71 patients, and was elevated in 67 (94%). According to the researchers, although an increased level of anti-TPO antibodies is not specific, it was considered as a criterion for the diagnosis of Hashimoto's encephalopathy.

It should be emphasized that the sensitivity of anti-TPO antibodies is 85.714%, whereas the specificity is 60.563% [21, 33, 47–50]. Thus, it is conceivable to conclude that the positive predictive value is 46.154%, and the negative predictive value is 91.489%. This, in turn, demonstrates that anti-TPO antibodies may constitute an extremely useful parameter, indicating that a person with a negative result does not actually suffer from Hashimoto's encephalopathy. However, anti-TPO level cannot be used to state conclusively that a patient with a positive result has Hashimoto's encephalopathy.

11.8.4.2 Thyroid-Stimulating Hormone (TSH) Antibodies

Thyroid-stimulating hormone (TSH) antibodies may also be present in patients with Hashimoto's encephalopathy. There are some reports of raised thyroid antibodies in the CSF, but the sensitivity and specificity are unclear.

11.8.4.3 Other Autoimmune Antibodies

Other autoimmune antibodies than *Anti-TPO* have also been observed in patients with Hashimoto's encephalopathy such as GABAAR (gamma-aminobutyric acid A receptor), NMDAR (N-methyl-D-aspartate receptor), Caspr2 (contactin-associated protein 2), leucine-rich glioma inactivated 1 (LGi1), α-amino-3-hydroxy-5-methylisoxazole-4-propionic acid receptor 1 and 2 (AMPAR1/2), or ANA (antinuclear antibodies) [33, 37, 39, 57].

11.8.4.4 Anti-NH2-Terminal-α-Enolase (Anti-NAE) Antibodies

Interestingly, a new antigen, alpha-enolase (α-enolase), has recently been discovered in the brains of Hashimoto's encephalopathy patients. In addition, high levels of α-enolase antibodies have been found in the serum and cerebrospinal fluid (CSF) of the same patient group [53]. As it seemed essential to find a specific parameter specifically characterizing Hashimoto's encephalopathy, researchers proposed antibodies directed against the amino-terminal domain of alpha enolase (NAE) as a potential reliable biomarker of Hashimoto's encephalopathy [18, 53]. However, it subsequently turned out that α-enolase was *not* specific to the blood vessels of the brain, and that it appeared in most cells of the human body [58]. It was demonstrated that increased values of α- and γ-enolases also occur in other autoimmune diseases, such as rheumatoid arthritis (RA), systemic lupus erythematosus (SLE), anti-neutrophil cytoplasmic antibodies (ANCAs) positive vasculitis, autoimmune nephritis, primary Sjögren's syndrome, systemic sclerosis, primary biliary cirrhosis (PBC), inflammatory bowel disease (IBD), and celiac disease [58–60]. Furthermore, one of the conducted studies has shown that the enolases have also been identified in a patient with Creutzfeldt–Jakob disease (CJD) [61], as well as in patients with limbic encephalitis [21]. Anti-NAEs are expressed in endothelial cells, which accounts for their presence in other vasculitic diseases, such as Kawasaki disease [62]. It is suggested that anti-NAE should be considered as a potential risk-modifying factor [63]. This, in turn, prompted the researchers to hypothesize that Hashimoto's encephalopathy may also constitute a form of immuno-pathological vasculitis [21, 31].

In their study, Kishitani et al. (2017) [21] measured the concentration of anti-NAE antibodies in 14 patients, and the results obtained were between 320 IU/mL and 40.960 IU/mL, which shows that the proposed parameter could be considered specific. In contrast, however, Mattozzi et al. (2020) [33] demonstrated an elevated level in just 1 patient out of the suspected 24 patients with Hashimoto's encephalopathy, and in 1 control. This, in turn, shows that anti-NAE is *not* a specific diagnostic indicator in all patients. It is highly likely that, due to different diagnostic criteria, Kishitani et al. [21] and Mattozzi et al. [33] received diverse results related to the specificity of anti-NAE antibodies. This highlights the particular need for a further, deeper understanding of the disease and a search for new diagnostic parameters [29].

11.8.5 Imaging Studies

11.8.5.1 Magnetic Resonance Imaging (MRI)

In their recent study (2023), Dumrikarnlert et al. [50] adopted brain MRI as a diagnostic criterion of Hashimoto's encephalopathy, and revealed non-specific white-matter changes in an area or areas that is/are non-specific to any other symptoms, such as in the corona radiata. None of the lesions were compatible with a diagnosis of multiple sclerosis, neuromyelitis optica, previous stroke, or brain injury [50]. The majority of patients with Hashimoto's encephalopathy have normal (approximately 60%) or non-specific magnetic resonance imaging (MRI) lesions [21, 64].

In the two cases of Hashimoto's encephalopathy described by Jegatheeswaran et al. (2021), the researchers described generalized brain atrophy or an increased signal in the subcortical white-matter area on a T2-weighted/fluid-attenuated inversion recovery (FLAIR) sequence [65]. Moreover, the authors emphasized that the changes in MRI did not disappear, despite the clinical improvement following the treatment [65]. Another case that co-existed with sensory ganglionopathy and painful neurological amyotrophy was reported by Kastrup et al. (2005) [66]. In general, abnormal MRI findings reported in the literature include ischemic lesions, demyelination, edema, atrophy, subcortical white matter high signal intensities, and increased signal in the medial temporal lobes (amygdala and hippocampus—a limbic encephalitis pattern) [67–71].

Bearing in mind that the range of the described changes is wide, they are not typical only for Hashimoto's encephalopathy, and therefore Hashimoto's encephalopathy may be mis-diagnosed as other autoimmune encephalitis. Nonetheless, MRI may be a valuable parameter in the diagnostic process, since it may also indicate other diseases that need to be excluded [71].

11.8.5.2 Other Imaging Studies

Single photon emission computed tomography (SPECT) scan shows focal and global hypoperfusion in approximately 75% of cases [43]. Cerebral angiography is normal.

11.8.6 Electro-encephalogram (EEG) Studies

EEG is almost always abnormal in over 90% of patients with Hashimoto's encephalopathy [19, 39]. However, EEG findings are usually non-specific and thus non-diagnostic [42]. The most common findings are diffuse or generalized slowing or frontal intermittent rhythmic delta activity (FIRDA), and theta-wave discharges [42]. Prominent tri-phasic waves, focal slowing, epileptiform abnormalities, and photo-paroxysmal and photo-myogenic responses may be seen. EEG may have some role in monitoring treatment response, and there are reports of EEG abnormalities improving rapidly with steroid treatment [72, 73]. The EEG also helps to exclude other conditions, such as CJD, in patients with rapidly progressive encephalopathy and myoclonus.

11.9 Diagnosis

It is vital to note that, to date, no clear diagnosis or treatment has been established for Hashimoto's encephalopathy, and the diagnosis itself is by exclusion. Therefore, firstly, it is essential to exclude all potential disorders of the central nervous system (CNS). Yet, in the available studies, different authors have used various criteria in the course of the diagnostic process of Hashimoto's encephalopathy.

The inclusion of "good response to corticosteroid treatment" as a necessary criterion in the diagnostic criteria of Hashimoto's encephalopathy remains controversial. Recent studies suggest that such a response is achieved in only 32% of patients [74]. A study by Castillo et al. (2006) suggested the following diagnostic criteria of Hashimoto's encephalopathy (Table 11.2).

In 2012, Tang et al. [47] applied certain criteria for the diagnosis of Hashimoto's encephalopathy: (1) clouding of consciousness, cognitive impairment, seizures, or neuro-psychiatric features, (2) elevated anti-TPO antibodies with euthyroid status (TSH 0.35–5.5 uIU/mL), and (3) no evidence of alternative infectious, toxic, metabolic, vascular, or neoplastic etiology in blood, urine, or CSF, or by neuro-imaging examinations. The researchers considered 13 patients but did not investigate the control group, which constitutes the most significant limitation of that study.

Table 11.2 Diagnostic criteria of Hashimoto's encephalopathy according to Castillo et al. [75]

1. Encephalopathy with cognitive impairment and at least one of the following features: (1) neuro-psychiatric symptoms such as hallucination, delusion, or paranoia, (2) myoclonus, generalized tonic-clonic or partial seizures, or (3) focal-neurological deficits
2. Elevated titers of thyroid tissue antibodies (TPO-ab or microsomal)
3. Euthyroidism (potentially achieved by replacement treatment with or mild hypothyroidism with TSH concentration below 20 mIU/L)
4. No evidence for infectious, toxic, metabolic, or neoplastic processes in blood, urine, or CSF
5. No serological evidence of neuronal antibodies (e.g., voltage-gated calcium channel, voltage-gated potassium channel, or other paraneoplastic antibodies) to support another diagnosis of vascular, neoplastic, or structural lesions that might explain the symptoms on imaging studies
6. Complete or nearly complete remission after initiation of glucocorticoid therapy

TPO-ab thyroid peroxidase antibody, *TSH* thyroid-stimulating hormone, *CSF* cerebrospinal fluid

Furthermore, all of the participants were Chinese. According to their medical history, five subjects presented with autoimmune diseases and three with thyroid disorders. Moreover, one patient reported systemic lupus erythematosus (SLE) and another suffered from Raynaud's syndrome.

In turn, Mamoudjy et al. (2013) [48] based their diagnosis on the clinical signs of hypothyroidism (goiter, fatigue, and/or stunted growth) and high serum anti-TPO antibody levels. The researchers compared the group of 8 children to 34 controls, and found that 4 of 8 children had a personal or familial history of autoimmune disease.

In another study, Sharma et al. (2015) [49] applied the following diagnostic criteria: (1) acute or subacute onset of altered mental status (AMS), (2) elevated anti-thyroid antibodies, (3) rapid response to the administration of corticosteroids reflected in patients' mental status, and (4) absence of structural, infectious, or other metabolic factors, which could account for the AMS and its response to steroids. Their study comprised 13 participants, yet they also failed to report the control group. In five patients, a history of hypothyroidism preceded the onset of neurological symptoms, and one presented with euthyroid goiter.

According to the diagnostic criteria suggested by Graus et al. (2016), the diagnosis of Hashimoto's encephalopathy is by exclusion [76]. In 2016, Graus et al. proposed the diagnostic criteria of Hashimoto's encephalopathy as summarized in Table 11.3 [76].

Kishitani et al. (2017) [21], in their research, relied merely on the presence of anti-thyroid antibodies and the responsiveness to immunotherapy. Their study involved 14 patients with Hashimoto's encephalopathy and 26 individuals who constituted the control group (12 healthy subjects and 14 participants with Hashimoto's thyroiditis who did not present with any neuropsychiatric symptoms). In three patients belonging to the study group, a history of Hashimoto's disease was present prior to the suspicion of Hashimoto's encephalopathy. The limitations of their study include the small number of patients and the inclusion of only Japanese subjects.

Mattozzi et al. (2020) [33] employed in their study of 24 patients and 13 controls the following criteria for the diagnosis of: (1) subacute onset of cognitive

Table 11.3 Diagnostic criteria of Hashimoto's encephalopathy

1. Encephalopathy with seizures, myoclonus, hallucinations, or stroke-like episodes
2. Subclinical or mild overt thyroid disease
3. Normal or non-specific brain MRI
4. Serum thyroid antibodies present (no specific disease—cut-off value)
5. Absence of other neuronal antibodies in serum or CSF
6. Exclusion of alternative causes of encephalopathy by differential diagnosis

MRI magnetic resonance imaging, *CSF* cerebrospinal fluid

impairment, psychiatric symptoms or seizures, (2) euthyroid status or mild hypothyroidism, (3) serum thyroid peroxidase antibodies (TPOAbs) > 200 IU/mL, and (4) absent neuronal antibodies in the serum or CSF and no other etiologies.

More recently, in 2023, a study by Dumrikarnlert et al. [50] included 13 patients and 91 control subjects. Interestingly, they applied the same Hashimoto's encephalopathy diagnostic criteria reported previously by Graus et al. in 2016 [76].

11.10 Differential Diagnosis

The most frequently reported clinical features of Hashimoto's encephalopathy are disturbances of consciousness, impaired memory, and sleep disturbance [36]. These symptoms are found in many neurological and psychiatric disorders, which makes the diagnosis of Hashimoto's encephalopathy even more challenging. Patients are often mis-diagnosed and need to be subsequently re-diagnosed. The issues related to mis-diagnosis prolong the waiting time for the optimal treatment.

Hashimoto's encephalopathy should be differentiated from the following disorders:

- Alzheimer's disease
- Cerebro-vascular accidents (CVA) (stroke)
- Creutzfeldt-Jakob disease (CJD)
- Epilepsy
- Migraine (including basilar, hemiplegic, and retinal types)
- Other forms of autoimmune encephalitis, including forms of limbic encephalitis such as anti-NMDA receptor encephalitis
- Schizophrenia
- Spontaneous cerebrospinal fluid leak

- Viral encephalitis
- Transient ischemic attack (TIA)

11.11 Treatment

There have been no controlled trials on the treatment of Hashimoto's encephalopathy, so there are no clearly established treatment guidelines and the optimal treatment is *not* exactly known.

11.11.1 First Choice: Corticosteroids

Because many patients with Hashimoto's encephalopathy respond to corticosteroids (the first choice) or immune-suppressant treatment, this condition is now also referred to as "steroid-responsive encephalopathy." Since Hashimoto's encephalopathy is rather rare, there are no guidelines regarding corticosteroid dose and/or duration. Initial treatment is usually with oral prednisone (50–150 mg/day) or high-dose intravenous (IV) methyl-prednisolone (1 g/day) for 3–7 days [75]. Most patients respond to steroid therapy with improvement occurring over weeks to months. Duration of therapy and tapering of steroids are adjusted according to the clinical response. Some patients require treatment to be continued for up to 2 years [14]. Although the effectiveness of glucocorticoid therapy is 60.94%, relapse occurs in 31.67% of patients after such treatment. It is vital to note that seizures may recur, particularly following a reduction in the steroid dose [39, 77].

11.11.2 Second-Line (Alternative) Treatments

A variety of alternative or second-line treatments have been proposed and tried in Hashimoto's encephalopathy patients who do not tolerate corticosteroids, do not respond, or relapse during steroid tapering. Such alternative treatments include azathioprine, cyclophosphamide, chloroquine, methotrexate, periodic IV immunoglobulin (IVIG), and plasma exchange [78]. Intravenous immunoglobulin treatment has been reported by several researchers to produce significant improvement in both adults and children, but the efficacy of plasma exchange is doubtful despite removal of anti-thyroid antibodies [34, 79–81].

11.11.3 Symptomatic Treatment

Thyroid hormone treatment is also included if required, and seizures, if present, are controlled with typical anti-epileptic agents [75, 78].

11.11.4 Treatment Complications

The treatment of patients with Hashimoto's encephalopathy results clearly demonstrate that in most cases, steroid therapy significantly improves the patients' condition. The majority of patients report complete recovery, or observe significant improvement; however, studies have described relapses, and some treated patients require further rounds of steroids and, at times, immunosuppressive therapy with other drugs. Corticosteroids are potentially more effective at the very onset of the disease; therefore, the delay in diagnosis may result in the need for another type of treatment. Interestingly, some studies describe cases of spontaneous recovery, as well [82].

Long-term steroid treatment is *not* risk-free, and hence it is worth bearing in mind that it may result in serious side effects. The patients who undergo such a treatment require frequent monitoring of clinical and laboratory parameters. Moreover, side effects may involve most major organ systems, such as musculo skeletal, gastrointestinal, cardiovascular, endocrine, neuro-psychiatric, dermatological, ocular, and immunological. All sorts of adverse reactions are possible, including joint necrosis, growth suppression, adrenal insufficiency, osteoporosis, gastrointestinal and hepatic effects, hyperlipidemia, or congenital malformations [82].

11.12 Prognosis

The prognosis of Hashimoto's encephalopathy is usually good. Patients can improve even if treatment is delayed for months or years after the onset of symptoms. Residual cognitive improvement occurs in around 25% of patients with long-standing, untreated disease. Patients usually remain disease-free after steroid tapering, but some relapse and require further courses of steroids and sometimes immunosuppressive therapy. There are some reports of spontaneous recovery as well [23, 83].

Duration of treatment is usually between 2 and 25 years. Earlier reports suggested that 90% of cases stay in remission after discontinuation of treatment; however, this is at odds with more recent studies which suggest that relapse commonly occurs after initial high-dose steroid treatment [75, 78]. Left untreated, this condition can result in coma and death.

11.13 Summary

Hashimoto's encephalopathy is a rare disease with non-specific clinical manifestations and uncertain pathogenesis. Furthermore, even the diagnostic criteria have not been clearly defined so far. Hashimoto's encephalopathy encompasses a wide spectrum of neurological features. Cerebellar involvement [84, 85] and extra-pyramidal features [19, 86] in the form of tremors and myoclonus, as well as autonomic features, have been reported [87]. It has been known to present with a pure, progressive cerebellar syndrome with normal cognitive function and intellectual performance [88]. Cognitive decline and psychosis/hallucinations would suggest a form of limbic encephalitis [33]. Stroke-like symptoms, myoclonus, and tremors are also frequently seen, either alone or as part of a syndrome [43]. Sometimes, Hashimoto's encephalopathy can present with an acute encephalopathy. Diagnosis is usually considered in patients with the above neurological symptoms, accompanied by either a euthyroid state or mild hypothyroidism [89, 90], normal or non-specific MRI and CSF findings, increased serum levels of thyroid antibodies (anti-TPO and/or anti-Tg) [91], a robust clinical response to steroids, and exclusion of other possible causes. Additionally, anti-NAE was also suggested as a parameter indicating Hashimoto's encephalopathy, yet it has been proven not to be specific.

Hashimoto's encephalopathy should be considered in the differential diagnosis in patients with acute or subacute features of encephalopathy, cerebellar and extrapyramidal features, autonomic failure, status epilepticus, non-convulsive status epilepticus (NCSE), as well as with rapidly progressive cognitive impairment and psychiatric symptoms of unclear etiology. Taking into account the possibility of the co-existence of various autoantibodies, Hashimoto's encephalopathy should, in some cases, be differentiated from other autoimmune encephalopathies and paraneoplastic syndromes. If elevated titers of antibodies to thyroid antigens are then demonstrated, corticosteroid treatment should be considered as soon as possible, along with treatment of the dysthyroid condition, if any. There are yet no guidelines regarding steroid dose and/or duration. Future large-scale research (randomized trials) should be conducted to look for more specific markers for Hashimoto's encephalopathy and to consider the need to take into account a potential genetic factor for the disease. Since Hashimoto's encephalopathy may also co-exist with other autoimmune diseases, it is of the essence to gain a deeper understanding with regard to the underlying processes involved in the development of this disorder [36].

References

1. Ferracci F, Bertiato G, Moretto G. Hashimoto's encephalopathy: epidemiological data and pathogenetic considerations. J Neurol Sci. 2004;217:165–8.
2. Genetic and Rare Diseases Information Center (GARD). Hashimoto's encephalitis – disease – overview. 2013. http://rarediseases.info.nih.gov/gard/8570/hashimotos-encephalitis/resources/1.
3. Ferracci F, Carnevale A. The neurological disorder associated with thyroid autoimmunity. J Neurol. 2006;253:975–84.
4. Gayatri NA, Whitehouse WP. Pilot survey of Hashimoto's encephalopathy in children. Dev Med Child Neurol. 2005;47:556–8.
5. Olmez I, Moses H, Sriram S, Kirshner H, Lagrange AH, Pawate S. Diagnostic and therapeutic aspects of Hashimoto's encephalopathy. J Neurol Sci. 2013;331:67–71.
6. Hamano H, Kawa S, Horiuchi A. High serum IgG4 concentrations in patients with sclerosing pancreatitis. N Engl J Med. 2001;344:732–8.
7. Kubo K, Yamamoto K. IgG4-related disease. Int J Rheum Dis. 2015;19:747–62.
8. Hosoi Y, Kono S, Terada T, Konishi T, Miyajima H. Hashimoto's encephalopathy associated with an elevated intrathecal IgG4 level. J Neurol. 2013;260:1174–6.

9. Fatourechi V. Hashimoto's encephalopathy: myth or reality? An endocrinologist's perspective. Best Pract Res Clin Endocrinol Metab. 2005;19:53–66.
10. Naga LN, Naveen KNR, Venkata RKC, Bhuvana BJN, Suresh KC, Siva RK, et al. A case report on Hashimoto's encephalopathy. World J Pharma Res. 2018;7(9):618–24.
11. Laurent C, Capron J, Quillerou B. Steroid-responsive encephalopathy associated with autoimmune thyroiditis (SREAT): characteristics, treatment and outcome in 251 cases from the literature. Autoimmun Rev. 2016;15:1129–33.
12. Kanazawa M, Shimohata T, Tanaka K, Nishizawa M. Clinical features of patients with myasthenia gravis associated with autoimmune diseases. Eur J Neurol. 2007;14:1403–4.
13. Brain L, Jellinek EH, Ball K. Hashimoto's disease and encephalopathy. Lancet. 1966;2:512–4.
14. Chaudhuri J, Mukherjee A, Chakravarty A. Hashimoto's encephalopathy: case series and literature review. Curr Neurol Neurosci Rep. 2023;23(4):167–75.
15. Mocellin R, Walterfang M, Velakoulis D. Hashimoto's encephalopathy: epidemiology, pathogenesis and management. Neurology. 2020;94:55–6.
16. Tamagno G, Federspil G, Murialdo G. Clinical and diagnostic aspects of encephalopathy associated with autoimmune thyroid disease (or Hashimoto's encephalopathy). Intern Emerg Med. 2006;1:15–23.
17. Lee J, Yu HJ. Hashimoto's encephalopathy in pediatric patients: homogeneity in clinical presentation and heterogeneity in antibody titers. Brain Dev. 2017;40(1):42–8.
18. Fujii A, Yoneda M, Ito T, Yamamura O, Satomi S, Higa H, et al. Autoantibodies against the amino terminal of alpha-enolase are a useful diagnostic marker of Hashimoto's encephalopathy. J Neuroimmunol. 2005;162(1–2):130–6.
19. Chong JY, Rowland LP, Utiger RD. Hashimoto encephalopathy: syndrome or myth? Arch Neurol. 2003;60:164–71.
20. Payer J, Petrovic T, Lisy L, Langer P. Hashimoto encephalopathy: a rare intricate syndrome. Int J Endocrinol Metab. 2012;10:506–14.
21. Kishitani T, Matsunaga A, Ikawa M, Hayashi K, Yamamura O, Hamano T, et al. Limbic encephalitis associated with anti-NH2-terminal of α-enolase antibodies: a clinical subtype of Hashimoto encephalopathy. Medicine (Baltimore). 2017;96:e6181.
22. Bertoni M, Falcini M, Sestini S, Niccoli L, Nannini C, Cantini F. Encephalopathy associated with Hashimoto's thyroiditis: an additional case. Eur J Intern Med. 2003;14:434–7.
23. Caselli RJ, Boeve BF, Scheithauer BW, O'Duffy JD, Hunder GG. Nonvasculitic autoimmune inflammatory meningoencephalitis (NAIM): a reversible form of encephalopathy. Neurology. 1999;53:1579–81.
24. Nolte KW, Unbehaun A, Sieker H, Kloss TM, Paulus W. Hashimoto encephalopathy: a brainstem vasculitis? Neurology. 2000;54:769–70.
25. Ishii K, Hayashi A, Tamaoka A, Usuki S, Mizusawa H, Shoji S. Case report: thyrotropin-releasing hormone-induced myoclonus and tremor in a patient with Hashimoto's encephalopathy. Am J Med Sci. 1995;310:202–5.
26. Blanchin S, Coffin C, Viader F, Ruf J, Carayon P, Potier F, et al. Anti-thyroperoxidase antibodies from patients with Hashimoto's encephalopathy bind to cerebellar astrocytes. J Neuroimmunol. 2007;192:13–20.
27. Popławska-Kita A, Kościuszko-Zdrodowska M, Siewko K, Telejko B, Hryniewicka J, Milewski H. High serum IgG4 concentrations in patients with Hashimoto's thyroiditis. Int J Endocrinol. 2015;2015:706843.
28. Zhang J, Zhao L, Gao Y, Liu M, Li T, Huang Y, et al. A classification of Hashimoto's thyroiditis based on immunohistochemistry for IgG4 and IgG. Thyroid. 2014;24:364–70.
29. Xie L, Gao Y, Li MR, Lu G, Guo XH. Distribution of immunoglobulin G subclasses of anti-thyroid peroxidase antibody in sera from patients with Hashimoto's thyroiditis with different thyroid functional status. Clin Exp Immunol. 2008;154:172–6.
30. Ihejirika DF. PASS program course notes: USMLE preparation. Lulu.com; 2014.
31. Grani G, Carbotta G, Nesca A, D'Alessandri M, Vitale M, Del Sordo M, et al. A comprehensive score to diagnose Hashimoto's thyroiditis: a proposal. Endocrine. 2015;49:361–5.

32. Zen Y, Nakanuma Y. Pathogenesis of IgG4-related disease. Curr Opin Rheumatol. 2011;23:114–8.
33. Mattozzi S, Sabater L, Escudero D, Ariño H, Armangue T, Simabukuro M, et al. Hashimoto encephalopathy in the 21st century. Neurology. 2020;94(2):e217–24.
34. Ragusa F, Fallahi P, Elia G, Gonnella D, Paparo SR, Giusti C, et al. Hashimoto's thyroiditis: epidemiology, pathogenesis, clinic and therapy. Best Pract Res Clin Endocrinol Metab. 2019;33:101367.
35. Chou KM, Huang BY, Chen CH, Lin JD, Lee CC. Correlation and presentation of thyroid functional status with thyroid autoantibodies in long-term follow-up of autoimmune thyroiditis: a study of 116 cases. J Formos Med Assoc. 2013;20:1039–46.
36. Pempera N, Miedziaszczyk M, Lacka K. Difficulties in the diagnostics and treatment of Hashimoto's encephalopathy—a systematic and critical review. Int J Mol Sci. 2024;25(13):7101–17.
37. Tzakas P, Sit SW. Progressive impairment of cognition and motor function: Hashimoto encephalopathy. CMAJ. 2011;183:495–7.
38. Das S, Reddy B. Hashimoto's encephalopathy presented with mutism: a case report. Gen Psychiatr. 2021;34:e100502.
39. Casciato S, Di Bonaventura C, Lapenta L, Fattouch J, Ferrazzano G, Fanella M, et al. Recurrent partial seizures with ictal yawning as atypical presentation of Hashimoto's encephalopathy. Epilepsy Behav. 2011;22:799–803.
40. Li J, Li F. Hashimoto's encephalopathy and seizure disorders. Front Neurol. 2019;10:440.
41. Tsai MH, Lee LH, Chen SD, Lu CH, Chen MT, Chuang YC. Complex partial status epilepticus as a manifestation of Hashimoto's encephalopathy. Seizure. 2007;16:713–6.
42. Ercoli T, Defazio G, Muroni A. Status epilepticus in Hashimoto's encephalopathy. Seizure. 2019;70:1–5.
43. Nagano M, Kobayashi K, Yamada-Otani M. Hashimoto's encephalopathy presenting with smoldering limbic encephalitis. Intern Med. 2019;58:1167–72.
44. Nissen MS, Blaabjerg M. Anti-IgLON5 disease: a case with 11-year clinical course and review of the literature. Front Neurol. 2019;10:1056.
45. Carta MG, Hardoy MC, Carpiniello B, Murru A, Marci AR, et al. A case control study on psychiatric disorders in Hashimoto disease and euthyroid goitre: not only depressive but also anxiety disorders are associated with thyroid autoimmunity. Clin Pract Epidemiol Ment Health. 2005;1:23.
46. Dardano A, Bazzzichi L, Bombardieri S, Monzani F. Symptoms in euthyroid Hashimoto's thyroiditis: is there a role for autoimmunity itself? Thyroid. 2012;22:334–5.
47. Tang Y, Xing Y, Lin MT, Zhang J, Jia J. Hashimoto's encephalopathy cases: Chinese experience. BMC Neurol. 2012;12:1–7.
48. Mamoudjy N, Korff C, Maurey H, Blanchard G, Steshenko D, Loiseau-Corvez MN, et al. Hashimoto's encephalopathy: identification and long-term outcome in children. Eur J Paediatr Neurol. 2013;17:280–7.
49. Sharma PMS, Javali M, Mahale R, Madhusudhan BK, Majeed AA, Srinivasa R. Hashimoto encephalopathy: a study of the clinical profile, radiological and electrophysiological correlation in a Tertiary Care Center in South India. J Neurosci Rural Pract. 2015;6:309–14.
50. Dumrikarnlert C, Thakolwiboon S, Senanarong V. Clinical presentations and treatment outcomes of Hashimoto encephalopathy at Siriraj Hospital–Thailand's largest national tertiary referral center. BMC Neurol. 2023;23:334.
51. Duffey P, Yee S, Reid IN, Bridges LR. Hashimoto's encephalopathy: postmortem findings after fatal status epilepticus. Neurology. 2003;61:1124–6.
52. Ferracci F, Moretto G, Candeago RM, Cimini N, Conte F, Gentile M, et al. Antithyroid antibodies in the CSF: their role in the pathogenesis of Hashimoto's encephalopathy. Neurology. 2003;60:712–4.
53. Ochi H, Horiuchi I, Araki N, Toda T, Araki T, Sato K. Proteomic analysis of human brain identifies alpha-enolase as a novel autoantigen in Hashimoto's encephalopathy. FEBS Lett. 2002;528:197–202.

54. Weetman AP. An update on the pathogenesis of Hashimoto's thyroiditis. J Endocrinol Invest. 2021;44:883–90.
55. Ahmed OM, El-Gareib AW, El-Bakry AM, Abd El-Tawab SM, Ahmed RG. Thyroid hormones states and brain development interactions. Int J Dev Neurosci. 2008;26:147–209.
56. Bernal J. Thyroid hormones and brain development. Vitam Horm. 2005;71:95–122.
57. Uy CE, Binks S, Irani SR. Autoimmune encephalitis: clinical spectrum and management. Pract Neurol. 2021;21:412–23.
58. Ji H, Wang JF, Guo J, Li Y, Lian S, Guo W, et al. Progress in the biological function of alpha-enolase. Anim Nutr. 2016;2:12–7.
59. Terrier B, Degand N, Duilpain P, Servettaz A, Guillevin L, Mouthon L. Alpha-enolase: a target of autoantibodies in infectious and autoimmune diseases. Autoimmun Rev. 2007;6:176–82.
60. Cheng JL, Beebe JD, Nepple KG, Zakharia Y, Mullins RF, Flamme-Wiese MJ, et al. Autoimmune retinopathy and optic neuropathy associated with enolase-positive renal oncocytoma. Am J Ophthalmol Case Rep. 2018;12:55–60.
61. Hayashi Y, Yamada M, Kimura M, Asano T, Satoh K, Kitamoto T, et al. Clinical findings of a probable case of MM2-cortical-type sporadic CJD with antibodies to anti-N-terminus of alpha-enolase. Prion. 2017;11:454–64.
62. Chun JK, Lee TJ, Choi KM, Lee KH, Kim DS. Elevated anti α enolase antibody levels in Kawasaki disease. Scand J Rheumatol. 2008;37:48–52.
63. Matsunaga A, Masamichi I, Makoto Y. Expanding clinical spectrum from Hashimoto's encephalopathy to anti-NAE antibody-associated disorders (NAEAD). Clin Exp Neuroimmunol. 2024;15:24–31.
64. Degnan AJ, Levy LM. Neuroimaging of rapidly progressive dementias, part 2: prion, inflammatory, neoplastic, and other etiologies. AJNR Am J Neuroradiol. 2014;35(3):424–31.
65. Jegatheeswaran V, Chan M, Chen YA. MRI findings of two patients with Hashimoto encephalopathy. Cureus. 2021;13:e15697.
66. Kastrup O, Maschke M, Schlamann K, Diener HC. Hashimoto encephalopathy and neuralgic amyotrophy-causal link or chance association? Eur Neurol. 2005;53:98–9.
67. Waliszewska-Prosół M, Bladowska J, Budrewicz S, Sasiadek M, Dziadkowiak E, Ejma M. The evaluation of Hashimoto's thyroiditis with event-related potentials and magnetic resonance spectroscopy and its relation to cognitive function. Sci Rep. 2021;11:2480.
68. Chen N, Qin W, Wei C, Li K. Time course of Hashimoto's encephalopathy revealed by MRI: report of two cases. J Neurol Sci. 2011;300:169–72.
69. Imperiale D, Guastamacchia G, Duca S, Appendino L, Marietti G, Romito A, et al. Regression of white matter MRI abnormalities in nonvasculitic autoimmune inflammatory meningoencephalitis following intravenous immunoglobulin. Eur Neurol. 2007;57:244–5.
70. Tang X, Liu X, Jing J, Jiang L, Liu P, Chen Y. Hashimoto's encephalopathy presenting as Wernekinck commissure syndrome: a case report. Clin Neuropathol. 2022;41:128–34.
71. Bladowska J, Waliszewska-Prosół M, Ejma M, Sasiadek M. The metabolic alterations within the normal appearing brain in patients with Hashimoto's thyroiditis are correlated with hormonal changes. Metab Brain Dis. 2019;34:53–60.
72. Muramatsu T, Hamano T, Shirafuji N, Matsunaga A, Ikawa M, Yoneda M. Hashimoto's encephalopathy presenting periodic synchronous discharge, as a differential diagnosis for Creutzfeldt-Jakob disease. Rinsho Shinkeigaku. 2013;53(9):716–20.
73. Waliszewska-Prosół M, Ejma M. Assessment of visual and brainstem auditory evoked potentials in patients with Hashimoto's thyroiditis. J Immunol Res. 2021;2021:3258942.
74. Ralli M, Angeletti D, Fiore M, D'Aguanno V, Lambiase A, Artico M, et al. Hashimoto's thyroiditis: an update on pathogenic mechanisms, diagnostic protocols, therapeutic strategies, and potential malignant transformation. Autoimmun Rev. 2020;19(10):102649.
75. Castillo P, Woodruff B, Caselli R, Vernino S, Lucchinetti C, Swanson J, et al. Steroid-responsive encephalopathy associated with autoimmune thyroiditis. Arch Neurol. 2006;63(2):197–202.
76. Graus F, Titulaer MJ, Balu R, Benseler S, Bien CG, Cellucci TJ. A clinical approach to diagnosis of autoimmune encephalitis. Lancet Neurol. 2016;15:391–404.

77. Smets I, Titulaer MJ. Antibody therapies in autoimmune encephalitis. Neurotherapeutics. 2022;19:823–31.
78. Flanagan EP, McKeon A, Lennon VA, Boeve BF, Trenerry MR, Tan KM, et al. Autoimmune dementia: clinical course and predictors of immunotherapy response. Mayo Clin Proc. 2010;85(10):881–7.
79. Cook MK, Malkin M, Karafin MS. The use of plasma exchange Hashimoto's encephalopathy: a case report and review of literature. J Clin Apher. 2015;30:188–92.
80. Zhu Y, Yang H, Xiao F. Hashimoto's encephalopathy: a report of three cases and relevant literature reviews. Int J Clin Exp Med. 2015;5(2):16817–26.
81. Horn S, Heuer H. Thyroid hormone action during brain development: more questions than answers. Mol Cell Endocrinol. 2010;315:19–26.
82. Caturegli P, De Remigis A, Rose NR. Hashimoto thyroiditis: clinical and diagnostic criteria. Autoimmun Rev. 2014;13:391–7.
83. Nunez J, Celi FS, Ng L, Forrest D. Multigenic control of thyroid hormone functions in the nervous system. Mol Cell Endocrinol. 2008;287:1–12.
84. Manto M. Hashimoto's associated ataxia. J Neurol Neurosurg Psychiatry. 2002;72:277–8.
85. Termsarasab P, Pitakpatapee Y, Frucht SJ, Srivanitchapoom P. Steroid-responsive encephalopathy associated with autoimmune thyroiditis (SREAT) presenting with pure cerebellar ataxia. Tremor Other Hyperkinet. 2018;8:585.
86. Sheetal SK, Mathew R, Peethambaran B. Hashimoto's encephalopathy as a treatable cause of corticobasal syndrome. Ann Indian Acad Neurol. 2016;19(2):285–6.
87. Inoeu K, Kitamura J, Yoneda M, Imamura E, Tokinobu H. Hashimoto's encephalopathy presenting with micrographia as a typical feature of parkinsonism. Neurol Sci. 2012;33(2):395–7.
88. Tomkins M, Cavalcoli F, Stanley E, O'Rourke K, Murphy S, Lynch T, et al. Autonomic alterations as a clinical manifestation of encephalopathy associated with autoimmune thyroid disease. Endocr J. 2018;65(8):869–75.
89. Shariff EM. Sudden-onset encephalopathy: do not ignore the possibility of Hashimoto's encephalopathy. Neurol India. 2020;68(3):681–3.
90. Hallowell JG, Staehling NW, Flanders WD, Hannon WH, Gunter EW, Spencer CA, et al. Serum TSH, T(4), and thyroid antibodies in the United States population (1998 to 1884): National Health and Nutrition Examination Survey (NHANES III). J Clin Endocrinol Metab. 2002;87:489–99.
91. Lee SW, Donlon S, Caplan JP. Steroid responsive encephalopathy associated with autoimmune thyroiditis (SREAT) or Hashimoto's encephalopathy: a case and review. Psychosomatics. 2011;52:99–108.

Chronic Thyroiditis: Hashimoto's Ophthalmopathy

12

12.1 Introduction

Autoimmune thyroid diseases comprise two main clinical presentations: Graves' disease (hyperthyroidism) and Hashimoto's thyroiditis (hypothyroidism), both characterized by antibodies that attack the thyroid gland. Indeed, these disorders are the opposite ends of the same underlying cause. Thyroid eye disease (TED), also known as "thyroid-associated ophthalmopathy or orbitopathy" (TAO), is an autoimmune disorder of the extraocular muscles and surrounding orbital connective tissue. It is characterized by an inflammatory orbital process and remodeling of surrounding connective tissue, with subsequent fat accumulation, myositis, and/or tissue scarring due to autoimmune activation of orbital fibroblasts [1, 2]. It is usually associated with Graves' disease, affecting approximately 25% of these patients, representing the most common extra-thyroidal manifestation of the disease; however, it can also be associated with Hashimoto's thyroiditis occurring in nearly 6% of those patients [3–7].

The close clinical relationship between hyperthyroidism (Graves' disease), Graves' ophthalmopathy, and thyroid dermopathy (peritibial myxedema) suggests that these conditions arise from a single underlying systemic process with variable expression in the thyroid gland, eyes, and skin. Elucidating the pathophysiology of TED is the cornerstone of evolving diagnostic criteria, drug development, and surgical management.

Bilateral ocular disease and hyperthyroidism usually occur simultaneously or within 18 months of each other, although occasionally Graves' ophthalmopathy precedes or follows the onset of hyperthyroidism by many years [8]. Approximately, 50% of patients with Graves' hyperthyroidism have symptoms of Graves' ophthalmopathy. These include a dry and gritty ocular sensation, photophobia, excessive tearing, double vision, and a pressure sensation behind the eyes. Typical clinical signs include upper eyelid retraction, periorbital edema and erythema, proptosis (Fig. 12.1), and impairment of eye motility [9]. Approximately 3%–5% of patients with Graves' ophthalmopathy have severe disease with intense pain, inflammation,

M. Sakr, *Thyroiditis*, https://doi.org/10.1007/978-3-032-19513-5_12

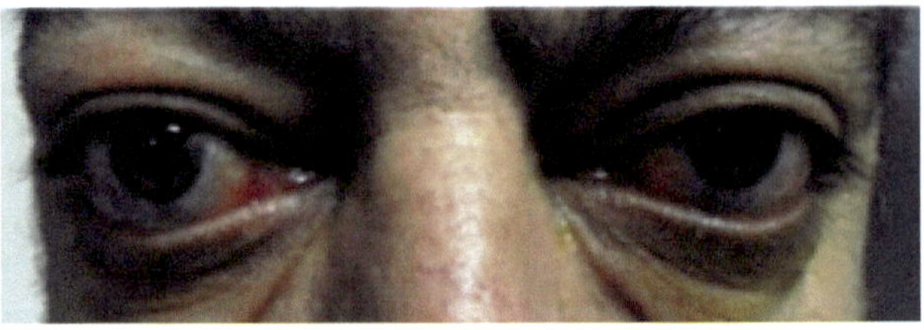

Fig. 12.1 A 35-year-old lady with thyroid-associated ophthalmopathy showing proptosis, periorbital edema, chemosis, and conjunctivitis

and sight-threatening corneal ulceration due to exposure keratopathy or compressive dysthyroid optic neuropathy (DON), therefore requiring surgical intervention in moderate to severe cases [10]. The presence of bothersome symptoms in TED patients was shown to severely impact their quality of life by being linked to feelings of depression and anxiety and a decline in self-confidence [11].

Subclinical eye involvement is common as revealed by magnetic resonance imaging (MRI) or computed tomographic (CT) scanning that show extraocular-muscle enlargement [12] in approximately 70% of adult patients with Graves' hyperthyroidism. Although clinically unilateral Graves' ophthalmopathy is not common, orbital imaging generally confirms the presence of asymmetric bilateral disease [13].

Thyroid dermopathy (nodular or diffuse thickening of pretibial skin) sometimes progresses to a debilitating disease. Although diagnosed on physical examination in only 13% of patients with severe Graves' ophthalmopathy, subclinical involvement of the skin of the legs and other regions of the body occurs more commonly [14]. Approximately 20% of patients with thyroid dermopathy have thyroid acropachy, manifesting as clubbing of fingers and toes.

12.2 Prevalence

Thyroid eye disease (TED) or thyroid-associated orbitopathy or ophthalmopathy (TAO) is believed to affect 25–50% of patients with Graves' disease and has an annual incidence of 20 cases per 100,000 people [15]. It may occur simultaneously with the manifestations of hyperthyroidism or later (approximately 70%), before the manifestation of hypothyroidism (approximately 25%), in the euthyroid state (<5%), and in hypothyroidism (3–5%) [16]. Ocular lesions in autoimmune thyroid diseases occur five times more often in women than in men (respectively, 16 and 2.9 cases per 100,000 annually); however, their course and prognosis are so far worse in men [17].

Although numerous studies have been reported about the prevalence of Graves' ophthalmopathy, similar studies about the prevalence of Hashimoto's ophthalmopathy are sparse. The first study about the prevalence of ophthalmopathy in Hashimoto's thyroiditis was reported in 2010 by Tjiang et al. [18]. They studied 91 patients with Hashimoto's thyroiditis and reported that the overall prevalence of any eye signs was 34%, and about one-third of patients had upper eyelid retraction. In addition to two patients who had eye muscle dysfunction, about a third of the patients had severe inflammatory changes such as periorbital swelling, chemosis, conjunctival injection, and proptosis.

In 2014, Kan and colleagues studied the prevalence of ophthalmopathy in 110 Hashimoto's thyroiditis for eye signs and compared them with healthy controls. They reported that the prevalence of eye signs was significantly ($p = 0.002$) higher than that of control subjects (22.7% versus 4.0%, respectively). In patients with Hashimoto's disease, 11.8% had upper eyelid retraction, 6.4% had proptosis, and 5.5% had ocular myopathy [19].

The levator palpebrae superioris and extraocular muscle involvement in Hashimoto's thyroiditis is rather common and has been emphasized in some studies. Grzesiuk et al. (2008) [20] reported a 36-year-old man with Hashimoto's thyroiditis who had enlargement of the medial and inferior rectus muscles bilaterally, with eye pain, conjunctivitis, edema of the eyelid, and exophthalmos. Hiraga et al. (2008) [21] reported a 76-year-old woman with Hashimoto's thyroiditis suffering from diplopia due to limitations of upper gaze in the right eye. She had enlargement of inferior rectus muscle unilaterally. In another study published in 2011 by Yoshihara and colleagues, they reported two patients with Hashimoto's thyroiditis with a high Clinical Activity Score (CAS). Their MRI images showed enlargement of the extraocular muscles, and both patients required systemic glucocorticoid therapy and orbital irradiation to manage the thyroid-associated ophthalmopathy [22].

12.3 Pathogenesis

A fundamental step in the management of TED is to better characterize the pathogenesis of TED and factors inducing the activation of orbital fibroblasts.

12.3.1 Autoantibodies

12.3.1.1 Autoantibodies Against TSH Receptor and Insulin-Like Growth Factor-1 Receptor

Although the pathogenesis of thyroid-associated ophthalmopathy (TAO) remains unclear, sensitized T-cells and autoantibodies against thyroid-stimulating hormone receptor (TSH-r) located on thyroid cells (thereby stimulating excess production of thyroid hormone), orbit muscles, and fibroblasts are targeted in patients developing ophthalmopathy [14, 23]. The production of autoantibodies directed towards TSH-r and insulin-like growth factor-1 receptor (IGF-1R) constitutes the main key factors involved in orbital fibroblast activation and proliferation [24, 25]. They may trigger an inflammatory process in the orbit tissues. As a result, leukocytes secrete cytokines, which stimulate fibroblasts [26]. Activated orbital fibroblasts can differentiate into two distinct phenotypes: lipid-rich adipocytes or scar-forming myofibroblasts [8]. This differential is crucial given that clinically, they form two distinct disease entities, which are type-I and type-II TED, respectively. The ensuing inflammatory process is a result of extra-cellular matrix production by activated orbital fibroblasts, as well as chemotaxis of B- and T-cells, mast cells, and macrophages to the orbital tissue [9, 27–29]. Throughout the body of molecular pathways that have been proposed to be involved in orbital fibroblast activation, immune dysregulations are the most important. Activated orbital fibroblasts lead to adipogenesis, which is involved in proptosis, orbital fat expansion, and swelling of extraocular tissues, as well as glycosaminoglycan, hyaluronan, and proteoglycan production, markers involved in scar formation.

Thus, the presence of anti-TSH-r antibodies in almost all patients with Graves' ophthalmopathy suggests that an immune reaction against TSH-r underlies both Graves' ophthalmopathy and hyperthyroidism [30]. Levels of anti-TSH-r antibodies correlate positively with the clinical features of Graves' ophthalmopathy [31]. Furthermore, a multicenter study by Diana et al. (2014), among pediatric patients, demonstrated that the level of TSH-r autoantibodies in individuals with Graves' disease correlated with disease severity and extra-thyroidal manifestation [32]. Anti-TSH-r antibody levels have been reported in the literature to influence also the prognosis [33]; these antibody levels are particularly elevated in patients with thyroid Dermopathy [34]. Conversely, immunoglobulins (Igs) were shown to stimulate IGF-1R in patients with Graves' disease; depletion of serum Igs significantly decreased IGF-1R in patients with Graves' disease [35]. However, the importance of IGF-1R in TED pathogenesis is yet controversial, with different works confirming or refuting the presence of IGF-1R autoantibodies in Graves' ophthalmopathy [36–39].

TSH-r is a G-protein-coupled trans-membrane receptor with major functions in cell proliferation [40]. Using orbital fibroblasts from patients with TED, it was shown that in vitro TSH stimulation significantly increased cell proliferation through the direct induction of the phosphoinositide 3-kinase (PI3K) pathway, and indirect up-regulation of the micro-RNAs (miRNA) miR-146a and miR-155 expression was also reported [41]. The activation of the PI3K pathway in orbital fibroblasts leads to cyclic adenosine monophosphate (cAMP) production and subsequent secretion of hyaluronan [42].

The IGF-1R is a member of the tyrosine kinase class of membrane receptors [43]. Its expression was shown to be significantly elevated in orbital fibroblasts and T- and B-cells of individuals with TED [44–47]. IGF-1R leads to downstream activation of the Ras/Raf/MEK and PI3K signaling pathways, therefore leading to cell proliferation, differentiation, inflammation, adipogenesis, and scar formations—hallmarks in TED [1]. Furthermore, once activated by its ligand, it was shown that IGF-1R localizes in the nucleus of orbital fibroblasts through ADAM17 signaling [44]. Recently, Wang et al. (2024) have demonstrated the crucial role of IGF-1R in cellular communication and interaction between orbital fibroblasts and B-cells [45]. Orbital fibroblasts highly expressive in IGF-1R were co-cultured with peripheral B-cells, resulting in an observed elevation in the expression of interleukin (IL)-6 and RANTES [45]. The authors also observed significant inhibition of the inflammatory process when pretreating the cells with rituximab [45]. Conversely, the role of IGF-1R in T-cell activation is yet to be fully elucidated in TED. A recent study performed by Kiernan et al. (2024) demonstrated that IGF-1R signaling through IGF-1 binding induces Th17 T cell subtype activation, with subsequent IL-17 production and a decrease in reactive oxygen species (ROS) production within Th17 cells [48]. The role of Th17 cells in Grave's ophthalmopathy pathogenesis has been underlined in the literature; Th17 cells promote orbital fibroblast and CD34+ fibroblast differentiation, adipogenesis, and orbital fibrosis in patients with Grave's ophthalmopathy [49, 50].

However, the TSH-r hypothesis cannot explain TAO in Hashimoto's thyroiditis, because patients with Hashimoto's thyroiditis are usually negative for TSH-r [51]. They generally have low titers of anti-thyrotropin-receptor antibodies, which are difficult to detect in some assays [52]. Although a few cases have been reported, the spectrum of eye signs and their prevalence in Hashimoto's thyroiditis are not well documented [12–14].

12.3.1.2 Anti-Tg, Anti-TPO Antibodies and LATS-P

Immunological cross-reactivity of sensitized T-lymphocytes and/or autoantibodies against thyroid and orbit may trigger the inflammatory process [53]. In both conditions, Graves' disease and Hashimoto's thyroiditis, anti-thyroglobulin (Tg), and anti-thyroid peroxidase (TPO) antibodies are detected in addition to the long-acting thyroid stimulator protector (LATS-P). Therefore, a transformation of Graves' disease into Hashimoto's thyroiditis disease and the reverse is also known, and is probably related to altered number of the respective blocking and stimulating antibodies [51].

12.3.1.3 Specific Antibodies Against Eye Muscle Antigens

Specific antibodies against eye muscle antigens such as calsequestrin, collagen XIII flavoprotein (Fp), and G2s, which are also shown to be good markers of eye muscle damage in Graves' patients, may be an alternative explanation for eye muscle damage in Hashimoto's thyroiditis [54–57]. In 2007, Gopinath et al. reported that calsequestrin and collagen XIII antibodies are also associated with chronic upper eyelid retraction as a dominant feature of ophthalmopathy in patients with Graves' disease and Hashimoto's thyroiditis [57]. In another study, Gopinath and colleagues (2007) [58] evaluated 11 patients with Hashimoto's thyroiditis for the presence of antibodies against eye muscle antigens and found that 7 patients (63.6%) were positive for at least one antibody, with calsequestrin and Fp antibodies being the most frequently detected. Five of these seven patients developed ophthalmopathy. Moreover, Gopinath et al. (2007) [59] presented a euthyroid lady with chronic upper eyelid retraction and positive calsequestrin and collagen XIII antibodies. She developed Hashimoto's thyroiditis and hypothyroidism 22 months later. Since the importance of eye muscle antibodies, particularly calsequestrin, was stated in the majority of the studies, it is conceivable that they may be used as indicators for prediction of the onset of eye muscle involvement, with the possibility of early treatment. A routine ophthalmic examination for patients with Hashimoto's thyroiditis seems reasonable to avoid missing the diagnosis of associated ophthalmopathy.

12.3.2 Immune Dysregulations

Immune dysregulations lead to inflammation, adipogenesis, myofibrillogenesis, hyaluronan synthesis, and scarring [60]. The role of lipid mediators (e.g., prostaglandins) and cytokines (e.g., IL-1β, IL-6, IL-15, IL-17, tumor necrosis factor alpha (TNF-α), platelet-derived growth factor (PDGF), and transforming growth factor beta (TGF-β)) in TED pathogenesis has been reported on numerous occasions in various comprehensive literature reviews and studies [1, 24, 61–65].

The underlying pathogenesis of TED involves an autoimmune response in which B-cells, T-cells, and CD34+ fibrocytes infiltrate the orbits following TSH-r and IGF-1R stimulation by autoantibodies [66]. The lymphocytes facilitate orbital fibroblast proliferation and differentiation through the release of pro-inflammatory cytokines and chemokines, ultimately leading to additional orbital fibroblast differentiation, adipogenesis, myofibrillogenesis, hyaluronan synthesis, and finally tissue scarring if left untreated [37].

Recently, in 2024, it was demonstrated that orbital fibroblast activation was under the regulation of SOX9; SOX9 was shown to activate orbital fibroblasts through the up-regulation of mitogen-activated protein kinase (MAPK)/extracellular signal-regulated kinase (ERK) 1/2 pathways [67]. Furthermore, orbital fibroblast adipogenesis was observed to be under the regulation of the Piezo1 receptor, a mechano-sensitive receptor. It is hypothesized that following increased intraorbital pressure due to extraocular muscle enlargement, Piezo1 receptors, found in orbital fibroblasts, are activated and inhibit adipogenesis of fibroblasts, as characterized by decreased expression of peroxisome proliferator-activated receptor gamma (PPARγ) and CEBPα mRNAs [68]. Conversely, Yes-associated protein (YAP), another mechano-sensitive receptor, was recently shown to be involved in chronic fibrosis in Grave's ophthalmopathy; pharmacological inhibition of YAP in primary cultured orbital fibroblasts was shown to significantly decrease TGFβ-induced myofibroblast differentiation and subsequent collagen formation [69].

12.4 Risk Factors

12.4.1 Metabolic and Environmental Risk Factors

Hyperthyroidism—and, to a much lesser extent, hypothyroidism—exacerbates TED; thus, achieving euthyroid status is essential to stabilizing the disease process. In fact, the onset of hyperthyroidism correlates with the onset of TED within 18 months before or after in 85% of cases [70]. Smoking is a significant modifiable risk factor—smokers with Graves' disease have nearly a tenfold higher risk of developing TED compared to non-smokers, tend to develop more severe forms of TED, and respond less favorably to immunosuppressive treatments; these sequelae are diminished in former smokers. Hypoxia and oxidative stress from active smoking are believed to be the culprits [50, 71, 72]. Recent studies have explored the role of hyper-cholesterolemia in TED development, with some suggesting a beneficial effect of statins, although the mechanism of both hyper-cholesterolemia and statins in the role of TED is not well understood [71]. Diabetes mellitus, obstructive sleep apnea, and vitamin D deficiency have also been implicated as potential risk factors [72].

12.4.2 Genetic Risk Factors

Ludgate et al. (2000) claimed that the occurrence of TAO depends on genetic predisposition and does *not* require the presence of antibodies stimulating the TSH receptor [73]. This discovery could explain the occurrence of ophthalmic symptoms in euthyroid state or in hypothyroidism associated with Hashimoto's thyroiditis. On account of differences between the immune systems of people and animals (mice), one should be careful in the interpretation of the results of these studies [74].

Although genetic predispositions have been stipulated to be involved in the differences observed for the susceptibility to TED development in different ethnic populations, until today, this aspect remains poorly understood [75]. Single-nucleotide polymorphisms (SNPs) in the genes coding for peroxisome proliferator-activated receptor gamma (PPARγ) and TSH-R were proposed as one of the mechanisms [76–78].

12.5 Clinical Implications

The records of 700 consecutive patients followed at the endocrine outpatient clinic and at the Joint Thyroid–Eye Clinic of the Johannes Gutenberg University Medical Center in Mainz, Germany, with a diagnosis of Hashimoto's thyroiditis were reviewed by Kahaly and colleagues (2016) [79]. All patients were screened for thyroid-associated eye disease, which was classified as clinically active or inactive, and as mild, moderate-to-severe, or sight-threatening. For comparison, a group of 53 patients with Graves' disease (26 without and 27 with eye disease) and 302 healthy control subjects were also included, making a total of 1055 subjects studied.

Thyroid-associated eye disease (thyroid-associated ophthalmopathy—TAO) was present in 44 of the 700 patients (6%) with Hashimoto's thyroiditis. Compared to the patients without thyroid-associated eye disease, those with Hashimoto's disease and TAO had higher levels of THS-r Ab and were more likely to be smokers ($p = 0.032$). They also tended to be older (49.3 years vs. 35.2 years, $p < 0.001$), have a longer duration of Hashimoto's thyroiditis (2.4 years vs. 0.9 years), and were less likely to have another associated autoimmune disease, i.e., thyroid disease only (75% versus 52.6%, $p = 0.005$). Associated type-1 diabetes mellitus was significantly less among those with Hashimoto's disease and TAO (2.3% vs. 16.3%) [79].

Moreover, TAO was inactive (i.e., non-inflammatory) and mild (i.e., not requiring glucocorticoid or radiation therapy) in two-thirds of Hashimoto's thyroiditis patients. Eye disease activity/severity was independent of gender, age, thyroid function, and smoking. No differences were noted in the prevalence of hypothyroidism or the rate of levothyroxine replacement [79]. Regarding immune reactivity, all healthy controls were TSH-r Ab negative. In contrast, serum was TSH-r Ab was positive in 30/44 (68.2%) of patients with TAO only and 36/656 (5.5%) of patients with Hashimoto's thyroiditis only, respectively ($p < 0.001$). Compared to patients with Hashimoto's thyroiditis, serum TSH-r Ab levels were significantly higher in patients with Hashimoto's thyroiditis and TAO ($p < 0.001$). Highest TSH-r Ab levels were noted in patients with active and severe TAO as compared to those with mild and inactive TAO ($p < 0.001$). In conclusion, TSH-r Ab is strongly associated with thyroid-associated ophthalmopathy in Hashimoto's thyroiditis and may contribute to the pathophysiology of the eye disease.

12.6 Clinical Manifestations

12.6.1 Introduction

Lid retraction, proptosis, and diplopia are hallmarks of TED, although many patients initially present with more elusive and milder signs and symptoms such as chemosis, dry eyes, or soft-tissue swelling [80]. Inflammation and expansion of the fibroadipose and extraocular muscle (EOM) tissues, facilitated by the TSHr-Ab/IGF-1R signaling complex, underlie the eyelid retraction, proptosis, diplopia, and the dreaded but rare dysthyroid optic neuropathy (DON) seen in TED [71, 81, 82]. Changes associated with thyroid disease beyond the orbit include an increase in peri-orbital and brow fat volume, lateral flare of the eyebrow, and malar and cheek swelling, signifying a diffuse facial soft tissue expansion [83]. Thyroid eye disease (TED) often presents bilaterally, but unilateral or asymmetric disease may occur as well. It is reported as having a higher incidence in women yet presents with greater severity and at an older age in men [44]. Pediatric patients are rare, with typically milder disease compared to adults [71].

Thyroid eye disease (TED) is classically described as "active" or "inactive." The active phase constitutes progressive inflammation lasting between 6 and 24 months, ultimately reaching a plateau, at which point the inactive phase commences with fibrosis and regression of inflammation [81]. Reactivation of TED can occur in certain circumstances. Several studies have shown that smoking constitutes one of the major risk factors for TED reactivation [84–86]. Smokers with TED were also shown to be at greater risk for TED progression, as well as poor treatment outcomes [84, 87]. Additional risk factors for disease reactivation encompass sustained TSH-r antibodies [25], radioactive iodine (RAI) treatment (risk of progression of 15–39%) [88, 89], and steroid treatment discontinuation in moderate-to-severe TED patients, in which up to 25% of reactivation rates were reported [90, 91].

12.6.2 Eyelid Retraction

The most common finding in TED is upper eyelid retraction, occurring in 90% of patients. The etiology of upper lid retraction is believed to be multifactorial, with sympathetic over-activity, inflammation, and fibrosis of Muller's muscle, enlargement and over-activity of the levator palpebrae superioris (LPS) secondary to inferior rectus restriction by way of Hering's law, and LPS overaction secondary to weakening of the orbicularis oculi muscle. The etiology of lower lid retraction is believed to be, in part, due to tension on the lid margin from inferior rectus enlargement [81]. Eyelid edema may be attributed to lymphatic dilatation and peri-vascular lymphocytic infiltrates in the dermis [81].

Depending on the severity of lid retraction, chronic eye exposure may develop, leading to dry eye disease (DES) and, if severe, exposure keratopathy with a risk of corneal scarring, ulceration, perforation, and endophthalmitis [92, 93]. This is further exacerbated by the presence of lagophthalmos, decreased blink frequency, and increased tear evaporation [92, 93]. In addition to an evaporative dry eye component, there are also aqueous and lipid deficiencies in TED, with decreased tear production and increased meibomian gland dropout [94]. Inflammatory changes in the ocular surface, including squamous cell metaplasia, superior limbic keratoconjunctivitis, and increased pro-inflammatory cytokines such as IL-1β, IL-6, IL-7, L-8, IL-10, IL-17A, TNF-α, lysozyme C, lacritin, and zinc-alpha-2 glycoprotein 1, with subsequently decreased tear break-up time and Schirmer's test, have been reported by several authors [94–99]. Occasionally, inflammatory DES may be an early symptom of TED; in fact, one single-center study found that nearly 4% of patients with refractory DES had occult TED [100]. Treatment options for DES secondary to TED include lubrication, topical cyclosporine, topical steroids, and tarsorrhaphy.

12.6.3 Proptosis

Proptosis affects 60% of patients with TED and is caused by the expansion of EOM and orbital fat, further increasing the risk of eye exposure [92, 93]. EOM dysfunction, observed in 40% of patients, manifests itself as diplopia and misalignment of the eyes [92]. The inferior rectus, then the medial rectus, and ultimately the superior rectus are most commonly involved, with only rare involvement of the lateral rectus or oblique muscles [101]. The resultant restrictive strabismus, occurring in 15% of patients, manifests as hypotropia and esotropia, which last beyond the active phase of TED due to eventual collagen deposition and fibrosis [102].

12.6.4 Diplopia

Diplopia in TED occurs mainly during upgaze due to inferior rectus muscle hypertrophy, but in some patients, diplopia during downgaze caused by superior rectus hypertrophy is particularly debilitating for daily activities [70]. Diplopia due to strabismus may be managed with prisms, monocular occlusion, and botulinum toxin A injection into the affected EOMs, and eventual strabismus surgery once the disease is rendered inactive [92, 93, 103]. Eye pain, described as dull and pressure-like, is reported in 30% of patients [92].

12.6.5 Dyschromatopsia, Visual Field Loss, and/or Visual Acuity Loss

Dyschromatopsia, visual field loss, and/or visual acuity loss due to DON occur in 6–15% of patients and are an emergency requiring immediate management, including surgical orbital decompression [72, 92]. The mechanism of action of DON includes mechanical compression of the optic nerve by the EOMs, an increase in orbital adipose tissue, crowding of the orbital apex, venous congestion, and resultant ischemia. A component of stretch optic neuropathy from proptosis has also been hypothesized. Older age, male gender, smoking, TSHr-Ab levels, and the presence of the cytotoxic T-lymphocyte-associated antigen-4 (CTLA-4) gene are identified as potential risk factors [104]. Additionally, Asian patients, who often present with more diffuse EOM involvement yet less prominent proptosis, may be at a greater risk of DON, possibly due to the shallower and more compact orbital anatomy [72]. Indeed, patients with minimal proptosis were found to be at higher risk of neuropathy due to the restrictive space within the bony walls, leading to a secondary "compartment syndrome effect" [93].

12.6.6 Glaucoma

A recent meta-analysis by Delavar et al. (2023) has demonstrated an association between patients with TED and the incidence of glaucoma; approximately 29% of patients with TED had glaucoma in comparison to non-TED patients [105]. However, previous results on this topic are conflicting. In 2018, Kim et al. previously reported a similar incidence of glaucoma in TED patients when compared to the general population but a greater prevalence (6.8%) of ocular hypertension in TED patients [106]. The increased risk of open-angle glaucoma (OAG) can partially be due to the elevated epi-scleral venous pressure and changes in ocular perfusion; thus, glaucomatous optic neuropathy must be distinguished from DON [104]. The pathophysiology of TED-associated glaucoma remains complex. Alongside changes in episcleral venous pressure, deposition of glycosaminoglycans within the trabecular meshwork was also hypothesized to be involved in its pathophysiology [107]. In addition, the treatment of TED can raise the intra-ocular pressure, thus establishing different pressure gradients within the lamina cribrosa and leading to glaucomatous changes [108]. Nevertheless, additional studies are required to better establish the relationship of TED with the prevalence or incidence of glaucoma in this population.

12.7 Assessment/Diagnosis

12.7.1 History-Taking

Patient history, including age, gender, ethnicity, co-morbidities, systemic associations, pregnancy or pregnancy potential, tobacco smoking, other environmental and psychological stressors, and likelihood of adherence to medical therapies, must be elicited in any new patient with TED [82].

It is important to ensure the absence of overt thyrotoxicosis, which can be life-threatening with complications including ischemia, atrial fibrillation, congestive heart failure, thromboembolism, stroke, psychosis, paralysis, and thyroid storm [82].

12.7.2 Ocular Examination

A comprehensive ocular examination includes (1) documentation of visual acuity, (2) presence or absence of a relative afferent pupillary defect, (3) intra-ocular pressure and color vision (the Hardy–Rand–Rittler plates may be more sensitive than the Ishihara plates for DON, given it would result in an acquired color vision deficiency), (4) Hertel exophthalmometry to document proptosis, and (5) extraocular movements to identify limitations [109] (Table 12.1) Eyelid changes, including the presence of lateral flare, lid lag, lagophthalmos, Bell's reflex, and upper and lower eyelid retraction, should also be noted. Ocular surface changes, including tear break-up time or Schirmer's test, presence of superior limbic kerato-conjunctivitis,

Table 12.1 Ocular eye exam and possible findings suggestive of thyroid eye disease (TED)

Ocular examination	Possible findings
Examination of the orbits and adnexa	
Eyelids	Lateral flare Lid lag Lagophthalmos and Bell's reflex Upper/lower eyelid retraction
Extraocular muscle assessment	Extraocular eye movement limitations Proptosis due to extraocular muscle enlargement
Anterior segment examination	
Cornea	Decreased tear breakup time Superior limbic kerato-conjunctivitis Exposure keratopathy Corneal ulceration
Posterior segment examination	
Optic nerve assessment	Increased cup-to-disc ratio Optic nerve head pallor Optic disc swelling Decreased color vision Relative afferent pupillary defect
Neurological investigations	
Visual field testing	Visual field defect secondary to optic nerve damage

exposure keratopathy, and corneal ulceration, and any related sequelae such as corneal perforation must be noted [70]. Many providers will obtain optical coherence tomography (OCT) of the macula and optic nerve as well as a formal visual field to document baseline structure and function; this is especially pertinent in cases where glaucomatous optic neuropathy and DON may be suspected.

12.7.3 Assessment of Clinical Activity: Classification Systems

One of the challenges in the management of TAO is to classify and grade its various clinical manifestations. Several classification systems to quantify the clinical activity and severity have been reported in the literature [70, 110].

12.7.3.1 NOSPECS Classification System

The NOSPECS (No signs or symptoms, Only signs, no symptoms, Soft tissue involvement, Proptosis, Extraocular muscle involvement, Corneal involvement, Sight loss) classification system is currently considered an *obsolete* classification system that was historically used to quantify clinical severity without information on clinical activity [72, 82, 110]. According to NOSPECS, mild disease encompasses grades I-III, whereas severe disease encompasses grades IV-VI (Table 12.2).

12.7.3.2 RELIEF Classification System

RELIEF (Resistance to retropulsion, Edema of the conjunctiva and caruncle, Lacrimal gland enlargement, Injection of horizontal rectus muscle insertions, Edema of the eyelids, and Fullness of the eyelids) classification system, similar to the NOSPECS classification system, is also currently considered an *obsolete* classification system that was used in the past to quantify clinical severity without information on clinical activity (Table 12.3) [72, 82, 110].

Table 12.2 NOSPECS classification system

Grade	Criteria
0	No physical signs or symptoms
I	Only signs, no symptoms
II	Soft tissue involvement Absent (II-0)—minimal (II-1)—moderate (II-2)—marked (II-3)
III	Proptosis (>2 mm of normal upper limit) 3–4 mm (III-1)—5–7 mm (III-2)—>8 (III-3)
IV	Extraocular muscle (EOM) involvement Absent (IV-0)–limitation of motion at extremes of gaze (IV-1)—evident restriction of movements (IV-2)—Fixed globe(s) (IV-3)
V	Corneal involvement due to lagophthalmos Absent (V-0)—stippling of cornea (V-1)—ulceration (V-2)—clouding, necrosis, and perforation (V-3)
VI	Sight loss due to optic nerve involvement Absent (VI-0)—disc pallor or visual field defect visual acuity 20/20 to 20/60 (VI-1)—disc pallor or visual field defect/visual acuity 20/70 to 20/200 (VI-2)—blindness/visual acuity less than 20/200 (VI-3)

Table 12.3 RELIEF classification system

Abbreviation	Description
R	Resistance to retropulsion
E	Edema of conjunctiva and caruncle
L	Lacrimal gland enlargement
I	Injection of horizontal rectus muscle insertions
E	Edema of eyelids
F	Fullness of eyelids

12.7.3.3 Clinical Activity Score (CAS) Grading System

The *CAS* (clinical activity score) grading system assesses clinical activity with a 7-point system for initial evaluation. Successive examinations are scored with a 10-point system. Each positive element is given one point. A score of 3 or less is considered as "inactive" while a score greater than 3/7 or 4/10 is considered an "active" disease and thus is supposedly more likely to respond to immunosuppression (Table 12.4). The CAS grading system is inexpensive and can be done instantly in a clinic.

12.7.3.4 EUGOGO Grading System

The EUGOGO (European Group of Graves' Orbitopathy) severity grading system assesses clinical activity and severity with mild, moderate-to-severe, and sight-threatening categories. Mild disease comprises one or more of the following: minor lid retraction <2 mm, mild soft-tissue involvement, exophthalmos <3 mm above normal for gender and race, and transient or no diplopia. Moderate-to-severe disease comprises one or more of the following: lid retraction >2 mm, moderate-to-severe soft-tissue involvement, exophthalmos >3 mm above normal for gender and race, and inconstant or constant diplopia. Finally, sight-threatening disease includes DON, or corneal breakdown (Table 12.5). This system is more commonly used in North America [70, 110].

12.7.3.5 The VISA Grading System

The VISA (Vision, Inflammation, Strabismus, and Appearance) grading system represents yet another classification system to assess clinical activity and severity. The primary goal of the section of "vision" is to rule out optic neuropathy in which the patient presents with episodes of graying out with and without color desaturation. The associated VISA "Inflammatory Index" is scored out of 10 such that a score <4/10 represents moderate disease and is managed conservatively, and severe disease with a score >5/10 is managed more aggressively [72, 82, 110]. Patients with evidence of disease progression and a score of 5/10 are also managed more aggressively. The symptoms of "strabismus" include (1) a progression from no diplopia, (2) diplopia in horizontal or vertical gaze, (3) intermittent diplopia in primary gaze, and (4) constant diplopia in primary gaze. Strabismus can be measured objectively by prism cover testing in different gaze directions. Objective measures of "appearance" change include eyelid retraction, proptosis, redundant skin and fat prolapse. Measures of "exposure" include corneal staining or ulceration (Table 12.6).

Table 12.4 Clinical activity score (CAS)

Initial evaluation (scored out of 7)	Successive evaluations (scored out of 10)
Spontaneous orbital pain	Increase of >2 mm proptosis
Gaze-evoked orbital pain	>8° decrease in ocular motility of one eye in any direction
Lid edema	Decrease in visual acuity of one Snellen line
Lid erythema	
Conjunctival erythema	
Chemosis	
Caruncle or plica inflammation	

Table 12.5 EUGOGO (European Group of Graves' Orbitopathy) severity grading system

Grade	Criteria
Soft tissue assessment	
Eyelid swelling	
1	Absent
2	Mild: none of the features defining moderate or severe categories
3	Moderate: definite swelling, no lower eyelid festoons or angulation of the upper eyelid skin fold in downgaze
4	Severe: lower eyelid festoons or upper eyelid fold becomes rounded at 45° in downgaze
Eyelid erythema	
1	Absent
2	Present
Conjunctival erythema	
1	Absent
2	Mild: equivocal or minimal
3	Moderate: <50%
4	Severe: >50%
Conjunctival edema	
1	Absent
2	Present
Caruncle or PSI	
1	Absent
2	Present
Lid margin assessment[a]*—palpebral aperture (mm)—lid retraction (mm)—levator function (mm)—lagophthalmos*	
1	Absent
2	Present
Bell's phenomenon	
1	Absent
2	Present

(continued)

Table 12.5 (continued)

Grade	Criteria
Proptosis assessment	
Hertel exophthalmometry to record inter-canthal distance and amount of proptosis	
Ocular motility assessment	
Prism cover test Monocular ductions Head posture Torsion Binocular single vision	
Corneal integrity assessment	
Normal Punctate keratopathy Ulcer Perforation	
Optic nerve assessment	
Visual acuity—color vision—visual field analysis—optic disc assessment: normal, atrophied, glaucomatous, or edematous—afferent pupil defect	
1	Absent
2	Present

PSI plica semilunaris inflammation
[a]At the mid-pupillary line

The VISA classification system tool is thus useful for assessing disease progression or response to therapy, as well as disease activity or quiescence. It is more commonly used in North America [70, 110].

Dolman and Rootman (2006) devised VISA classification system based on four disease endpoints that can be used in the office setting to record changes and to guide and assess therapy [111]. These include Vision, Inflammation, Strabismus, and Appearance (VISA)/exposure, which help direct appropriate management in a logical sequence where non-severe cases, whether active or inactive, would require supportive measures only, while severe cases would require glucocorticoid therapy or orbital radiotherapy if active, and strabismus surgery or eyelid retraction surgery, if inactive. In either case, orbital decompression is only indicated if compressive optic neuropathy has not resolved with maximal medical treatment [112].

12.7.4 Orbital Imaging

12.7.4.1 Computerized Tomography (CT) Scan

Computerized tomography (CT) scan is the most commonly utilized imaging technique for evaluating TAO. It is more sensitive than magnetic resonance imaging (MRI) in identifying enlarged extraocular muscles [113]. Imaging studies may be particularly helpful when radiation therapy or decompressive surgery is planned, as they define the degree of extraocular muscle and orbital fat involvement and delineate clearly sinus and skull base anatomy before intervention. Findings on CT

Table 12.6 VISA (Vision, Inflammation, Strabismus, and Appearance) grading system

Grade	Criteria
1 Point	Vision
	Visual acuity
	Pupillary reflex
	Color vision
	Visual fields
	Optic nerve examination
	Visual evoked potentials
10 Points	*Inflammation/congestion*
Caruncular edema	
0	Absent
1	Present
Chemosis	
0	Absent
1	Conjunctiva lies behind the gray line of the lid
2	Conjunctiva extends anterior to the gray line of the lid
Conjunctival erythema	
0	Absent
1	Present
Lid redness	
0	Absent
1	Present
Lid edema	
0	Absent
1	Present, without redundant tissues
2	Present, with lower lid festoon and bulging palpebral skin
Retrobulbar ache at rest	
0	Absent
1	Present
Retrobulbar ache with gaze	
0	Absent
1	Present
Diurnal variation	
0	Absent
1	Present
6 Points	*Strabismus/motility restriction*
Diplopia	
0	Absent
1	Diplopia with horizontal or vertical gaze
2	Intermittent diplopia in primary gaze
3	Constant diplopia in primary gaze

(continued)

Table 12.6 (continued)

Grade	Criteria
Ocular restriction	
0	Duction >45°
1	Duction 30–45°
2	Duction 15–30°
3	Duction <15°
3 Points	*Appearance/exposure*
	Appearance concerns (i.e., proptosis, lid retraction, and fat pockets)
	Symptoms from ocular exposure (i.e., foreign body sensation, photophobia, dryness, and secondary tearing)
	Measurements including eyelid retraction, scleral show, LPS function, lagophthalmos, and proptosis with Hertel exophthalmometer
	Signs of corneal exposure, including punctate epithelial erosions, ulcerations, corneal thinning, and corneal perforation

LPS levator palpebrae superioris

scanning may include EOM belly enlargement that typically spares the tendinous insertions (tendon-sparing enlargement) (Fig. 12.2) [70, 92, 102]. Imaging with CT scan may be especially helpful in clarifying the diagnosis of TED by revealing bilateral radiographic disease in cases where the presence of only unilateral disease is suspected clinically [70]. The order of muscle involvement is inferior rectus, medial rectus, and finally, the superior rectus; involvement of the lateral rectus or oblique muscles is *not* typically seen. Although this is the most frequent finding, it is worth noting that any single or combination of muscle involvement can occur.

Other signs include apical crowding and increased angle of the orbital apex (i.e., a deviation from the normal positioning or the orbital apex, which is the point where the optic nerve enters the orbit), increased angle of the medial orbital wall (i.e., the medial orbital wall angles are usually parallel to each other), enlarged superior ophthalmic vein (SOV), orbital fat prolapse, peri-neural fat effacement, enlarged lacrimal gland, and a taut optic nerve in cases with significant proptosis.

Orbitopathy may be radiographically classified as primarily lipogenic (type-I), primarily myogenic (type-II), or mixed (type-III) [70]. CT imaging exophthalmometry should also be measured, as it is more reliable than Hertel exophthalmometry; in cases of lateral orbital decompression where the inter-zygomatic method of exophthalmometry cannot be utilized, the measurement from the posterior clinoid process to the anterior corneal surface may suffice instead [70, 114].

12.7.4.2 Magnetic Resonance Imaging (MRI)

Magnetic resonance imaging (MRI) can provide additional soft tissue resolution, further aiding in the assessment of disease activity [92]. There is a positive correlation between the T1 signal intensity ratio, T1 post-gadolinium signal intensity ratio, and apparent diffusion coefficient with the CAS. T1-weighted images of inactive TED show isointense EOM and facial muscles, with the enhancement of EOMs post-gadolinium. T2-weighted images of inactive TED show hypointense EOMs, whereas active TED has hyperintense EOMs. Barrett's index, used to assess for the

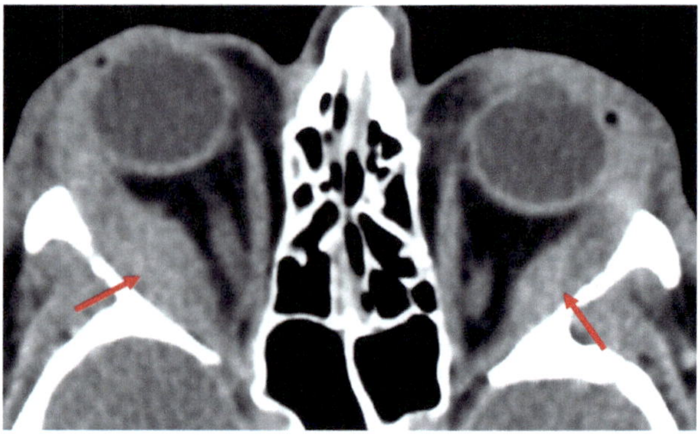

Fig. 12.2 Computed tomography (CT) scan in axial plane showing bilateral extraocular muscle enlargement (red arrows) in thyroid eye disease (TED)

presence of DON, may be derived from CT imaging or MRI—the vertical index is the sum of the vertical muscle diameters divided by the height of the orbit through the optic nerve; the horizontal index is the sum of the horizontal muscle diameters divided by the width of the orbit through the optic nerve. A Barrett's index greater than 60% is suggestive of DON [70, 115].

12.7.4.3 Orbital Color Doppler Imaging

Orbital color Doppler imaging (CDI) is emerging as an important radiographic tool to assess the hemodynamic changes that occur with TED [70]. Orbital and ocular perfusion may be sequentially monitored for prognostication and to assess treatment response [104, 116]. Blood flow velocities are measured in the SOV, ophthalmic artery (OA), central retinal artery (CRA), and posterior ciliary artery (PCA). The active phase of TED demonstrates high peak systolic and end-diastolic velocities in the OA and CRA. Reduction or reversal in SOV maximum velocity is noted due to elevation in cone pressure following soft tissue expansion in the orbit; these findings, in addition to the CRA-resistivity index, are improved after orbital decompression [104]. Furthermore, changes in choroidal thickness and the retino-choroidal micro-vasculature have been noted on OCT with and without angiography [104].

12.7.5 Serologic Studies and Molecular Biomarkers

In 2018, Li et al. [93] reported that TED is associated with hyperthyroidism in 90% of cases, hypothyroidism in 5%, and occurs in euthyroid individuals in the remaining 5%. TED is most commonly linked to disease which is caused by autoantibody stimulation of the TSHr with the TSHr-Ab [92]. TSHR-Ab levels correlate with the CAS, representing the only known biomarker for TED and specifically for Graves' ophthalmopathy [71, 117]. TSHr expression was shown to be elevated in the orbital fat of patients with TED; the activity of TSHr-Ab through TSHR binding stimulates the release of pro-inflammatory cytokines in the orbital tissues, leading to the accumulation of mucopolysaccharides and glycosaminoglycans with resultant soft tissue swelling [118]. TSHr-stimulating immunoglobulins (TSI), a subtype of

TSHr-Ab, have also been found to correlate with disease activity and specifically with DON [119, 120].

Competitive-binding assays and cell-based bioassays for the diagnosis of thyroid eye disease (TED) may be used to assess different types of TSHr-Ab throughout the disease course (Table 12.7).

Competitive-binding assays provide information on the presence and concentration of TSHR-Ab through the measurement of TSHr-binding inhibitory immunoglobulins (TBII) and are available globally, whereas cell-based bioassays provide functional information through the measurement of TSI, including whether the antibody is stimulatory or inhibitory [117, 118]. Both TBII and TSI represent subtypes of the TSHr-Ab.

The latest, third-generation competitive-binding assays measure the inhibitory ability of TBII on M22, a labeled F(ab)2 human TSHR-stimulating monoclonal antibody, on the TSHr. TSHr-Ab is detected in 95–98% of patients with Graves' disease using third-generation competitive binding assays. Cell-based bioassays utilize stably transfected cell lines or chimeric cell lines expressing TSHr to measure the stimulatory activity in patients with Graves' disease, with 99–100% sensitivity and 100% specificity values for antibody function [118]. In contrast, anti-thyroid peroxidase (TPO) and anti-thyroglobulin (anti-Tg) antibodies have *not* shown a correlation with TED [92].

12.7.6 Liquid Biopsy: A Novel Approach

Liquid biopsy is a novel technology that has gained great interest in the past few years for disease diagnosis and monitoring given its non-invasive nature, low cost, highly sensitive nature, and the possibility to provide real-time monitoring of diseases [124]. Although the application of liquid biopsy has been thoroughly discussed in the diagnosis and monitoring of cancers [124–126], Kulbay et al. discussed recently (2024) the possibility of translating liquid biopsy technology to TED diagnosis and disease monitoring, a tool not yet applicable, given the lack of well-defined, sensitive, and proven biomarkers [60].

Traditionally, liquid biopsy consists of isolating and analyzing tumor-derived moieties, which encompass circulating tumor cells (CTCs), circulating tumor DNA (ctDNA), tumor-derived extra-cellular vesicles (EVs), and circulating cell-free RNA (cfRNA) [124]. It was demonstrated that the serological expression of numerous miRNAs, such as miR-130a [127, 128] miR-484, and miR-192-5p [129], is

Table 12.7 Current competitive-binding assays and cell-based bioassays

Assay	Example
TSHr-binding inhibitory immunoglobulin assay [121]	IMMULITE TSI [121] EliA™ [122] Elecsys® [122]
Cell-based bioassays with TSI measurement	Thyretain™ [123]

TSH-r thyroid-stimulating hormone receptor, *TSI* TSHr-stimulating immunoglobulins

altered in TED. The expression of miR-130a was shown to be elevated in patients with TED, and it modulated adipogenesis through the inhibition of AMPK activity [127, 128]. Furthermore, miR-103a-3p was shown to be elevated in TGFβ-activated orbital fibroblasts, where it was shown to promote cell proliferation and differentiation through the ERK-Jun N-terminal kinase (JNK) and TGFβ/Smad signaling pathways [130].

Numerous challenges exist for the implementation of liquid biopsies in the diagnosis, management, and treatment response monitoring of TED. A major drawback is the lack of evidence-based biomarkers. Although several cytokines, miRNAs, and protein expression modifications have been reported in TED, the sensitivity in detecting their serological expression through liquid biopsy has yet to be fully established. Furthermore, technical limitations, such as the lack of resources and well-trained technicians, limit the translation of liquid biopsy into clinical practice for TED management. However, with the growing body of literature on this topic, it is conceivable that liquid biopsies can offer a rapid method of screening, diagnosis, and disease monitoring for treatment of TED in the near future [60].

12.8 Treatment

12.8.1 General Considerations

The management of TED currently involves a dynamic and multidisciplinary approach. In mild cases, pharmacological treatment may not be required. However, in moderate or severe disease, medical intervention, predominantly pharmacological but also surgical, is required in order to prevent sight-threatening complications [60].

From the endocrine perspective, the goal of treatment of patients with TAO is the achievement of a euthyroid state. In addition, patients should be counseled regarding the risks of smoking and benefits of cessation. The decision of treatment relies on the activity and severity of the disease. *Vision* dysfunction from optic neuropathy is the first priority and, depending on whether inflammation is present, might be treated with corticosteroids, radiotherapy (RT), and/or orbital decompression. *Inflammation* is the next priority and may be treated with conservative measures, corticosteroids, steroid-sparing immuno-suppressives and/or RT. *Strabismus* and appearance changes are usually managed medically and expectantly (with patching or Fresnel prisms) until signs of inflammation and disease progression have subsided. Strabismus can then be managed with ground-in prisms or surgery, whereas proptosis, eyelid retraction, dermatochalasis, and fat prolapse can be managed surgically.

It is noteworthy that there is no current universal gold-standard treatment for TED nor a consensus on an optimal treatment plan. Thus, current management is mainly guided by individual expert opinion. Studies that aim at establishing a gold-standard treatment approach would be highly beneficial to the field. In 2021, the EUGOGO published a clinical guideline for the management of TED to help address this issue; however, it has not been widely adopted in clinical practice globally [131]. However, most patients with Hashimoto's disease usually have mild ocular manifestations. Simple local supportive measures are usually sufficient to obtain symptomatic relief.

Pharmaceutical intervention is considered when TED progresses to moderate, severe, or sight-threatening stages. The absence of medical intervention in mild cases is due to the high frequency of spontaneous resolution. For these patients, it is sufficient to treat local symptoms and monitor the progression carefully [131, 132]. However, it is important to note that selenium has been demonstrated to be beneficial in a subset of patients with mild TED [131, 133]. Selenium has an important anti-oxidative effect in the thymus, where it exists in high concentrations. RCT evidence supports selenium supplementation for the improvement in quality of life and ophthalmic outcomes in mild cases of TED [15, 131, 133]. Even though selenium was only studied in mild cases, EUGOGO recommended a 6-month selenium regimen for those with active disease or mild TED due to its positive impact on ophthalmic outcomes [131].

12.8.2 Pharmacotherapy: First-Line Treatments

12.8.2.1 Glucocorticoids

The current first-line treatment of thyroid eye disease (TED) is glucocorticoids. However, biological agents, notably teprotumumab, which was FDA approved in 2020, are increasingly being used as first-line treatment options (Table 12.8). One meta-analysis compared these two options, concluding that teprotumumab is more likely to reduce proptosis and diplopia than glucocorticoids [134]. However, the lack of direct comparison limits conclusive evidence of clinical superiority, and thus glucocorticoids are still widely the preferred first-line treatment in many countries. Furthermore, the greater cost of teprotumumab compared to glucocorticoids makes its selection as a first-line treatment less likely in certain countries where the medical financial budget is limited [60].

Glucocorticoids are employed for their anti-inflammatory and immunosuppressive actions [135]. In a review by Rajendram et al. (2008), the response to glucocorticoids ranged from 63% to 77% [136]. Among to glucocorticoids, there are two clinically relevant therapies: intravenous methylprednisolone (IVMP) and oral prednisone. Both share common mechanisms of action, which include increasing anti-inflammatory processes and suppressing pro-inflammatory aspects of TED [15, 137]. Although IVMP is more laborious to administer, it is preferred to oral prednisone owing to its higher effectiveness and fewer side-effects as compared to oral glucocorticoids [15, 138–142]. Thus, IVMP is considered the gold standard first-line treatment for moderate-to-severe TED. However, the cumulative dose of IVMP should be *not* exceed 6–8 g [143]. Routine liver assessment during treatment to rule out liver toxicity is recommended by some centers. Recurrences are not infrequent, thus repeated dosing is often required.

Table 12.8 First-line medications used to treat thyroid-associated ophthalmopathy

First-line treatment	Posology	Advantages	Disadvantages
Intravenous methyl-prednisolone (IVMP) [131, 140, 149, 150]	EUGOGO regimen: 6 weekly infusions of 500 mg Additional 6 weekly infusions of 250 mg in moderate-to-severe disease Doses can be adjusted between 4.5 and 7.5 g/cycle according to severity	Gold standard: effectively controls disease activity Induces rapid anti-inflammatory response Higher response rates than oral prednisone Well-tolerated with fewer serious side-effects compared to oral steroids	IV administration Safety concerns with cumulative high doses (>8 g/cycle) Monitoring for adverse events (arrhythmias, hyperglycemia, infections, etc.). Requires gastric and bone protection
Oral prednisone [151]	0.5–1 mg/kg/day tapered based on response Lowest effective dose over prolonged periods	Oral administration Effective in mild to moderate cases	Slower onset of action Higher risk of systemic adverse effects than IVMP
Teprotumumab [134]	Initial dose: 10 mg/kg, IV Maintenance dose: 20 mg/kg, IV every 3 weeks for seven additional infusions	Effective in reducing TED clinical activity Reduce proptosis and CAS (to 0 or 1)	High cost Lack of rigorous scientific evidence so far

12.8.2.2 Teprotumumab

Teprotumumab has emerged as a promising treatment of moderate-to-severe TED. It is a humanized monoclonal antibody that partially antagonizes IGF-1R by binding its alpha subunit and is demonstrated to be effective in reducing TED clinical activity, and reducing the severity of diplopia and proptosis. Teprotumumab was shown to reduce proptosis by 2.31 mm on average (range 1.17–3.45 mm), and to reduce the CAS to 0 or 1 [144]. However, its use was shown to induce ototoxicity [145]. Teprotumumab is the first of several promising biologics to be approved for TED and provides an alternative treatment option for patients with moderate-to-severe TED who cannot tolerate or fail to respond to glucocorticoids. In adults, the initial dose is 10 mg/kg, IV, while the maintenance dose is 20 mg/kg, IV, every 3 weeks for seven additional infusions. Some clinicians now support the use of teprotumumab as first-line treatment, especially in chronic TED, but its clinical use is limited by its high cost (5000 times more than IVMP) [146, 147], and a lack of rigorous scientific evidence directly comparing it to IVMP [148].

12.8.3 Pharmacotherapy: Second-Line Treatments

In refractory cases of TED, there are several second-line treatment options, such as biologics and immuno-suppressants (as well as orbital radiation). Yet, there is a lack of direct evidence supporting one second-line treatment over the other. As a result, the clinical use of these drugs is individualized for the patients through shared decision-making. There are several options a physician can choose from, including immunomodulators, notably tocilizumab targeting IL-6 and rituximab targeting CD-20. Additionally, there are a multitude of steroid-sparing immunosuppressive agents, such as mycophenolate, azathioprine, cyclosporine, methotrexate, and sirolimus, which are used at the discretion of the physician and patient (Table 12.9). Altogether, these immunosuppressive agents serve as viable alternatives to IVMP or

Table 12.9 Second-line medications used to treat thyroid-associated ophthalmopathy

Second-line treatment	Posology	Advantages	Disadvantages
Azathioprine [155–157]	Initial dose of 1–2 mg/kg/day orally + RT or corticosteroids	Can reduce risk of relapse following steroid taper Beneficial outcomes in combination with glucocorticoids	Effective only as a combination therapy
Cyclosporine [158–160]	2–5 mg/kg/day orally + prednisone	Fast onset of action Effective in combination with prednisone	Requires therapeutic drug monitoring Serious side-effects: (nephro- and neuro-toxicity, hypertension)
Mycophenolate [15]	Mycophenolate mofetil 1 g/day orally or Mycophenolate sodium 0.72 g/day orally for 24 weeks + IVMP	Improved clinical outcomes when used in combination with IVMP Less severe adverse effects than corticosteroids	Requires monitoring for gastrointestinal disturbances and systemic adverse effects Lack of long-term data
Sirolimus [161]	2 mg orally on Day 1 followed by 0.5 mg/day for 12 weeks	Superior response rate compared to IVMP in moderate-to-severe cases Anti-fibrotic properties in renal and pulmonary transplant patients	Significant adverse effect profile requiring careful monitoring
Methotrexate [162, 163]	Typically initiated at 7.5–10 mg orally weekly	Effective in reducing inflammation by suppressing lymphocytes Promising results in combination with glucocorticoids for sight-threatening cases	Lack of robust randomized controlled trials limits evidence of efficacy Potential adverse effects include fatigue, nausea, and hair loss

teprotumumab, but with the limited evidence available in the literature, it is frequently unclear when one specific agent is superior to another [60].

Cyclosporine affects both cell-mediated and humoral immune reactions; however, its effect when given as a monotherapy is inferior to prednisone. Several controlled studies reported that the use of cyclosporine in combination with prednisone was more effective than prednisone alone [152, 153]. Regular monitoring for side-effects during the course of cyclosporine treatment is required. Methotrexate is given in doses of 5–25 mg once per week and may prove to be promising [154].

12.8.4 Radiotherapy (RT)

The rationale for the use of radiotherapy (RT) for TAO resides both in its non-specific anti-inflammatory effect and in the high radio-sensitivity of lymphocytes infiltrating the orbit [164]. Orbital RT is effective in patients who have active eye disease with recent progression. Patients with inactive TAO do *not* respond to irradiation [165]. The most common delivered dose is 20 Gy per eye, fractionated over a 2-week period. Side-effects include transient exacerbations of inflammation, but this can be avoided with glucocorticoid coverage. With modern techniques, there seems to be no increased risk of cataract, or secondary malignancies, and only a remote risk of retinopathy [166]. In patients with diabetes mellitus, irradiation should be considered as a relative contraindication. Even though the efficacy of RT has been recently questioned, it remains widely used [167].

12.8.5 Surgical Treatment

12.8.5.1 Indications

Indications of surgical intervention in TAO include optic neuropathy, diplopia, corneal exposure, and cosmesis. *Surgical procedures* may be directed toward orbital decompression, strabismus repair, and the correction of eyelid abnormality. Traditionally, orbital decompression, if required, is performed initially, followed by strabismus surgery and then eyelid repair. This is because the nature and degree of strabismus may change after orbital surgery, and lid position may be altered following strabismus repair.

The timing of surgery is important. Decompression may be necessary urgently for compressive optic neuropathy or severe proptosis with corneal ulceration refractory to other treatment measures. Yet, most decompression surgery is performed when a patient has been stable in the inactive state for at least 6–8 months [143].

12.8.5.2 Orbital Decompression

Any surgical procedure that enlarges the bony orbit and/or removes the orbital fat is defined as orbital decompression. At present, the medial wall, the orbital floor, and/or the lateral wall continue to be addressed during bony decompression surgery [143]. Preserving the medial orbital strut between the ethmoid cavity and the orbital floor may minimize the risk of globe dystopia and diplopia [168]. The combination of bony decompression and fat removal has gained popularity due to the low risks associated with fat decompression [169, 170].

12.8.5.3 Eye Muscle Surgery

Ocular motility disorders in TAO are typically due to a restrictive myopathy, and extraocular muscle involvement is characterized by accumulation of inflammatory cells and fluid. Later, the muscle is replaced by fibrous tissue, which makes the muscle stiff and inextensible. Due to the often incomitant nature of strabismus, surgery in TAO is often aimed at the resolution of diplopia in primary position and downgaze. Surgery should be performed on a patient who does not have active thyroid disease for at least 6 months, and typically involves release of the restricted muscle by recession rather than resection.

12.8.5.4 Eyelid Surgery

The most common indication for lid surgery is upper lid retraction. Treatment consists of a graded Muller's and levator aponeurosis weakening. Criterion for successful correction is covering of 1–2 mm of the superior cornea. Lower lid lengthening is indicated in lower lid retraction. Recession of lower lid retractors alone is insufficient to correct more than 1 mm of lid retraction and an interposition graft or spacer is needed if there is significant lower lid retraction.

12.8.5.5 Blepharoplasty

Blepharoplasty is the final surgical procedure in the rehabilitation of the TAO patient. Skin excision in the lower lid should be done carefully to avoid ectropion and/or lower lid retraction.

12.8.6 Novel Therapeutic Approaches

The cutting-edge advances in TED pathogenesis, as well as in the field of pharmaceutics, have led to the establishment of numerous clinical trials over the past years, with a goal of developing targeted immunotherapy for the treatment of TED.

12.8.6.1 Teprotumumab and IGF-1R Inhibitors

Teprotumumab is a monoclonal antibody that was initially developed as an oncology drug [15]. However, it was repurposed as a treatment for TED. It functions by partially antagonizing IGF-1R, which co-localizes with TSHr on orbital fibroblasts. By binding IGF-1R's alpha subunit, teprotumumab inhibits IGF-1R through three mechanisms: (1) internalization and degradation of IGF-1R, (2) IGF-1R activation blockade, and (3) IGR-1R and TSHr complex formation inhibition [171–173]. Consequently, teprotumumab prevents IGF-1R-mediated activation of IL-6 and IL-8 synthesis by TSH, ultimately having an anti-inflammatory effect [171–173]. Teprotumumab is currently administered intravenously (IV), with current regimens requiring patients to receive 8 infusions, which are 60–90 min in length every 3 weeks, a time-consuming and expensive process [148].

In preliminary phase II and III OPTIAC trials, teprotumumab was compared to placebo in active moderate and severe TED. The primary endpoint was a decrease in CAS of greater than 2, which was achieved in 69% of patients receiving teprotumumab compared to 20% in the placebo arm at 24 weeks. Along with a strong improvement in quality of life, diplopia, and proptosis (decrease of 2 mm or greater) in patients with Graves' ophthalmopathy, these data supported its FDA approval in 2020 for use in TED, irrespective of its severity [174].

Although Teprotumumab is a promising therapy for TED, it is difficult to administer due to its requirement for IV delivery [15, 175]. As a result, new IGF-1R antagonists have been sought. VRDN-001 is a full IGF-1R antagonist that was studied in a phase I/II clinical trial at doses of 3, 10, and 20 mg/kg. Key outcomes included an 83% overall responder rate and significant reductions in both proptosis (by 2.4 mm) and CAS (by 4.3 points) [176]. A phase III study is currently being conducted to assess the clinical outcomes of VRDN-001 compared to placebo in patients with moderate to severe TED (NCT05176639). Two other actively recruiting phase III trials are assessing VRDN-001 in specific populations, such as chronic TED patients, and assessing adverse effects over a longer time frame (NCT06021054, NCT06384547). Two new IGF-R1 monoclonal antibodies, VRDN-002 and VRDN-003, are also being studied. They are distinct as they have modified Fc fragments of VRDN-001 to increase the half-life of the drug [177–180]. In pre-clinical studies, both VRDN-002 and VRDN-003 were administered to non-human primates IV and subcutaneously (SC), with the latter presenting a clinical advantage over teprotumumab. In healthy volunteers, IV administration of VRDN-002 was well tolerated with an increased half-life [178]. The results of these preclinical studies are promising and may fuel future VRDN-002 and VRDN-003 clinical investigations [174]. A notable advantage of these drugs is SC administration, which is less laborious than IV administration. Lonigutamab is another IGF-1R inhibitor administered SC currently in phase I/II clinical study evaluating its safety and efficacy in patients with TED (NCT05683496).

Linsitinib is a small-molecule dual inhibitor of both IGF-1R and insulin receptors. Linsitinib inhibits the tyrosine kinase domain of IGF-1R, preventing autophosphorylation and downstream signaling [181, 182]. In pre-clinical studies in murine models of Graves' ophthalmopathy, researchers successfully prevented the development and progression of TED, serving as foundational evidence for clinical studies of linsitinib [181]. A key advantage of linsitinib is its oral route of administration. Currently, a phase IIb RCT (LIDS) is underway to assess the safety and efficacy of linsitinib compared to placebo in patients with active moderate-to-severe TED (NCT05276063).

12.8.6.2 Tocilizumab and IL-6 Receptor Antagonists

Tocilizumab is a monoclonal antibody widely used in the treatment of autoimmune conditions. It targets interleukin-6 receptors (IL-6R), which recruit gp-130 that then dimerizes to activate a pro-inflammatory cascade involved in B- and T-cell activation [15]. IL-6R exists in both soluble and membrane forms in a multitude of immune cells, both of which are inhibited by tocilizumab, resulting in the prevention of downstream homodimer formation with gp-130. The end-result is the inhibition of IL-6R-mediated pro-inflammatory pathways such as antibody and acute phase protein synthesis [183].

Prior to its study in TED, tocilizumab was mainly used to treat rheumatoid arthritis. The foundation for its use in TED came from a small RCT that included 32 patients with Graves' ophthalmopathy who had failed IV corticosteroid therapy. In patients receiving IV tocilizumab, there were greater reductions in CAS (86% achieving CAS lower than 3 vs. 39% in the placebo) at 0, 4, 8, and 12 weeks [184]. Other small observational studies [185, 186], as well as a systematic review [187], have also supported the use of tocilizumab as a second-line therapy. However, a larger, long-term RCT would be needed to favor widespread clinical implementation of tocilizumab [185–187].

12.8.6.3 Rituximab (RTX) and Targeting B-Cells

Initially developed as the first molecule to treat non-Hodgkin's lymphoma (NHL), rituximab (RTX) is now increasingly used to treat various autoimmune diseases. RTX is a monoclonal antibody directed against CD20 surface antigen, which is involved in B-cell differentiation and activation [188, 189]. RTX inhibits B-cells through several pathways. Firstly, RTX activates intracellular signaling pathways, resulting in cell apoptosis. Its Fc domain activates the classical pathway of the complement system by activating C1, leading to the formation of membrane attack complexes (MAC), causing cell lysis [188, 189]. Another pathway mediated by RTX's Fc domain is the activation of NK-cells through their fragment crystallizable receptor (FCR), which results in the release of granzymes and perforins, causing cytotoxic death of B-cells [188, 189]. Finally, through FCRs of phagocytes, such as macrophages, RTX induces phagocytosis of B-cells, resulting in their intracellular degradation [188, 189].

The use of RTX to treat TED is based on two RCTs: one conducted in Italy and the other in the United States. However, these two small single-center studies provided conflicting results. In the American study, patients with moderate-to-severe TED were given either RTX or placebo, and no advantage or reduction in CAS was seen in the experimental arm [190]. However, the Italian study compared RTX (1000 mg 2 weeks apart) to IVMP and found that RTX outperformed IVMP, with all patients showing inactivation of Graves' ophthalmopathy at 24 weeks in the RTX arm, compared to 69% in the IVMP arm [191]. Despite the conflicting results, RTX is used as a second-line treatment; however, future studies could aim to elucidate which subset of TED patients would benefit most from RTX.

Another strategy to target B-cells has also been investigated. Belimumab, an immune-modulator approved for treatment of systemic lupus erythematosus (SLE), is a monoclonal antibody that targets B-lymphocyte stimulator protein (BLyS, aka. BAFF), a cytokine involved in B-cell differentiation [192]. By binding its target BLyS, belimumab inhibits BLyS interaction with BCR as well as other proteins, ultimately inhibiting B-cell differentiation into plasma cells and triggering apoptosis [192]. Belimumab is being studied as a treatment for TED on the basis that BLyS levels are elevated in TED patients.

12.8.7 Future Therapeutic Possibilities: TSHr Inhibitors

Thyroid-stimulating hormone receptor (TSHr) inhibitors are an emerging, promising therapeutic strategy for the treatment of TED. This is largely due to past evidence demonstrating that TSHr has a synergistic relationship with IGF-R1 and has been seen to be over-expressed in TED, leading to adipogenesis [15, 193]. Even though TSHr's involvement in TED is not fully understood, drugs targeting it are under study.

In pre-clinical studies, one such drug, K1–70 (a recombinant human antibody), has been shown to interfere with TSHr signaling by interfering with ligand binding [194]. These findings led to a phase 1 clinical trial that demonstrated tolerable IV and intra-muscular (IM) administration in patients with Grave's disease [195]. It is not yet used for TED treatment, as no further clinical trials have yet been conducted. Other TSHr antagonists are being investigated as potential therapies. S37A is a small molecule that interferes with signal transduction by inhibiting TSHr signaling in the presence of its ligand in cell lines and has shown promising results in studies [15, 196]. These studies have not yet been translated into practice, but nevertheless, they show that TSHr is a potential target for TED treatments.

12.8.8 Future Therapeutic Strategies

12.8.8.1 Targeting Cytokines

The promising results of recently FDA-approved immune-modulating agents have further driven the exploration of novel immune markers, cytokines, and cells as targets. Most of the drug candidates have been validated in pre-clinical models and are currently being investigated in clinical trials. The first notable target being studied is IL-17. IL-17 has been associated with TED pathophysiology, and thus a group is examining vunakizumab (SHR-1314), an SC administered monoclonal antibody targeting IL-17a, preventing its interaction with its receptor. A phase I study in psoriasis patients demonstrated that vunakizumab is tolerable in human subjects, and this study is being translated into a phase II clinical trial for patients with moderate-to-severe TED (NCT05394857). Another group conducted a phase III clinical trial for secukinumab, another monoclonal antibody targeting IL-17a, in patients with TED (NCT04737330). However, this study was terminated early due to the low probability of meeting the primary endpoint. Therefore, targeting IL-17a as a therapy for TED still remains unconfirmed [197].

Another cytokine being targeted in phase I and II clinical trials in patients with TED and pulmonary fibrosis is IL-11 (NCT05331300, NCT0622545, respectively). Although the role of IL-11 in TED is *not* well understood, it is postulated that IL-11 may play a role in the altered phenotype of orbital fibroblasts [15, 198]. Thus, researchers are currently striving to inhibit the IL-11 receptor (IL-11R) with LASN01, a fully human antibody. The goal of this strategy is to prevent signaling and pro-inflammatory activity mediated by IL-11R, which would act as a potential therapy for TED.

12.8.8.2 Neonatal Fragment Crystallizable Receptor: Batoclimab

The neonatal fragment crystallizable receptor (FcRn) plays a crucial role in transporting immunoglobulin G (IgG) across barriers and protecting it from degradation. FcRn inhibitors have recently emerged as a potential treatment for various autoimmune diseases, including Myasthenia Gravis [199]. Batoclimab is a monoclonal antibody that targets FcRn, preventing it from recycling IgG [174]. In TED, this may enhance the breakdown of pathogenic autoantibodies targeting TSHR and IGF-R1 [174]. In a phase IIa trial (ASCEND-GO 1), seven patients with active moderate-to-severe TED received SC batoclimab as weekly injections. The results showed a 64.8% decrease in serum IgG levels and a 56.7% reduction in anti-TSHR antibodies [200]. However, the subsequent phase IIb trial (ASCEND-GO 2) was terminated due to increased serum cholesterol levels in participants [15, 174]. It is unclear if batoclimab will be used in TED clinically.

12.8.8.3 Sirolimus

Sirolimus is an immune-suppressive agent that has recently been studied in clinical trials to treat TED. It acts by suppressing the sensitivity of lymphocytes to cytokines, predominantly to IL-2, thus reducing lymphocyte activation [15]. In a preliminary observational study comparing sirolimus to IVMP, the sirolimus cohort outperformed IVMP at 24 weeks (86.6% versus 26.6%, respectively).

12.8.8.4 Statins

Statins are used to reduce cholesterol levels by inhibiting 3-hydroxy-3-methylglutaryl-coenzyme A (HMG-CoA). In recent studies, statins have been shown to be effective in treating TED. This is due to their anti-inflammatory and anti-immunomodulatory properties. Their anti-inflammatory effects include inhibiting the induction of pro-inflammatory cytokines released from T lymphocytes. One recent phase II clinical trial evaluated the effects of adding atorvastatin to intravenous glucocorticoids in patients with and hyper-cholesterolemia. Results showed that adding a statin to IVMP improved outcomes in patients with Graves' ophthalmopathy, although a bigger population is needed to confirm the results found in this study [201].

12.9 Role of Artificial Intelligence in Thyroid Eye Disease

Artificial intelligence (AI) is rapidly becoming immersed in medical practices. Its application within the field of ophthalmology has grown quickly as it presents the possibility to optimize diagnostics, prognostics, and disease management. TED is a highly complex and variable disease, reliant on a thorough diagnosis from imaging, clinical assessment, and thyroid function assessment. AI can be a valuable tool in managing TED, aiding every step of the way, from diagnosis and tracking disease progression to personalizing treatments.

12.9.1 Diagnostic Applications

12.9.1.1 Measuring Proptosis

Traditionally, diagnosis of TED relies on the physician's expertise, which can lead to inconsistencies in diagnosis and can limit the early detection of disease [202]. To address current limitations, AI modalities are being developed to facilitate the diagnosis and screening of TED through the accurate identification of early-stage clinical markers of TED. For example, current methods of measuring proptosis are limited by their lack of reproducibility and unreliability, largely due to the high degree of subjectivity involved [203]. To objectify this measurement, one study developed an AI model that can quickly and reliably identify clinically relevant proptosis based on orbital CT scans. Their model measured proptosis at a concordance correlation coefficient (CCC) of 0.9895 on axial CT images and a CCC of 0.9902 on sagittal CT images, which were both comparable to the results of clinician-based measurements [203]. With more advancements, an improved model would be a promising alternative to current standards that would optimize the reliability and accuracy of proptosis measurements.

12.9.1.2 Assessing Facial Symptoms

Another group of researchers applied their machine learning model to facial scans of TED. They trained their model to recognize specific symptoms, including, but not limited to, eyelid retraction, ocular dyskinesia, and conjunctival congestion. They concluded that their model could reliably identify patients with facial symptoms of TED with an average area under the curve (AUC) of 0.85 [204].

12.9.1.3 Screening

Beyond identifying and quantifying symptoms of TED, AI-based modalities have been explored for the purpose of screening for TED. One study developed an AI-powered tool aimed at diagnosing TED without clinician input based on orbital CT scans [205]. The researchers concluded that their model could diagnose TED (85.67%) as accurately as residents (84.33%), whose clinical interpretation is the current benchmark in TED diagnosis [205]. If such a model could be perfected to outperform clinicians, it could be used to screen patients at risk, providing a valid, reliable, and automated diagnostic tool [202, 205].

12.9.2 Disease Monitoring

Artificial intelligence (AI) could also aid in the management of TED by quantifying the severity of the disease to track progression and assist in the selection of an optimal treatment plan. To explore this application, one study, by Li et al. (2024), developed an AI-powered program that could quantify inflammation of extraocular muscles based on contrast-enhanced MRI in order to evaluate the activity stage of TED [206]. Another study, by Moon et al. (2022), examined a machine learning model's ability to assess CAS. They reported that their model could predict the CAS based on patients' facial scans with an accuracy of 84.6% when training the model with an unfiltered data set, and that the accuracy increased to 89.0% when trained with filtered data sets with consistent results [207]. Additionally, an AI-based model was trained by Lee et al. without orbital CT scans, to differentiate between active and inactive TED, achieving an AUC (area under curve) of 0.871 [208]. Altogether, these studies all developed AI-based modalities with the potential to be used clinically to analyze images to quickly provide clinicians with clinically relevant information that could assist in monitoring disease progression and activity.

12.9.3 Decision-Making Tool

The information acquired from AI-driven systems can also help clinicians guide their treatment selection. This was demonstrated by a group of researchers whose convolutional neural network (CNN), specifically tailored for image-centric tasks, could analyze orbital CT scans to quantify proptosis and identify patients that required surgical drainage [209]. Although this model's measurements of proptosis differed significantly from those made by physicians, it still showed promise, as the linear and volumetric measurements of proptosis made by the CNN were more predictive of the requirement of surgery as compared to those measured by physicians (AUC of 0.78 and 0.79, respectively) [209].

Another group of researchers examined the use of AI models in predicting responses to treatment in patients with TED. Their model, XGBoost, analyzed clinical characteristics and laboratory results, predicting the response of TED patients to steroid treatment with an accuracy of 0.861 [191]. The authors reported that the specific patterns of both thyroid-stimulating immunoglobulin and low-density lipoprotein cholesterol were the most significant factors in predicting the XGBoost's ability to predict response [191]. These results further demonstrate the use of AI-based modalities in identifying specific clinical patterns that can impact a patient's response to treatment or guide a physician in choosing the optimal treatment.

12.9.4 Significant Barriers in Clinical Application of AI in TED Patients

Altogether, the data that the AI tool can acquire from facial scans, imaging modalities (e.g., CT scans and MRI), and laboratory diagnostics can open the possibility of quicker and improved clinical decision-making. Recent efforts to integrate AI in the clinical management of TED have demonstrated its potential to improve diagnosis, progression assessment, and clinical decision-making. As these systems continue to advance, their clinical integration will grow, offering clinicians valuable tools to deliver optimal and comprehensive care. However, major challenges constitute drawbacks to the translation of AI-based deep learning models for the management of TED to clinical practice [202]. The complexity of TED and the variability in its clinical manifestations are significant barriers. Greater training data sets are required to achieve excellent performance of deep learning models and enable their generalization to different populations. Furthermore, such models come with a great cost—high costs in their development and future application to clinical medicine. Additional technical limitations are also faced, such as the ethical aspects surrounding data privacy and the necessity for validation steps to filter and manage potential AI-derived medical errors.

12.10 Current Challenges and Future Perspectives of TED

Autoimmune diseases, such as TED, have strikingly varying phenotypes and encompass complex pathogenesis. A current limitation in the management of TED is the lack of reliable markers to diagnose, assess the severity of disease, and establish treatment response [160]. Currently, ocular examination, repetitive laboratory investigations, and imaging modalities form the backbone of TED diagnosis. However, numerous efforts have been deployed in recent years to develop less invasive, cost-friendly, and rapid diagnostic tools such as "liquid biopsy" and "AI-derived deep learning models." However, their translation to clinical practice is yet to be optimized. The limited understanding of disease pathology currently limits the exploitation of biological agents for TED treatment. For example, although TED patients do have IGF-1R autoantibodies, the presence of such markers has not been associated with the severity of the disease nor with susceptibility to specific treatments [160]. Further studies are thus required to close the fundamental science knowledge gap regarding TED pathogenesis.

Management of patients with TED involves a multidisciplinary approach that may require input from several specialists. Currently, the lack of consensus on the optimal treatment plan results in varying treatment approaches. IVMP and glucocorticoids have been used as the gold standard, followed by immune-suppressive agents. However, new biological agents have emerged that may offer enhanced therapeutic benefits with fewer adverse events [160].

Teprotumumab is now viewed as a first-line treatment in TED patients in the United States [210], but its use is limited worldwide in the same setting, given its greater cost compared to glucocorticoids. We believe that through rigorous studies and the development of alternative options by pharmaceutical companies, these medications will offer specialists more diverse options to combat TED. Overall, biological agents will be most effective in an era of personalized medicine, whereby specific diagnostic markers can guide clinicians to optimal treatment regimens. Thus, linking specific markers to susceptibility to biologics may be required to fully reach the potential of biologics in treating TED.

12.11 Summary

Thyroid-associated ophthalmopathy (TAO), also known as thyroid eye disease (TED) is a self-limiting autoimmune disease associated mainly with Graves' disease, but also with Hashimoto's disease and euthyroid states. There are two distinct stages of the disease, an active inflammatory stage followed by an inactive quiescent stage. The pathophysiology of TAO remains unclear. There are no effective means of preventing the disease or reliably altering its course. Current therapeutic options include local supportive measures, corticosteroids, steroid-sparing immunosuppressive agents, and external beam radiation for reducing the inflammation during active disease, and surgery for correcting the residual abnormalities secondary to fibrosis in the inactive state of the disease.

References

1. Gupta V, Hammond CL, Roztocil E, Gonzalez MO, Feldon SE, Woeller CF. Thinking inside the box: current insights into targeting orbital tissue remodeling and inflammation in thyroid eye disease. Surv Ophthalmol. 2022;67:858–74.
2. Smith TJ. New advances in understanding thyroid-associated ophthalmopathy and the potential role for insulin-like growth factor-I receptor. F1000Res. 2018;7:134.
3. Boulos PR, Hardy I. Thyroid-associated orbitopathy: a clinicopathologic and therapeutic review. Curr Opin Ophthalmol. 2004;15(5):389–400.
4. Yamada M, Wu Li A, Wall J. Thyroid-associated ophthalmopathy: clinical features, pathogenesis, and management. Crit Rev Clin Lab Sci. 2000;37(6):523–49.
5. Maheshwari R, Weis E. Thyroid associated orbitopathy. Indian J Ophthalmol. 2012;60(2):87–93.
6. Dagi LR, Elliott AT, Roper-Hall G, Cruz OA. Thyroid eye disease: honing your skills to improve outcomes. J AAPOS. 2010;14(5):425–31.
7. El-Kaissi S, Frauman AG, Wall JR. Thyroid-associated ophthalmopathy: a practical guide to classification, natural history and management. Intern Med J. 2004;34(8):482–91.
8. Wiersinga WM, Smit T, van der Gaag R, Koornneef L. Temporal relationship between onset of Graves' ophthalmopathy and onset of thyroidal Graves' disease. J Endocrinol Investig. 1988;11:615–9.
9. Bahn RS. Graves' ophthalmopathy. N Engl J Med. 2010;362(25):726–38.
10. Wiersinga WM, Bartalena L. Epidemiology and prevention of Graves' ophthalmopathy. Thyroid. 2002;12:855–60.
11. Smith TJ, Hegedüs L, Lesser I, Perros P, Dorris K, Kinrade M, et al. How patients experience thyroid eye disease. Front Endocrinol. 2023;14:1283374.

12. Enzmann DR, Donaldson SS, Kriss JP. Appearance of Graves' disease on orbital computed tomography. J Comput Assist Tomogr. 1979;3:815–9.
13. Wiersinga WM, Smit T, van der Gaag R, Mourits M, Koornneef L. Clinical presentation of Graves' ophthalmopathy. Ophthalmic Res. 1989;21:73–82.
14. Fatourechi V. Pretibial myxedema: pathophysiology and treatment options. Am J Clin Dermatol. 2005;6:295–309.
15. Moledina M, Damato EM, Lee V. The changing landscape of thyroid eye disease: current clinical advances and future outlook. Eye. 2024;38:1425–37.
16. Shirakawa H, Amemiya T, Kasagi K, et al. Hashimoto disease with hyperthyroid ocular signs. Metab Pediatr Ophthalmol. 1981;5:213–8.
17. Krassas GE, Wiersinga WM. Thyroid eye disease: current concepts and the EUGOGO perspective. Thyroid Int. 2005;4:3–4.
18. Tjiang H, Lahooti H, McCorquodale T, Parmar KR, Wall JR. Eye and eyelid abnormalities are common in patients with Hashimoto's thyroiditis. Thyroid. 2010;20(3):287–90.
19. Kan E, Kan EK, Ecemis G, Colak R. Presence of thyroid-associated ophthalmopathy in Hashimoto's thyroiditis. Int J Ophthalmol. 2014;7(4):644–7.
20. Grzesiuk W, Szydlarska D, Pragacz A, Bar-Andziak E. Thyroid associated orbitopathy in patients with Hashimoto's thyroiditis: a case report. Pol Arch Med Wewn. 2008;118(5):318–21.
21. Hiraga A, Mimura M, Kamitsukasa I. Isolated inferior rectus muscle myopathy due to Hashimoto's thyroiditis. Intern Med. 2008;47(13):1283–4.
22. Yoshihara A, Yoshimura Noh J, Nakachi A, Ohye H, Sato S, Sekiya K, et al. Severe thyroid associated orbitopathy in Hashimoto's thyroiditis. Report of 2 cases. Endocr J. 2011;58(5):343–8.
23. Bahn RS. Pathophysiology of Graves' ophthalmopathy: the cycle of disease. J Clin Endocrinol Metab. 2003;88(5):1939–46.
24. Łacheta D, Miśkiewicz P, Głuszko A, Nowicka G, Struga M, Kantor I, et al. Immunological aspects of Graves' ophthalmopathy. Biomed Res Int. 2019;2019:7453260.
25. Roos JCP, Paulpandian V, Murthy R. Serial TSH-receptor antibody levels to guide the management of thyroid eye disease: the impact of smoking, immunosuppression, radio-iodine, and thyroidectomy. Eye. 2019;33:212–7.
26. Khoo TK, Bahn RS. Pathogenesis of Graves' ophthalmopathy: the role of autoanti-bodies. Thyroid. 2007;17:1013–8.
27. Guo N, Woeller CF, Feldon SE, Phipps RP. Peroxisome proliferator-activated receptor γ ligands inhibit transforming growth factor-β-induced, hyaluronan-dependent, T cell adhesion to orbital fibroblasts. J Biol Chem. 2011;286:18856–67.
28. Pawlowski P, Wawrusiewicz-Kurylone N, Eckstein A, Reszec J, Luczynski W, Johnson K, et al. Disturbances of modulating molecules (FOXP3, CTLA-4/CD28/B7, and CD40/CD40L) mRNA expressions in the orbital tissue from patients with severe Graves' ophthalmopathy. Mediat Inflamm. 2015;2015:340934.
29. Yang I-H, Rose GE, Ezra DG, Bailly M. Macrophages promote a profibrotic phenotype in orbital fibroblasts through increased hyaluronic acid production and cell contractility. Sci Rep. 2019;9:9622.
30. Khoo DH, Eng PH, Ho SC, Tai ES, Morgenthaler NG, Seah LL, et al. Graves' ophthalmopathy in the absence of elevated free thyroxine and triiodothyronine levels: prevalence, natural history, and thyrotropin receptor antibody levels. Thyroid. 2000;10:1093–00.
31. Gerding MN, van der Meer JW, Broenink M, Bakker O, Wiersinga WM, Prummel MF. Association of thyrotrophin receptor antibodies with the clinical features of Graves' ophthalmopathy. Clin Endocrinol. 2000;52:267–71.
32. Diana T, Brown RS, Bossowski A, Segni M, Niedziela M, König J, et al. Clinical relevance of thyroid-stimulating autoantibodies in pediatric Graves' disease—a multicenter study. J Clin Endocrinol Metab. 2014;99:1648–55.
33. Eckstein AK, Plicht M, Lax H, Neuhäuser M, Mann K, Lederbogen S, et al. Thyrotropin receptor autoantibodies are independent risk factors for Graves' ophthalmopathy and help to predict severity and outcome of the disease. J Clin Endocrinol Metab. 2006;91:3464–70.

34. Morris JC III, Hay ID, Nelson RE, Jiang NS. Clinical utility of thyrotropin-receptor antibody assays: comparison of radioreceptor and bioassay methods. Mayo Clin Proc. 1988;63:707–17.
35. Varewijck AJ, Boelen A, Lamberts SWJ, Fliers E, Hofland LJ, Wiersinga WM, et al. Circulating IgGs may modulate IGF-I receptor stimulating activity in a subset of patients with Graves' ophthalmopathy. J Clin Endocrinol Metab. 2013;98:769–76.
36. Minich W, Dehina N, Welsink T, Schwiebert C, Morgenthaler NG, Köhrle J, et al. Autoantibodies to the IGF1 receptor in Graves' orbitopathy. J Clin Endocrinol Metab. 2013;98:752–60.
37. Gontarz-Nowak K, Szychlińska M, Matuszewski W, Stefanowicz-Rutkowska M, Bandurska-Stankiewicz E. Current knowledge on Graves' orbitopathy. J Clin Med. 2020;10:16.
38. Weightman DR, Perros P, Sherif IH, Kendall-Taylor P. Autoantibodies to IGF-1 binding sites in thyroid associated ophthalmopathy. Autoimmunity. 1993;16:251–7.
39. Wu Y, Zhang J, Deng W, Mo C, Liang Y, Huang K, et al. Comparison of orbital fibroblasts from Graves' ophthalmopathy and healthy control. Heliyon. 2024;10:e28397.
40. Tuncel M. Thyroid stimulating hormone receptor. Mol Imaging Radionucl Ther. 2017;26(Suppl. S1):87–91.
41. Woeller CF, Roztocil E, Hammond C, Feldon SE. TSHR signaling stimulates proliferation through PI3K/Akt and induction of miR-146a and miR-155 in thyroid eye disease orbital fibroblasts. Investig Ophthalmol Vis Sci. 2019;60:4336–45.
42. Krieger CC, Kahaly GJ, Azam A, Klubo-Gwiezdzinska J, Neumann S, Gershengorn MC. Graves' autoantibodies exhibit different stimulating activities in cultures of thyrocytes and orbital fibroblasts not reflected by clinical assays. Thyroid. 2022;32:90–6.
43. LeRoith D, Holly JMP, Forbes BE. Insulin-like growth factors: ligands, binding proteins, and receptors. Mol Metab. 2021;52:101245.
44. Hoa N, Tsui S, Afifiyan NF, Sinha Hikim A, Li B, Douglas RS, et al. Nuclear targeting of IGF-1 receptor in orbital fibroblasts from Graves' disease: apparent role of ADAM17. PLoS One. 2012;7:e34173.
45. Wang R, Song D, Zhong LH. Potential role of IGF-1R in the interaction between orbital fibroblasts and B lymphocytes: an implication for B lymphocyte depletion in the active inflammatory phase of thyroid-associated ophthalmopathy. BMC Immunol. 2024;25:31.
46. Mohyi M, Smith TJ. IGF1 receptor and thyroid-associated ophthalmopathy. J Mol Endocrinol. 2018;61:T29–43.
47. Paik JS, Kim S-E, Kim JH, Lee J-Y, Yang S-W, Lee S-B. Insulin-like growth factor-1 enhances the expression of functional TSH receptor in orbital fibroblasts from thyroid-associated ophthalmopathy. Immunobiology. 2020;225:151902.
48. Kiernan K, Alwarawrah Y, Nichols AG, Danzaki K, MacIver NJ. Insulin and IGF-1 have both overlapping and distinct effects on CD4+ T cell mitochondria, metabolism, and function. Sci Rep. 2024;14:4331.
49. Fang S, Huang Y, Zhong S, Li Y, Zhang Y, Li Y, et al. Regulation of orbital fibrosis and adipogenesis by pathogenic Th17 cells in Graves orbitopathy. J Clin Endocrinol Metab. 2017;102:4273–83.
50. Buonfiglio F, Ponto KA, Pfeiffer N, Kahaly GJ, Gericke A. Redox mechanisms in autoimmune thyroid eye disease. Autoimmun Rev. 2024;23:103534.
51. Wall JR, Bernard N, Boucher A, Salvi M, Zhang ZG, Kennerdell J, et al. Pathogenesis of thyroid-associated ophthalmopathy: an autoimmune disorder of the eye muscle associated with Graves' hyperthyroidism and Hashimoto's thyroiditis. Clin Immunol Immunopathol. 1993;68(1):1–8.
52. Eckstein AK, Lösch C, Glowacka D, Schott M, Mann K, Esser J, et al. Euthyroid and primarily hypothyroid patients develop milder and significantly more asymmetrical Graves' ophthalmopathy. Br J Ophthalmol. 2009;93:1052–6105.
53. Iyer S, Bahn R. Immunopathogenesis of Graves' ophthalmopathy: the role of the TSH receptor. Best Pract Res Clin Endocrinol Metab. 2012;26(3):281–9.

54. Wescombe L, Lahooti H, Gopinath B, Wall JR. The cardiac calsequestrin gene (CASQ2) is up-regulated in the thyroid in patients with Graves' ophthalmopathy--support for a role of autoimmunity against calsequestrin as the triggering event. Clin Endocrinol. 2010;73(4):522–8.
55. Gopinath B, Wescombe L, Nguyen B, Wall JR. Can autoimmunity against calsequestrin explain the eye and eyelid muscle inflammation of thyroid eye disease? Orbit. 2009;28(4):256–61.
56. Gopinath B, Musselman R, Beard N, Tani J, Adams C, Wall JR. Antibodies targeting the calcium binding skeletal muscle protein calsequestrin are sensitive and specific markers of ocular myopathy in patients with Graves' disease. Clin Exp Immunol. 2006;145(1):56–62.
57. Gopinath B, Adams CL, Musselman R, Tani J, Wall JR. Antibodies against calsequestrin and type XIII collagen are good markers for chronic upper eyelid lag and retraction. Ocul Immunol Inflamm. 2007;15(2):81–8.
58. Gopinath B, Ma G, Wall JR. Eye signs and serum eye muscle and collagen XIII antibodies in patients with transient and progressive thyroiditis. Thyroid. 2007;17(11):1123–9.
59. Gopinath B, Ma G, Lahooti H, Wall JR. A case of Hashimoto's thyroiditis presenting with chronic upper eye lid retraction and positive calsequestrin and collagen XIII antibodies. Int J Endocrinol Metab. 2007;6(2):34–7.
60. Kulbay M, Tanya SM, Tuli N, Dahoud J, Dahoud A, Alsaleh F, et al. A comprehensive review of thyroid eye disease pathogenesis: from immune dysregulations to novel diagnostic and therapeutic approaches. Int J Mol Sci. 2024;25(21):11628.
61. Dik WA, Virakul S, van Steensel L. Current perspectives on the role of orbital fibroblasts in the pathogenesis of Graves' ophthalmopathy. Exp Eye Res. 2016;142:83–91.
62. Rapoport B, Pillarisetty RJ, Herman EA, Congco EG. Evidence for prostaglandin production by human lymphocytes during culture with human thyroid cells in monolayer: a possible role for prostaglandins in the pathogenesis of graves' disease. Biochem Biophys Res Commun. 1977;77:1245–50.
63. Aoun T, Danielova Gueorguieva D, Wu KY. Orbital inflammation in thyroid eye disease: stess responses and their implications. Stresses. 2024;4:54–78.
64. Ahsanuddin S, Wu AY. Single-cell transcriptomics in thyroid eye disease. Taiwan J Ophthalmol. 2023;14(4):554–64.
65. Patrick C, Roztocil E, Husain F, Feldon SE, Woeller C. Activating the aryl hydrocarbon receptor with naturally occurring compounds to mitigate thyroid eye disease orbital fibroblast activation. Invest Ophthalmol Vis Sci. 2024;65:3052.
66. Girnita L, Smith TJ, Janssen JA. It takes two to tango: IGF-I and TSH receptors in thyroid eye disease. J Clin Endocrinol Metab. 2022;107(Suppl S1):S1–S12.
67. Zhou M, Lin B, Wu P, Ke Y, Huang S, Zhang F, et al. SOX9 induces orbital fibroblast activation in thyroid eye disease via MAPK/ERK1/2 pathway. Investig Ophthalmol Vis Sci. 2024;65:25.
68. Galgoczi E, Orsos I, Molnar Z, Ujhelyi B, Steiber Z, Szabo L, et al. Modelling of mechanical stimuli through piezo1 receptor activation and its effect on adipogenic differentiation of orbital fibroblasts. In: Endocrine abstracts, vol. 101. Bristol: Bioscientifica; 2024.
69. Ko J, Kim YJ, Choi SH, Lee CS, Yoon JS. Yes-associated protein mediates the transition from inflammation to fibrosis in Graves' orbitopathy. Thyroid. 2023;33:1465–75.
70. Shah SS, Patel BC. Thyroid eye disease. In: StatPearls. Treasure Island: StatPearls Publishing; 2024. http://www.ncbi.nlm.nih.gov/books/NBK582134/.
71. Bartalena L, Gallo D, Tanda ML, Kahaly GJ. Thyroid eye disease: epidemiology, natural history, and risk factors. Ophthalmic Plast Reconstr Surg. 2023;39:S2–8.
72. Yu CY, Ford RL, Wester ST, Shriver EM. Update on thyroid eye disease: regional variations in prevalence, diagnosis, and management. Indian J Ophthalmol. 2022;70:2335–45.
73. Ludgate M. Animals models of Graves' disease. Eur J Endocrinol. 2000;142:1–8.
74. Ludgate ME. Animal models of thyroid-associated ophthalmopathy. Thyroid. 2002;12:205–8.
75. Lee MH, Chin YH, Ng CH, Nistala KRY, Ow ZGW, Sundar G, et al. Risk factors of thyroid eye disease. Endocr Pract. 2021;27:245–53.
76. Yin X, Latif R, Bahn R, Tomer Y, Davies TF. Influence of the TSH receptor gene on susceptibility to Graves' disease and Graves' ophthalmopathy. Thyroid. 2008;18:1201–6.

77. Pawlak-Adamska E, Daroszewski J, Bolanowski M, Oficjalska J, Janusz P, Szalinski M, et al. PPARg2 Ala 12 variant protects against Graves' orbitopathy and modulates the course of the disease. Immunogenetics. 2013;65:493–500.
78. Alevizaki M, Mantzou E, Cimponeriu A, Saltiki K, Philippou G, Wiersinga W. The Pro12Ala PPARγ gene polymorphism: possible modifier of the activity and severity of thyroid-associated orbitopathy (TAO). Clin Endocrinol. 2009;70:464–8.
79. Kahaly GJ, Diana T, Glang J, Kanitz M, Pitz S, König J. Stimulating antibodies are highly prevalent in Hashimoto's thyroiditis and associated orbitopathy. J Clin Endocrinol Metab. 2016;101(5):1998–2004.
80. Chin YH, Ng CH, Lee MH, Koh JWH, Kiew J, Yang SP, et al. Prevalence of thyroid eye disease in Graves' disease: a meta-analysis and systematic review. Clin Endocrinol. 2020;93:363–74.
81. Osaki TH, Monteiro LG, Osaki MH. Management of eyelid retraction related to thyroid eye disease. Taiwan J Ophthalmol. 2022;12(1):12–21.
82. Hoang TD, Stocker DJ, Chou EL, Burch HB. 2022 Update on clinical management of Graves disease and thyroid eye disease. Endocrinol Metab Clin N Am. 2022;51(2):287–304.
83. Ugradar S, Goldberg RA, Douglas RS. Changing the face of thyroid eye disease. Eye (Lond). 2023;37(2):197–9.
84. Thornton J, Kelly SP, Harrison RA, Edwards R. Cigarette smoking and thyroid eye disease: a systematic review. Eye (Lond). 2007;21(9):1135–45.
85. Patel P, Khandji J, Kazim M. Recurrent thyroid eye disease. Ophthalmic Plast Reconstr Surg. 2015;31:445–8.
86. Kimball LE, Kulinskaya E, Brown B, Johnston C, Farid NR. Does smoking increase relapse rates in Graves' disease? J Endocrinol Investig. 2002;25(2):152–7.
87. Subramaniam DL, Yadalla D, Rajagopalan J. Are severe forms of thyroid eye disease common in the Indian population? Clinical characteristics of 136 patients from a tertiary eye care centre. Indian J Endocrinol Metab. 2023;27(1):56–61.
88. Rashad R, Pinto R, Li E, Sohrab M, Distefano AG. Thyroid eye disease. Life. 2022;12:2084.
89. Stan MN, Bahn RS. Risk factors for development or deterioration of Graves' ophthalmopathy. Thyroid. 2010;20:777–83.
90. Zang S, Ponto K, Kahaly G. Intravenous glucocorticoids for Graves' orbitopathy: efficacy and morbidity. J Clin Endocrinol Metab. 2011;96:320–32.
91. Park J, Kim J, Ryu D, Choi H. Factors related to steroid treatment responsiveness in thyroid eye disease patients and application of SHAP for feature analysis with XGBoost. Front Endocrinol. 2023;14:1079628.
92. Szelog J, Swanson H, Sniegowski MC, Lyon DB. Thyroid eye disease. Mo Med. 2022;119(4):343–50.
93. Li Z, Cestari DM, Fortin E. Thyroid eye disease: what is new to know? Curr Opin Ophthalmol. 2018;29:528.
94. Rana HS, Akella SS, Clabeaux CE, Skurski ZP, Aakalu VK. Ocular surface disease in thyroid eye disease: a narrative review. Ocul Surf. 2022;24:67–73.
95. Kim YS, Kwak AY, Lee SY, Yoon JS, Jang SY. Meibomian gland dysfunction in Graves' orbitopathy. Can J Ophthalmol. 2015;50(4):278–82.
96. Gürdal C, Saraç O, Genç I, Kırımlıoğlu H, Takmaz T, Can I. Ocular surface and dry eye in Graves' disease. Curr Eye Res. 2011;36(1):8–13.
97. Aass C, Norheim I, Eriksen EF, Børnick EC, Thorsby PM, Pepaj M. Comparative proteomic analysis of tear fluid in Graves' disease with and without orbitopathy. Clin Endocrinol. 2016;85(5):805–12.
98. Bajkowska D, Szelachowska M, Buczyńska A, Krętowski AJ, Siewko K. Tears as a source of biomarkers in the diagnosis of Graves' orbitopathy. Biomolecules. 2022;12(11):1620.
99. Khazaei H, Khazaei D, Verma R, Ng J, Wilmarth PA, David LL, Rosenbaum JT. The potential of tear proteomics for diagnosis and management of orbital inflammatory disorders including Graves' ophthalmopathy. Exp Eye Res. 2021;213:108813.

100. Gupta A, Sadeghi PB, Akpek EK. Occult thyroid eye disease in patients presenting with dry eye symptoms. Am J Ophthalmol. 2009;147:919–23.
101. Rana K, Juniat V, Patel S, Selva D. Extraocular muscle enlargement. Graefes Arch Clin Exp Ophthalmol. 2022;260:3419–35.
102. Glatt HJ. Optic nerve dysfunction in thyroid eye disease: a clinician's perspectve. Radiology. 1996;200:26–7.
103. Akbari MR, Mirmohammadsadeghi A, Mahmoudzadeh R, Veisi A. Management of thyroid eye disease-related strabismus. J Curr Ophthalmol. 2020;32(1):1–13.
104. Goel R, Shah S, Sundar G, Arora R, Gupta S, Khullar T. Orbital and ocular perfusion in thyroid eye disease. Surv Ophthalmol. 2023;68(3):481–506.
105. Delavar A, Radha Saseendrakumar B, Lee TC, Topilow NJ, Ting MA, Liu CY, et al. Associations between thyroid eye disease and glaucoma among those enrolled in the National Institutes of Health all of US research program. Ophthalmic Plast Reconstr Surg. 2023;39(4):336–40.
106. Kim JW, Ko J, Woo YJ, Bae HW, Yoon JS. Prevalence of ocular hypertension and glaucoma as well as associated factors in Graves' orbitopathy. J Glaucoma. 2018;27:464–9.
107. Knepper PA, Goossens W, Hvizd M, Palmberg PF. Glycosaminoglycans of the human trabecular meshwork in primary open-angle glaucoma. Invest Ophthalmol Vis Sci. 1996;37(7):1360–7.
108. Wu J, Du Y, Li J, Fan X, Lin C, Wang N. The influence of different intraocular pressure on lamina cribrosa parameters in glaucoma and the relation clinical implication. Sci Rep. 2021;11(1):9755.
109. Huna-Baron R, Glovinsky Y, Habot-Wilner Z. Comparison between Hardy–Rand–Rittler 4th edition and Ishihara color plate tests for detection of dyschromatopsia in optic neuropathy. Graefes Arch Clin Exp Ophthalmol. 2013;251:585–9.
110. Barrio-Barrio J, Sabater AL, Bonet-Farriol E, Velázquez-Villoria Á, Galofré JC. Graves' ophthalmopathy: VISA versus EUGOGO classification, assessment, and management. J Ophthalmol. 2015;2015:249125.
111. Dolman PJ, Rootman J. VISA classification for Graves' orbitopathy. Ophthalmic Plast Reconstr Surg. 2006;22:319–24.
112. Bartalena L, Pinchera A, Marcoocci G. Management of Grave's ophthalmopathy: reality and perspectives. Endocr Rev. 2000;21(2):168–99.
113. Polito E, Leccisotti A. MRI in Graves' orbitopathy: recognition of enlarged muscles and prediction of steroid response. Ophthalmologica. 1995;209:182–6.
114. Tiong TYV, Sundar G, Young SM, Makmur A, Yong HRC, Wong YLJ, et al. A novel method of CT exophtalmometry in patients with thyroid eye disease. Asia Pac J Ophthalmol (Phila). 2020;9(1):39–43.
115. Monteiro ML, Gonçalves AC, Silva CT, Moura JP, Ribeiro CS, Gebrim EM. Diagnostic ability of Barrett's index to detect dysthyroid optic neuropathy using multidetector computed tomography. Clinics (Sao Paulo). 2008;63(3):301–6.
116. Shah SS, Khanam S. Orbital color Doppler imaging. In: StatPearls. Treasure Island: StatPearls Publishing; 2024. Available online: http://www.ncbi.nlm.nih.gov/books/NBK572120/.
117. Kahaly GJ, Diana T, Olivo PD. TSH receptor antibodies: relevance & utility. Endocr Pract. 2020;26:97–106.
118. Diana T, Kahaly GJ. Thyroid stimulating hormone receptor antibodies in thyroid eye disease—methodology and clinical applications. Ophthalmic Plast Reconstr Surg. 2018;34:S13.
119. Diana T, Ponto KA, Kahaly GJ. Thyrotropin receptor antibodies and Graves' orbitopathy. J Endocrinol Investig. 2021;44:703–12.
120. Ponto KA, Diana T, Binder H, Matheis N, Pitz S, Pfeiffer N, Kahaly GJ. Thyroid-stimulating immunoglobulins indicate the onset of dysthyroid optic neuropathy. J Endocrinol Investig. 2015;38(7):769–77.
121. Bitcon V, Donnelly J, Kiaei D. Sensitivity of assays for TSH-receptor antibodies. J Endocrinol Investig. 2016;39:1195–6.

122. López Ortega JM, Martínez PS, Acevedo-León D, Capell NE. Anti-TSH receptor antibodies (TRAb): comparison of two third generation automated immunoassays broadly used in clinical laboratories and results interpretation. PLoS One. 2022;17(7):e0270890.
123. Lee JI, Jang HW, Kim SK, Choi JY, Kim JY, Hur KY, et al. Diagnostic value of a chimeric TSH receptor (Mc4)-based bioassay for Graves' disease. Korean J Intern Med. 2011;26(2):179–86.
124. Lone SN, Nisar S, Masoodi T, Singh M, Rizwan A, Hashem S, et al. Liquid biopsy: a step closer to transform diagnosis, prognosis and future of cancer treatments. Mol Cancer. 2022;21(1):79.
125. Halawa T, Baeesa S, Fadul MM, Badahdah AA, Enani M, Fathaddin AA, et al. The role of liquid biopsy in the diagnosis and prognosis of WHO grade 4 astrocytoma. Cureus. 2023;15(6):e41221.
126. Kulbay M, Marcotte E, Remtulla R, Lau THA, Paez-Escamilla M, Wu KY, Burnier MN Jr. Uveal melanoma: comprehensive review of its pathophysiology, diagnosis, treatment, and future perspectives. Biomedicine. 2024;12(8):1758.
127. Douglas CF, Roztocil E, Hammond C, Gonzalez M, Feldon SE, Woeller C. Investigating the role of circulating microRNAs as potential biomarkers for thyroid eye disease. Investig Ophthalmol Vis Sci. 2021;62:3349.
128. Hammond CL, Roztocil E, Gonzalez MO, Feldon SE, Woeller CF. MicroRNA-130a is elevated in thyroid eye disease and increases lipid accumulation in fibroblasts through the suppression of AMPK. Invest Ophthalmol Vis Sci. 2021;62(1):29.
129. Kim N, Choung H, Kim YJ, Woo SE, Yang MK, Khwarg SI, et al. Serum microRNA as a potential biomarker for the activity of thyroid eye disease. Sci Rep. 2023;13(1):234.
130. Xie B, Xiong W, Zhang F, Wang N, Luo Y, Chen Y, et al. The miR-103a-3p/TGFBR3 axis regulates TGF-β-induced orbital fibroblast activation and fibrosis in thyroid-eye disease. Mol Cell Endocrinol. 2023;559:111780.
131. Bartalena L, Kahaly GJ, Baldeschi L, Dayan CM, Eckstein A, Marcocci C, et al. The 2021 European Group on Graves' orbitopathy (EUGOGO) clinical practice guidelines for the medical management of Graves' orbitopathy. Eur J Endocrinol. 2021;185(4):G43–67.
132. Bartalena L, Baldeschi L, Boboridis K, Eckstein A, Kahaly GJ, Marcocci C, et al. The 2016 European Thyroid Association/European Group on Graves' orbitopathy guidelines for the management of Graves' orbitopathy. Eur Thyroid J. 2016;5(1):9–26.
133. Marcocci C, Kahaly GJ, Krassas GE, Bartalena L, Prummel M, Stahl M, et al. Selenium and the course of mild Graves' orbitopathy. N Engl J Med. 2011;364(20):1920–31.
134. Douglas RS, Dailey R, Subramanian PS, Barbesino G, Ugradar S, Batten R, et al. Proptosis and diplopia response with teprotumumab and placebo vs the recommended treatment regimen with intravenous methylprednisolone in moderate to severe thyroid eye disease: a meta-analysis and matching-adjusted indirect comparison. JAMA Ophthalmol. 2022;140:328.
135. Bartalena L, Marocci C, Bogazzi F, Bruno-Bossio G, Pinchera A. Glucocorticoid therapy of Graves' ophthalmopathy. Exp Clin Endocrinol. 1991;97:320–7.
136. Rajendram R, Lee RW, Potts MJ, Rose GE, Jain R, Olver JM, et al. Protocol for the combined immunosuppression and radiotherapy in thyroid eye disease (CIRTED) trial: a multi-centre, double-masked, factorial randomised controlled trial. Trials. 2008;9:6.
137. Längericht J, Krämer I, Kahaly GJ. Glucocorticoids in Graves' orbitopathy: mechanisms of action and clinical application. Ther Adv Endocrinol Metab. 2020;11:204201882095833.
138. Kahaly GJ, Pitz S, Hommel G, Dittmar M. Randomized, single blind trial of intravenous versus oral steroid monotherapy in Graves' orbitopathy. J Clin Endocrinol Metab. 2005;90:5234–40.
139. Macchia PE, Bagattini M, Lupoli G, Vitale M, Vitale G, Fenzi G. High-dose intravenous corticosteroid therapy for Graves' ophthalmopathy. J Endocrinol Investig. 2001;24:152–8.
140. Marcocci C, Bartalena L, Tanda ML, Manetti L, Dell'Unto E, Rocchi R, et al. Comparison of the effectiveness and tolerability of intravenous or oral glucocorticoids associated with orbital radiotherapy in the management of severe Graves' ophthalmopathy: results of a prospective, single-blind, randomized study. J Clin Endocrinol Metab. 2001;86(8):3562–7.

141. Stiebel-Kalish H, Robenshtok E, Hasanreisoglu M, Ezrachi D, Shimon I, Leibovici L. Treatment modalities for Graves' ophthalmopathy: systematic review and metaanalysis. J Clin Endocrinol Metab. 2009;94(8):2708–16.
142. Aktaran S, Akarsu E, Erbağci I, Araz M, Okumuş S, Kartal M. Comparison of intravenous methylprednisolone therapy vs. oral methylprednisolone therapy in patients with Graves' ophthalmopathy. Int J Clin Pract. 2007;61(1):45–51.
143. Wiersinga WM, Kahaly GJ. Graves' orbitopathy: a multidisciplinary approach. Basel: Karger; 2007.
144. Lin F, Yao Q, Yu B, Deng Z, Qiu J, He R. The efficacy and safety of teprotumumab in thyroid eye disease: evidence from randomized controlled trials. Int J Clin Pract. 2023;2023:6638089.
145. Najjar W, Yu J. Audiologic demonstration of ototoxicity from teprotumumab treatment in a patient with thyroid eye disease. OTO Open. 2022;6(2):2473974X221097097.
146. Perros P, Hegedüs L. Teprotumumab in thyroid eye disease: wonder drug or great divider? Eur Thyroid J. 2023;12:e230043.
147. Burch HB, Perros P, Bednarczuk T, Cooper DS, Dolman PJ, Leung AM, et al. Management of thyroid eye disease: a consensus statement by the American Thyroid Association and the European Thyroid Association. Thyroid. 2022;32(12):1439–70.
148. Douglas RS, Wang Y, Dailey RA, Harris GJ, Wester ST, Schiffman JS, Tang RA, Fowler B, Fleming J, Smith TJ. Teprotumumab in clinical practice: recommendations and considerations from the OPTIC Trial Investigators. J Neuroophthalmol. 2021;41(4):461–8.
149. van Geest RJ, Sasim IV, Koppeschaar HP, Kalmann R, Stravers SN, Bijlsma WR, et al. Methylprednisolone pulse therapy for patients with moderately severe Graves' orbitopathy: a prospective, randomized, placebo-controlled study. Eur J Endocrinol. 2008;158(2):229–37.
150. Bartalena L. Prevention of Graves' ophthalmopathy. Best Pract Res Clin Endocrinol Metab. 2012;26:371–9.
151. Strianese D, Iuliano A, Ferrara M, Comune C, Baronissi I, Napolitano P, et al. Methotrexate for the treatment of thyroid eye disease. J Ophthalmol. 2014;2014:128903.
152. Kahaly G, Schrezenmeir J, Krause U, Schweikert B, Meuer S, Muller W, et al. Cyclosporine and prednisone v. prednisone in treatment of Graves' ophthalmopathy: a controlled, randomized and prospective study. Eur J Clin Investig. 1986;16:415–22.
153. Prummel MF, Mourits MP, Berghout A, Krenning EP, van der Gaag R, Koornneef L, et al. Prednisone and cyclosporine in the treatment of severe Graves' ophthalmopathy. N Engl J Med. 1989;321:1353–9.
154. Smith JR, Rosenbaum JT. A role for methotrexate in the management of non-infectious orbital inflammatory disease. Br J Ophthalmol. 2001;85:1220–4.
155. Strianese D. Efficacy and safety of immunosuppressive agents for thyroid eye disease. Ophthalmic Plast Reconstr Surg. 2018;34(Suppl. S1):S56–9.
156. Perros P, Weightman DR, Crombie AL, Kendall-Taylor P. Azathioprine in the treatment of thyroid-associated ophthalmopathy. Acta Endocrinol. 1990;122(1):8–12.
157. Rajendram R, Taylor PN, Wilson VJ, Harris N, Morris OC, Tomlinson M, et al. Combined immunosuppression and radiotherapy in thyroid eye disease (CIRTED): a multicentre, 2 × 2 factorial, double-blind, randomised controlled trial. Lancet Diabetes Endocrinol. 2018;6(4):299–309.
158. Matsuda S, Koyasu S. Mechanisms of action of cyclosporine. Immunopharmacology. 2000;47(2–3):119–25.
159. Prummel MF, Mourits MP, Berghout A, Krenning EP, van der Gaag R, Koornneef L, Wiersinga WM. Prednisone and cyclosporine in the treatment of severe Graves' ophthalmopathy. N Engl J Med. 1989;321(20):1353–9.
160. Barbesino G, Salvi M, Freitag SK. Future projections in thyroid eye disease. J Clin Endocrinol Metab. 2022;107(Suppl. S1):S47–56.
161. Lanzolla G, Maglionico MN, Comi S, Menconi F, Piaggi P, Posarelli C, et al. Sirolimus as a second-line treatment for Graves' orbitopathy. J Endocrinol Investig. 2022;45(11):2171–80.

162. Yong KL, Chng CL, Ming Sie N, Lang S, Yang M, Looi A, et al. Methotrexate as an adjuvant in severe thyroid eye disease: does it really work as a steroid-sparing agent? Ophthalmic Plast Reconstr Surg. 2019;35(4):369–73.
163. Rivera-Grana E, Lin P, Suhler EB, Rosenbaum JT. Methotrexate as a corticosteroid-sparing agent for thyroid eye disease. J Clin Exp Ophthalmol. 2015;6:422.
164. Kahaly GJ, Roesler HP, Kutzner J, Kutzner J, Pitz S, Müller-Forell W, et al. Radiotherapy for thyroid-associated orbitopathy. Exp Clin Endocrinol Diabetes. 1999;107(Suppl 5):S201–7.
165. Bartalena L, Marcocci C, Pinchera A. Orbital radiotherapy for Graves' ophthalmopathy. J Clin Endocrinol Metab. 2004;89:13–4.
166. Marcocci C, Bartalena L, Rocchi R, Marino M, Menconi F, Morabito E, et al. Long term safety of orbital radiotherapy for Grave's ophthalmopathy. J Clin Endocrinol Metab. 2003;88:3561–6.
167. Bartley GB, Gorman CA. Perspective—part 1: then Mayo orbital radiotherapy for Graves' ophthalmopathy (ORGO) study: lessons learnt. Ophthalmic Plast Reconstr Surg. 2002;18:170–2.
168. Goldberg RA, Shorr N, Cohen MS. The medical orbital strut in the prevention of postdecompression dystopia in dysthyroid ophthalmopathy. Ophthalmic Plast Reconstr Surg. 1992;8:32–4.
169. Goldberg RA. The evolving paradigm of orbital decompression surgery. Arch Ophthalmol. 1998;116:95–6.
170. Unal M, Leri F, Konuk O, Hasanreisoglu B. Balanced orbital decompression combined with fat removal in Graves' ophthalmopathy: do we really need to remove the third wall? Ophthalmic Plast Reconstr Surg. 2003;19:112–8.
171. Yvon C, Khong JJ, Malhotra R, Patel BC. Teprotumumab. In: StatPearls. Treasure Island: StatPearls Publishing; 2024.
172. Ugradar S, Kang J, Kossler AL, Zimmerman E, Braun J, Harrison AR, Bose S, Cockerham K, Douglas RS. Teprotumumab for the treatment of chronic thyroid eye disease. Eye (Lond). 2022;36(8):1553–9.
173. Chen H, Mester T, Raychaudhuri N, Kauh CY, Gupta S, Smith TJ, et al. Teprotumumab, an IGF-1R blocking monoclonal antibody inhibits TSH and IGF-1 action in fibrocytes. J Clin Endocrinol Metab. 2014;99(9):E1635–40.
174. Kamboj A, Harrison AR, Mokhtarzadeh A. Emerging therapies in the medical management of thyroid eye disease. Front Ophthalmol. 2023;3:1295902.
175. Douglas RS, Kahaly GJ, Ugradar S, Elflein H, Ponto KA, Fowler BT, et al. Teprotumumab efficacy, safety, and durability in longer-duration thyroid eye disease and re-treatment: OPTIC-X study. Ophthalmology. 2022;129(4):438–49.
176. Moster M, Douglas R, Cockerham K, Turbin R, Nijhawan N, Schiffman J, et al. Phase 1/2 clinical study of VRDN-001, a full antagonist antibody to the insulin-like growth factor-1 receptor (IGF-1R), in patients with thyroid eye disease (TED) (P3-9.001). Neurology. 2023;100(Suppl. S2):2098.
177. Dickinson B. VRDN-002, a second-generation insulin like growth factor-1 receptor (IGF-1R) inhibitory antibody for thyroid eye disease: preclinical pharmacokinetics and clinical promise. Investig Ophthalmol Vis Sci. 2022;63:3995–A0337.
178. Foster K, She A, Summerfelt RM, Dickinson B, Katz B, Wiczling P, et al. VRDN-002, a next-generation half-life extended antagonist antibody to IGF-1 receptor for thyroid eye disease (TED): safety and pharmacokinetic/pharmacodynamic (PK/PD) results in healthy volunteers. Invest Ophthalmol Vis Sci. 2023;64:4038.
179. Dickinson B, Foster K, Bedian V. Preclinical pharmacokinetics of VRDN-003, a next-generation half-life extended antibody to the IGF-1 receptor for thyroid eye disease. Investig Ophthalmol Vis Sci. 2023;64:4043.
180. Newell R, Zhao Y, Bedian V. Design and preclinical characterization of VRDN-003, a next-generation, half-life extended antibody to IGF-1 receptor in development for thyroid eye disease (TED). Investig Ophthalmol Vis Sci. 2023;64:4044.

181. Gulbins A, Horstmann M, Daser A, Flögel U, Oeverhaus M, Bechrakis NE, et al. Linsitinib, an IGF-1R inhibitor, attenuates disease development and progression in a model of thyroid eye disease. Front Endocrinol (Lausanne). 2023;14:1211473.
182. Puzanov I, Lindsay CR, Goff L, Sosman J, Gilbert J, Berlin J, et al. A phase I study of continuous oral dosing of OSI-906, a dual inhibitor of insulin-like growth factor-1 and insulin receptors, in patients with advanced solid tumors. Clin Cancer Res. 2015;21(4):701–11.
183. Okuda Y. Review of tocilizumab in the treatment of rheumatoid arthritis. Biol Targets Ther. 2008;2:75–82.
184. Perez-Moreiras JV, Gomez-Reino JJ, Maneiro JR, Perez-Pampin E, Romo Lopez A, Rodríguez Alvarez FM, et al. Tocilizumab in Graves Orbitopathy Study Group. Efficacy of tocilizumab in patients with moderate-to-severe corticosteroid-resistant Graves orbitopathy: a randomized clinical trial. Am J Ophthalmol. 2018;195:181–90.
185. Ceballos-Macías José J, Rivera-Moscoso R, Flores-Real Jorge A, Vargas-Sánchez J, Ortega-Gutiérrez G, Madriz-Prado R, et al. Tocilizumab in glucocorticoid-resistant graves orbitopathy. A case series report of a mexican population. Ann Endocrinol. 2020;81:78–82.
186. Sánchez-Bilbao L, Martínez-López D, Revenga M, López-Vázquez Á, Valls-Pascual E, Atienza-Mateo B, et al. Anti-IL-6 receptor tocilizumab in refractory Graves' orbitopathy: National Multicenter Observational Study of 48 patients. J Clin Med. 2020;9:2816.
187. Duarte AF, Xavier NF, Sales Sanz M, Cruz AAV. Efficiency and safety of tocilizumab for the treatment of thyroid eye disease: a systematic review. Ophthalmic Plast Reconstr Surg. 2024;40:367–73.
188. Randall KL. Rituximab in autoimmune diseases. Aust Prescr. 2016;39:131–4.
189. Ravani P, Bonanni A, Rossi R, Caridi G, Ghiggeri GM. Anti-CD20 antibodies for idiopathic nephrotic syndrome in children. Clin J Am Soc Nephrol. 2016;11(4):710–20.
190. Stan MN, Garrity JA, Carranza Leon BG, Prabin T, Bradley EA, Bahn RS. Randomized controlled trial of rituximab in patients with Graves' orbitopathy. J Clin Endocrinol Metab. 2015;100(2):432–41.
191. Salvi M, Vannucchi G, Currò N, Campi I, Covelli D, Dazzi D, et al. Efficacy of B-cell targeted therapy with rituximab in patients with active moderate to severe Graves' orbitopathy: a randomized controlled study. J Clin Endocrinol Metab. 2015;100(2):422–31.
192. Blair HA, Duggan ST. Belimumab: a review in systemic lupus erythematosus. Drugs. 2018;78:355–66.
193. Zhang L, Baker G, Janus D, Paddon CA, Fuhrer D, Ludgate M. Biological effects of thyrotropin receptor activation on human orbital preadipocytes. Invest Ophthalmol Vis Sci. 2006;47(12):5197–203.
194. Núñez Miguel R, Sanders P, Allen L, Evans M, Holly M, Johnson W, et al. Structure of full-length TSH receptor in complex with antibody K1-70™. J Mol Endocrinol. 2022;70(1):e220120.
195. Furmaniak J, Sanders J, Sanders P, Li Y, Rees SB. TSH receptor specific monoclonal autoantibody K1-70™ targeting of the TSH receptor in subjects with Graves' disease and Graves' orbitopathy—results from a phase I clinical trial. Clin Endocrinol. 2022;96:878–87.
196. Marcinkowski P, Hoyer I, Specker E, Furkert J, Rutz C, Neuenschwander M, et al. A new highly thyrotropin receptor-selective small-molecule antagonist with potential for the treatment of Graves' orbitopathy. Thyroid. 2019;29(1):111–23.
197. Cieplińska K, Niedziela E, Kowalska A. Immunological processes in the orbit and indications for current and potential drug targets. J Clin Med. 2023;13:72.
198. Wu P, Lin B, Huang S, Meng J, Zhang F, Zhou M, et al. IL-11 is elevated and drives the profibrotic phenotype transition of orbital fibroblasts in thyroid-associated ophthalmopathy. Front Endocrinol (Lausanne). 2022;13:846106.
199. Yan C, Duan RS, Yang H, Li HF, Zou Z, Zhang H, et al. Therapeutic effects of batoclimab in Chinese patients with generalized myasthenia gravis: a double-blinded, randomized, placebo-controlled phase II study. Neurol Ther. 2022;11(2):815–34.

200. Janes J, Kahaly G, Liang S, Tedeschi P. ODP509 proof-of-concept, multicenter, open-label phase 2a study of batoclimab in active and moderate-to-severe thyroid eye disease. J Endocr Soc. 2022;6(Suppl. S1):A778–9.
201. Lanzolla G, Sabini E, Leo M, Menconi F, Rocchi R, Sframeli A, et al. Statins for Graves' orbitopathy (STAGO): a phase 2, open-label, adaptive, single centre, randomised clinical trial. Lancet Diabetes Endocrinol. 2021;9(11):733–42.
202. Yi C, Niu G, Zhang Y, Rao J, Liu G, Yang W, et al. Advances in artificial intelligence in thyroid-associated ophthalmopathy. Front Endocrinol (Lausanne). 2024;15:1356055.
203. Zhang Y, Rao J, Wu X, Zhou Y, Liu G, Zhang H. Automatic measurement of exophthalmos based orbital CT images using deep learning. Front Cell Dev Biol. 2023;11:1135959.
204. Huang X, Ju L, Li J, He L, Tong F, Liu S, et al. An intelligent diagnostic system for thyroid-associated ophthalmopathy based on facial images. Front Med (Lausanne). 2022;9:920716.
205. Song X, Liu Z, Li L, Gao Z, Fan X, Zhai G, et al. Artificial intelligence CT screening model for thyroid-associated ophthalmopathy and tests under clinical conditions. Int J Comput Assist Radiol Surg. 2021;16(2):323–30.
206. Li Y, Ma J, Xiao J, Wang Y, He W. Use of extreme gradient boosting, light gradient boosting machine, and deep neural networks to evaluate the activity stage of extraocular muscles in thyroid-associated ophthalmopathy. Graefes Arch Clin Exp Ophthalmol. 2024;262:203–10.
207. Moon JH, Shin K, Lee GM, Park J, Lee MJ, Choung H, et al. Machine learning-assisted system using digital facial images to predict the clinical activity score in thyroid-associated orbitopathy. Sci Rep. 2022;12:22085.
208. Lee J, Lee S, Lee WJ, Moon NJ, Lee JK. Neural network application for assessing thyroid-associated orbitopathy activity using orbital computed tomography. Sci Rep. 2023;13:13018.
209. Fu R, Bandos A, Leader JK, Melachuri S, Pradeep T, Bhatia A, et al. Artificial intelligence automation of proptosis measurement: an indicator for pediatric orbital abscess surgery. Ophthalmol Ther. 2023;12(5):2479–91.
210. Douglas RS, Kossler AL, Abrams J, Briceño CA, Gay D, Harrison A, et al. Expert consensus on the use of teprotumumab for the management of thyroid eye disease using a modified-Delphi approach. J Neuroophthalmol. 2022;42(3):334–9.

Chronic Thyroiditis: Hashimoto's Anxiety and Depression

13

13.1 Introduction

Autoimmune thyroiditis (AIT) is considered a major health problem with implications for both patients and physicians as it causes somatic and psychiatric disorders, the extent of which is not fully known so far. Hashimoto's thyroiditis (chronic lymphocytic thyroiditis) denotes an autoimmune thyroid condition, characterized by T-cell infiltration and progressive destruction of thyroid tissue, leading to hypothyroidism [1–3], with diagnosis typically involving the detection of thyroid-specific antibodies and diffuse changes in the thyroid gland observed through ultrasonography [4, 5].

During destruction of thyroid gland cells, it is possible to experience increase in hormone levels temporarily resulting in transient hyperthyroidism (Hashitoxicosis or thyrotoxicosis). When the high level of hormones is managed by the body, the thyroid function starts to decline resulting in hypothyroidism, which causes depression and anxiety.

In parallel, depressive and anxiety disorders are prevalent mental health conditions [6], whose incidence has been further heightened by the global COVID-19 pandemic [7]. Emerging evidence points to a potential link between Hashimoto's thyroiditis and an increased risk of depressive and anxiety disorders [8], a relationship largely attributed to hypothyroidism, as thyroid hormone deficiencies often result in emotional disturbances such as depression and anxiety [9]. It is conceivable that both conditions are caused by the same aberrancy present in the immuno-endocrinal center, which is difficult to correct.

Interestingly, recent studies have proposed that thyroid antibodies may be independently linked to depression and anxiety disorders, regardless of thyroid function [8, 9]. This hypothesis is supported by clinical studies in euthyroid patients [10–13], as well as neuro-imaging research [14], and animal studies involving euthyroid mice [15], all of which have reported similar findings. Nevertheless, some studies hold a differing view, finding no direct association between depression and thyroid antibodies [16]. Similarly, the relationship between thyroid antibodies and anxiety

M. Sakr, *Thyroiditis*, https://doi.org/10.1007/978-3-032-19513-5_13

disorders remains contentious, with conflicting results across the literature [17, 18]. Thus, the role of thyroid antibodies in the development of depression and anxiety remains a subject of ongoing debate.

Although a recent meta-analysis (2018) has indicated that patients with Hashimoto's thyroiditis have an elevated risk of developing depression and anxiety disorders [8], this analysis did not specifically compare euthyroid Hashimoto's thyroiditis patients with healthy controls. Given that depression and anxiety are significant global public health concerns, each affecting approximately 300 million people worldwide [19], it becomes increasingly crucial to further investigate their underlying causes.

13.2 Effect of Thyroid Hormones on the Central Nervous System (CNS)

Thyroid hormone affects and governs the central nervous system (CNS) both during the development phase and also during the entire life. It regulates gene expression in myelination, differentiation of neuronal and glial cells, and neuronal viability and function. The effect of thyroid hormones on serotonin (5-hydroxytryptamine [5-HT]) is explained by desensitization of 5-HT1A auto-receptor at the site of raphe nuclei, which probably results in an increase in the release of serotonin from the raphe neurons [20–22].

The mechanism of thyroid hormone activity in the brain is unclear due to the complexity of neuro-transmission interaction with the thyroid. One hypothesis stated that thyroid hormone modulates post-synaptic beta-adrenergic receptors in the cerebral cortex and cerebellum, while others stated that the modulation of 5-HT and its receptors is responsible, causing reduction in 5-HT levels [23, 24].

Both the hyper- and hypo-thyroid states have co-morbidity with psychiatric conditions. Similarly, patients with mood disorders show derangement in TSH and thyrotropin-releasing hormone (TRH), whereas T3 and T4 may remain normal [20, 21, 25, 26].

13.3 Prevalence

Autoimmune thyroiditis (AIT) is a common disease with a prevalence of approximately 4–13% in the United States [27, 28]. It generally affects more women than men [27], and its frequency increases with age, reaching up to 20% among elderly women [29–31].

Depression and anxiety disorders are pervasive psychiatric diseases with prevalence rates of 6.6% for depression [32, 33] and 18.1% for anxiety disorders [33] in the United States. Thus, approximately 23.8% of patients with AIT experience depression and nearly 41.6% of patients with AIT experience anxiety disorders. This implies that 3% of the US population (approximately 9.7 million people) has depression, and 5.4% (approximately 17.5 million people) has anxiety disorders concomitantly with AIT. This also implies that about 45.5% of depressive disorders and 29.8% of anxiety disorders are associated with this endocrine disease.

Prevalence rates for autoimmune thyroiditis in Europe vary between 5% and 14% [34, 35], emphasizing the global nature of the disease. Assuming that depression and anxiety disorders are illnesses that often appear together [36] with a co-morbidity of up to 57.5% [37], patients with AIT have a high risk of suffering from both depression and anxiety (e.g., depression and panic disorder) [38]. Notably, the COVID-19 pandemic exacerbated this trend, leading to a 27.6% rise in cases of major depressive disorder and a 25.6% increase in anxiety disorder cases worldwide [39].

13.4 Link Between Autoimmune Thyroiditis and Psychiatric Disorders

Recently, the connection between autoimmunity and psychiatric disorders has been discovered for various autoimmune diseases including Hashimoto's thyroiditis. For example, N-methyl-d-aspartate receptor hypo-function caused by immunoglobulin antibodies has been reported to be associated with the development of schizophrenia and psychoses [40, 41]. Tic disorders were also found to be associated with a significant increase in anti-streptolysin O titers [42]. Furthermore, bipolar disorders [43] and Alzheimer's disease [44] could be explained by autoimmune explanatory approaches.

Autoimmune thyroiditis (AIT) results in hypothyroidism, which leads to alterations in cardiovascular function such as hypertension due to increased systemic vascular resistance [45], and advanced atherosclerosis [32]. Furthermore, it contributes to a higher risk of infertility and early miscarriage [46], in addition to weight gain even after treatment with thyroxine [47].

Less is known about specific psychiatric burden of symptoms in autoimmune thyroiditis patients. Several authors reported a cumulative occurrence of mood disorders and symptoms of depression among hypothyroid patients, as well as frequent thyroid diseases among patients with depression [48–51]. Moreover, many studies described symptoms of anxiety in patients with AIT [10, 48, 51–53] in addition to other neuro-psychological symptoms such as attentional and executive disturbances [54], fatigue [47], or general reduction in the quality of life [55, 56].

13.5 Association Between Hashimoto's Thyroiditis and Anxiety/Depression Disorders

Although numerous studies have explored the potential causal relationship between Hashimoto's thyroiditis and psychiatric disorders, the association remains contentious and inconclusive. Autoimmune thyroid disease may be linked to depression [57] and anxiety [58]. However, there are only a few qualitative reviews (and no quantitative studies) describing an association between Hashimoto's thyroiditis and the development of depression and anxiety disorders [13, 41, 49, 50].

Marangell and Callahan (1998) [59] described the first studies investigating a link between thyroid disease and the brain using positron emission tomography (PET) paradigms, and Hendrick et al. (1998) [60] reported a high occurrence of hypothyroidism among depression patients resistant to treatment. Despite these indications, no direct association between particular alterations in brain regions because of AIT and the development of a *depressive disorder* was found [49, 61]. Regarding *anxiety*, the first symptoms among patients with hypothyroidism are often generalized agitation or extreme restlessness [10]. As some of the symptoms of hypothyroidism are caused by hypertension [45] and sensations of nightly tachycardia [62, 63], it is presumable that this condition leads to a facilitated development of generalized anxiety disorder.

A meta-analysis by Siegmann et al. (2018) [8] reviewed psychiatric disorders among patients with hypothyroidism. The study examined 19 studies with a total of 36,174 participants. Results showed that patients with AIT have a higher chance of showing symptoms of depression and anxiety, irrespective of gender and age, compared with healthy controls [8].

Given the critical role thyroid hormones play in the central nervous system (CNS)—impacting the production of neurotrophic factors, learning and memory mechanisms, and the regulation of brain stem cell fate [64–70], as well as mood regulation [71]—the association between Hashimoto's thyroiditis and psychiatric disorders is frequently attributed to hypothyroidism induced by Hashimoto's thyroiditis [72, 73].

In addition to the psychiatric disorders attributed to hypothyroidism in Hashimoto's thyroiditis, emerging evidence suggests that thyroid antibodies may be independently associated with depression and anxiety disorders, irrespective of thyroid function. This hypothesis is supported by findings from research on Hashimoto's encephalopathy, where auto-antibodies have been shown to exert significant effects on the CNS. Further, the detection of anti-thyroid peroxidase (anti-TPO) and anti-thyroglobulin (anti-Tg) auto-antibodies in the cerebrospinal fluid (CSF) of patients with unipolar depression reinforces the potential role of immune mechanisms in psychiatric conditions beyond thyroid dysfunction [74]. However, some studies have challenged the role of thyroid antibodies in anxiety and depression, raising questions about their independent influence [16, 18]. Notably, Hashimoto's thyroiditis can manifest across a spectrum of thyroid states, ranging from overt hypothyroidism to subclinical hypothyroidism, and even in euthyroid individuals [10–13, 75–80]. This diversity of clinical presentations offers valuable opportunities for further research into the complex interactions between Hashimoto's thyroiditis and psychiatric disorders.

Recently, Wang et al. [81] in 2024 presented the first meta-analysis to systematically review anxiety and depression in euthyroid patients with HT. This review included 11 articles [10–13, 75–80, 82], all of which were related to depression (1365 patients—694 Hashimoto's thyroiditis vs. 671 controls), and 8 of which also addressed anxiety (1009 patients—516 Hashimoto's thyroiditis vs. 493 controls).

The authors concluded that euthyroid Hashimoto's thyroiditis patients exhibit a higher prevalence of anxiety disorders compared to healthy control groups and are more susceptible to anxiety and depression symptoms. They added that thyroid antibodies themselves are also associated with depression and anxiety disorder. Some animal studies and imaging evidence also support these findings. Cai et al. (2018) [15] discovered that in an euthyroid Hashimoto's thyroiditis mouse model, mice exhibited more anxiety-like behavior in open field and elevated plus maze tests, and more depressive-like behavior in forced swimming and tail suspension tests compared to controls. Piga et al. (2004) [14] reported a high prevalence of brain perfusion abnormalities in euthyroid HT, similar to those observed in severe Hashimoto's encephalopathy.

13.6 How Hypothyroidism Triggers Anxiety/Depression

Thyroid hormone exerts direct control over several major neurotransmitters including norepinephrine, serotonin, and gamma-aminobutyric acid (GABA) receptors. In fact, the hormone is involved in creation of these neurotransmitters. In case of hypothyroidism, these neurotransmitters do not function properly resulting in *anxiety* and panic attacks. Physical symptoms associated with hypothyroidism further increases anxiety, not due to the hormone defect, but by the fear triggered by the symptoms.

A slight reduction in thyroid hormone secretion such as that found in sub-clinical hypothyroidism may affect cognition and mood [83]. At variance with other tissues which mainly rely on peripherally generated tri-iodothyronine (T3), the brain utilizes preferentially circulating thyroxine (T4) directly secreted by the thyroid gland and may become hypothyroid before other organs [84, 85].

However, it must be emphasized that despite being reported in hypothyroidism, panic attacks and anxiety are seen more prevalently in hyperthyroidism, where excessive amount of thyroid hormone is secreted. In hypothyroidism, the most common symptoms may be fatigue and depression instead of anxiety.

The link between thyroid autoimmunity and "depression" may, however, involve other mechanisms related to the autoimmune pathogenesis of thyroid disease rather than hypothyroidism. Since several neuroendocrine secretory systems are involved in the control of immune reaction, a common neuroendocrine dysregulation involving cytokines might concur towards the pathogenesis of both affective disorders and autoimmune disease. Recent studies suggested that thyroid autoimmunity may be affected by the hypothalamic-pituitary-adrenal axis (HPA) through the balance of pro-inflammatory and anti-inflammatory cytokines [86]. In accordance with this view, the increased frequency of post-partum depression, contributed to the fact that pregnancy would seem to be a "protected" period, could explain at least in part the consequences on thyroid autoimmunity elicited by HPA-related modifications to the immunity axis. Indeed, similar phenomena are observed in rheumatoid arthritis and multiple sclerosis [87, 88].

13.7 Clinical Implications

Psychiatric manifestations usually appear first in cases of hypothyroidism. They form about 2–12% of the initial symptoms in about all of the reported cases. Initially, it starts with anxiety, memory lapses, progressive mental slowing, and speech deficits [89, 90]. In cases of acute hypothyroidism, anxiety disorders occur in about 30–40% of patients with subclinical hypothyroidism (SCH). Patients can present with anxiety, irritability, poor concentration, slow information processing, and poor learning in comparison to normal subjects [91–94].

Hypothyroidism impacts certain aspects of cognitive functioning (slowed information processing speed, reduced efficiency in executive functions, and poor learning) and mood. More severe hypothyroidism can mimic melancholic depression and dementia, thus causing reduction in health-related quality of life. Before prescribing any antidepressant, physicians must go for thyroid function tests. Even mild cases of hypothyroid state can cause depression [95, 96]. Although the results are inconsistent, data do suggest that the neuropsychiatric symptoms tend to improve with treatment for both overt hypothyroidism and subclinical hypothyroidism and normalization to a euthyroid state [97].

13.8 Treatment

13.8.1 Introduction

Societal and economic costs caused by depression and anxiety disorders are high [98, 99] and can be lowered by appropriate and early treatment. However, depression and anxiety are multifactorial issues—there is not a single cure for these. By awareness of the association between these disorders and AIT, proper thyroid and anti-depressant treatment can be implemented beyond psychotherapy. Furthermore, screening tests for symptoms of depression and anxiety in patients with AIT, and for AIT in patients with depression and anxiety, could be established.

Patients often seek medical attention owing to psychiatric symptoms but are unaware of autoimmune thyroiditis. As AIT is a chronic disease [100], so are the symptoms of depression and anxiety associated with it. Both anxiety and depression have persistent courses owing to, among other factors, helplessness [101] and classical fear conditioning [102]. Autoimmune thyroiditis, however, can appear in phases (hyperthyroid vs. hypothyroid) [103] and is thus not always traceable as the root cause of these symptoms, which impedes proper diagnoses and appropriate therapy.

13.8.2 Thyroidectomy

Depression and anxiety disorders associated with Hashimoto's thyroiditis require a different treatment than usual. Occasionally, there are conditions when a thyroidectomy is indicated, such as persistence of significant pain, cosmetic symptoms, or pressure complaints after a fair trial of thyroid therapy [104].

13.8.3 Pharmacotherapy

Regarding pharmacotherapy, an extension of possible medication must be taken into consideration. Besides typical levothyroxine (L-T4) treatment, selenium supplementation can help to reduce the amount of thyroid antibodies and improve mood or well-being [105]. Furthermore, an early administration of anti-depressants could be indicated to attenuate the chronic course of AIT. Thyroid metabolism is associated with the brain serotonin system [20]; thus, selective serotonin re-uptake inhibitors are appropriate medications to treat depression in patients with AIT [106].

Classical, tricyclic antidepressants, however, are *not* suited for patients with hypothyroidism. On the one hand, patients with hypothyroidism do not respond as well to tricyclic antidepressants as patients with depression who are euthyroid [38, 60] and, on the other hand, typical adverse effects of tricyclic antidepressants such as weight gain already occur in patients with hypothyroidism [47] and can be further enhanced. Thus, it is important to administer modern antidepressants with a neutral effect on weight.

A 2016 study by Bathla and colleagues [107] revealed the difficulties associated with the presence of anxiety and depression symptoms in hypothyroid patients. This study used Hamilton scale for measuring anxiety and depression in 100 patients with hypothyroidism and showed that if thyroid hormone treatment is not working for hypothyroid patients, they should be checked for the presence of anxiety and depression symptoms and the symptoms managed accordingly. Likewise, in case of patients who are under treatment for anxiety or depression, if the anti-anxiety or anti-depressive medications do not work, they should be screened for thyroid disorder. The study suggested that even in euthyroid cases, the use of thyroxine could alleviate anxiety and depression.

Moreover, patients with AIT and no symptoms of depression or anxiety must be aware of the vulnerability to develop psychiatric issues. As a consequence, both a screening for psychiatric symptoms is advisable in patients with AIT, and a test for AIT is recommended in patients with depression and anxiety disorders. This test must not be narrowed down to thyroid-stimulating hormone (TSH) (thyrotropin) levels and free triiodothyronine (FT3) and free thyroxine (FT4), but should comprise thyroid peroxidase antibodies (TPO) as well. In population-based studies, only 4–5% of patients show elevated TSH levels, whereas 13–23% are positive for TPO antibodies [27, 28, 34, 35, 106]. If only the TSH level is measured, the clinician will miss many patients with AIT detectable by assessment of TPO antibodies and ultrasonography [108].

13.8.4 Psychotherapy

Working with a skilled mental health professional is an essential part of a holistic approach to overcoming depression. There are many evidence-based approaches to helping with depression, such as [109] (1) cognitive behavioral therapy (CBT), (2) inter-personal therapy, (3) behavioral therapy, (4) mindfulness-based cognitive therapy, and (5) psychodynamic therapies.

Exercise is a powerful way to enhance mood. Except those with severe depression, exercise may work as well as antidepressant medications [110]. Walking just for 20–40 min a day for three times per week can be effective to enhance mood [111]. Whether doing aerobic or non-aerobic exercise, the scientific consensus is that any movement and exercises more supportive in depression than none [112].

13.8.5 Supplements

Mental health can be supported by providing the brain with supportive nutrients and herbs. Supplements that help with inflammation, immune balance, sleep, and stress are also beneficial.

13.8.5.1 Psychobiotics

Psychobiotics are probiotics that support mental health through the gut-brain axis. These help with mood by [113] (1) balancing the hypothalamic-pituitary-adrenal (HPA) axis, (2) modulating the immune response, (3) regulating inflammation, and producing neuro-hormones and neuro-transmitters.

13.8.5.2 Omega-3 Fatty Acids

Omega-3 fatty acids (DHA [docosahexaenoic acid] and EPA [eicosapentaenoic acid]) are necessary for healthy brain metabolism and function. Omega-3s support healthy cell membranes and cell signaling between neurons which can balance mood [114]. Omega-3 fatty acids also modulate whole-body inflammation. Countries in which the population has lower Omega-3 fatty acid intake have higher rates of depression [114].

13.8.5.3 Vitamin D3

Healthy vitamin D3 levels are associated with lower levels of depression. Vitamin D helps balance mood in three ways: (1) regulating "mood" through vitamin D receptors in areas of the brain, such as the prefrontal cortex, (2) modulating the immune system, and (3) modulating neuro-inflammation [115].

13.8.5.4 Magnesium

Magnesium is required for healthy nervous system function. Magnesium deficiency can contribute to mood issues and neuronal damage [116]. Magnesium glycinate or magnesium taurate supplementation may promote significant improvements in overall mood [116].

13.8.5.5 Saffron

Saffron is an herbal supplement that improves resilience to stress and enhances mood. In a 2021 study of 56 people, saffron supplementation reduced negative physiological responses to stress and improved mood. The saffron-treated group also reported improvements in social relationships [117].

13.9 Future Perspectives

Future research should focus on more specific analyses, such as differentiating the various forms of hypothyroidism shown in Table 13.1 or investigating its association with sub-forms of anxiety. Moreover, it is important to examine the influence of autoimmune thyroiditis on concrete symptoms of depression and thus clarify the causal relationship behind this association [8].

The interaction of thyroid hormones and brain regions responsible for depression or anxiety should also be further studied. Overall, it is necessary to develop a biopsychosocial model about the origin of depression and anxiety that also comprises autoimmune thyroiditis [8].

13.10 Summary

It is an established entity that thyroid hormones play an important role in mood and behavior, and cognition. Autoimmune thyroiditis, including Hashimoto's thyroiditis, can lead to depression and anxiety disorders. It is thus important to enhance awareness among physicians about this connection to accelerate the diagnostic process. In patients with depression and anxiety disorders, a test for autoimmune thyroiditis should be performed, and in patients with autoimmune thyroiditis, a screening for psychiatric symptoms is necessary. Thus, patients presenting with anxiety or depression disorders should be treated and monitored by both an

Table 13.1 Current terminology concerning autoimmune thyroiditis

Term	Definition
Hashimoto's thyroiditis	Elevated TSH values FT4 within normal range Presence of thyroid peroxidase antibodies (TPO-Ab)
Autoimmune thyroiditis	Elevated TSH values FT4 within normal range Presence of TPO-Ab comprising Hashimoto's and atrophic thyroiditis
Subclinical hypothyroidism	Elevated TSH values FT4 within normal range
Latent hypothyroidism	Elevated TSH values FT4 within normal range
Overt hypothyroidism	Elevated TSH values

TSH thyroid-stimulating hormone, *FT4* serum free T4, *TPO-Ab* thyroid peroxidase-antibody

endocrinologist and a psychiatrist in liaison with each other so as to optimize their management. Moreover, an early recognition of an endocrine condition will help minimize psychiatric morbidity and hence improve health.

References

1. Merakchi K, Djerbib S, Dumont JE, Miot F, De Deken X. Severe autoimmune thyroiditis in transgenic NOD.H2^{h4} mice expressing Interleukin-4 in the thyroid. Thyroid. 2023;33(3):351–64.
2. Ralli M, Angeletti D, Fiore M, D'Aguanno V, Lambiase A, Artico M, et al. Hashimoto's thyroiditis: an update on pathogenic mechanisms, diagnostic protocols, therapeutic strategies, and potential malignant transformation. Autoimmun Rev. 2020;19(10):102649.
3. Antonelli A, Ferrari SM, Corrado A, Di Domenicantonio A, Fallahi P. Autoimmune thyroid disorders. Autoimmun Rev. 2015;14(2):174–80.
4. Pearce EN, Farwell AP, Braverman LE. Thyroiditis. N Engl J Med. 2003;348(26):2646–55.
5. Dayan CM, Daniels GH. Chronic autoimmune thyroiditis. N Engl J Med. 1996;335(2):99–107.
6. Castelpietra G, Knudsen AKS, Agardh EE, Armocida B, Beghi M, Iburg KM, et al. The burden of mental disorders, substance use disorders and self-harm among young people in Europe, 1990–2019: findings from the Global Burden of Disease Study 2019. Lancet Reg Health Eur. 2022;16:100341.
7. GBD 2019 Diseases and Injuries Collaborators. Global burden of 369 diseases and injuries in 204 countries and territories, 1990–2019: a systematic analysis for the Global Burden of Disease Study 2019. Lancet. 2020;396(10258):1204–22.
8. Siegmann EM, Müller HHO, Luecke C, Philipsen A, Kornhuber J, Grömer TW. Association of depression and anxiety disorders with autoimmune thyroiditis: a systematic review and meta-analysis. JAMA Psychiatry. 2018;75(6):577–84.
9. Carta MG, Loviselli A, Hardoy MC, Massa S, Cadeddu M, Sardu C, et al. The link between thyroid autoimmunity (antithyroid peroxidase autoantibodies) with anxiety and mood disorders in the community: a field of interest for public health in the future. BMC Psychiatry. 2004;4:25–33.
10. Yalcin MM, Altinova AE, Cavnar B, Bolayir B, Akturk M, Arslan E, et al. Is thyroid autoimmunity itself associated with psychological well-being in euthyroid Hashimoto's thyroiditis? Endocr J. 2017;64(4):425–9.
11. Giynas Ayhan M, Uguz F, Askin R, Gonen MS. The prevalence of depression and anxiety disorders in patients with euthyroid Hashimoto's thyroiditis: a comparative study. Gen Hosp Psychiatry. 2014;36(1):95–8.
12. Stanić G, Marinković S, Milin Lazović J, Ignjatović Ristić D. Association between affective temperaments and psychosomatic symptoms in women with Hashimoto's thyroiditis. PLoS One. 2023;18(8):e0290066.
13. Kirim S, Keskek SO, Köksal F, Haydardedeoglu FE, Bozkirli E, Toledano Y. Depression in patients with euthyroid chronic autoimmune thyroiditis. Endocr J. 2012;59(8):705–8.
14. Piga M, Serra A, Deiana L, Loi GL, Satta L, Di Liberto M, et al. Brain perfusion abnormalities in patients with euthyroid autoimmune thyroiditis. Eur J Nucl Med Mol Imaging. 2004;31(12):1639–44.
15. Cai YJ, Wang F, Chen ZX, Li L, Fan H, Wu ZB, et al. Hashimoto's thyroiditis induces neuroinflammation and emotional alterations in euthyroid mice. J Neuroinflammation. 2018;15(1):299.
16. Delitala AP, Terracciano A, Fiorillo E, Orrù V, Schlessinger D, Cucca F. Depressive symptoms, thyroid hormone and autoimmunity in a population-based cohort from Sardinia. J Affect Disord. 2016;191:82–7.

17. Martino G, Caputo A, Vicario CM, Feldt-Rasmussen U, Watt T, Quattropani MC, et al. Alexithymia, emotional distress, and perceived quality of life in patients with Hashimoto's thyroiditis. Front Psychol. 2021;12:667237.
18. Engum A, Bjøro T, Mykletun A, Dahl AA. Thyroid autoimmunity, depression and anxiety; are there any connections? An epidemiological study of a large population. J Psychosom Res. 2005;59(5):263–8.
19. Chodavadia P, Teo I, Poremski D, Fung DSS, Finkelstein EA. Prevalence and economic burden of depression and anxiety symptoms among Singaporean adults: results from a 2022 web panel. BMC Psychiatry. 2023;23(1):104.
20. Bauer M, Heinz A, Whybrow PC. Thyroid hormones, serotonin and mood: of synergy and significance in the adult brain. Mol Psychiatry. 2002;7:140–56.
21. Smith JW, Evans AT, Costall B, Smythe JW. Thyroid hormones, brain function and cognition: a brief review. Neurosci Biobehav Rev. 2002;26:45–60.
22. Bernal J, Nunez J. Thyroid hormones and brain development. Eur J Endocrinol. 1995;133:390–8.
23. Atterwill CK, Bunn SJ, Atkinson DJ, Smith SL, Heal DJ. Effects of thyroid status on presynaptic alpha 2-adrenoceptor function and beta-adrenoceptor binding in the rat brain. J Neural Transm. 1984;59:43–55.
24. Belmaker RH, Agam G. Mechanisms of disease: major depressive disorder. N Engl J Med. 2008;358:55–68.
25. Linkowski P, Brauman H, Mendlewicz J. Thyrotrophin response to thyrotrophin-releasing hormone in unipolar and bipolar affective illness. J Affect Disord. 1981;3:9–16.
26. Loosen PT. The TRH-induced TSH response in psychiatric patients: a possible neuroendocrine marker. Psychoneuroendocrinology. 1985;10:237–60.
27. Forman-Hoffman V, Philibert RA. Lower TSH and higher T4 levels are associated with current depressive syndrome in young adults. Acta Psychiatr Scand. 2006;114:132–9.
28. Hollowell JG, Staehling NW, Flanders WD, Hannon WH, Gunter EW, Spencer CA, et al. Serum TSH, T4, and thyroid antibodies in the United States population (1988 to 1994): National Health and Nutrition Examination Survey (NHANES III). J Clin Endocrinol Metab. 2002;87(2):489–99.
29. Canaris GJ, Manowitz NR, Mayor G, Ridgway EC. The Colorado thyroid disease prevalence study. Arch Intern Med. 2000;160(4):526–34.
30. Surks MI, Ortiz E, Daniels GH, Sawin CT, Col NF, Cobin RH, et al. Subclinical thyroid disease: scientific review and guidelines for diagnosis and management. JAMA. 2004;291(2):228–38.
31. Chaudhary R, Chabra S, Singla M, Mishra BP, Sharma A. Psychiatric morbidity among hypothyroid patients—a hospital based study. Delhi Psychiatry J. 2014;17:35–8.
32. Pies RW. Women, mood, and the thyroid. Women Psychiatry Health. 1995;4:4–10.
33. Kessler RC, Berglund P, Demler O, Jin R, Koretz D, Merikangas KR, et al. National Comorbidity Survey Replication. The epidemiology of major depressive disorder: results from the National Comorbidity Survey Replication (NCS-R). JAMA. 2003;289(23):3095–105.
34. Kessler RC, Chiu WT, Demler O, Merikangas KR, Walters EE. Prevalence, severity, and comorbidity of 12-month DSM-IV disorders in the National Comorbidity Survey Replication. Arch Gen Psychiatry. 2005;62(6):617–27.
35. Bjoro T, Holmen J, Krüger O, Midthjell K, Hunstad K, Schreiner T, The Health Study of Nord-Trondelag (HUNT), et al. Prevalence of thyroid disease, thyroid dysfunction and thyroid peroxidase antibodies in a large, unselected population. Eur J Endocrinol. 2000;143(5):639–47.
36. Vanderpump MPJ. The epidemiology of thyroid disease. Br Med Bull. 2011;99(1):39–51.
37. Sartorius N, Ustün TB, Lecrubier Y, Wittchen HU. Depression comorbid with anxiety: results from the WHO study on psychological disorders in primary health care. Br J Psychiatry Suppl. 1996;30(30):38–43.
38. Belzer K, Schneier FR. Comorbidity of anxiety and depressive disorders: issues in conceptualization, assessment, and treatment. J Psychiatr Pract. 2004;10(5):296–306.

39. COVID-19 Mental Disorders Collaborators. Global prevalence and burden of depressive and anxiety disorders in 204 countries and territories in 2020 due to the COVID-19 pandemic. Lancet. 2021;398(10312):1700–12.
40. Joffe RT, Levitt J. Major depression and subclinical (grade 2) hypothyroidism. Psychoneuroendocrinology. 1992;17(2–3):215–21.
41. Pollak TA, McCormack R, Peakman M, Nicholson TR, David AS. Prevalence of anti–N-methyl-d-aspartate (NMDA) receptor antibodies in patients with schizophrenia and related psychoses: a systematic review and meta-analysis. Psychol Med. 2014;44(12):2475–87.
42. Coyle JT, Tsai G, Goff D. Converging evidence of NMDA receptor hypofunction in the pathophysiology of schizophrenia. Ann N Y Acad Sci. 2003;1003:318–27.
43. Pozzi M, Pellegrino P, Carnovale C, Perrone V, Antoniazzi S, Perrotta C, et al. On the connection between autoimmunity, tic disorders and obsessive-compulsive disorders: a meta-analysis on anti-streptolysin O titres. J Neuroimmune Pharmacol. 2014;9(5):606–14.
44. Eaton WW, Pedersen MG, Nielsen PR, Mortensen PB. Autoimmune diseases, bipolar disorder, and non-affective psychosis. Bipolar Disord. 2010;12(6):638–46.
45. Nagele E, Han M, Demarshall C, Belinka B, Nagele R. Diagnosis of Alzheimer's disease based on disease-specific autoantibody profiles in human sera. PLoS One. 2011;6(8):e23112.
46. Biondi B, Cooper DS. The clinical significance of subclinical thyroid dysfunction. Endocr Rev. 2008;29(1):76–131.
47. Poppe K, Velkeniers B, Glinoer D. The role of thyroid autoimmunity in fertility and pregnancy. Nat Clin Pract Endocrinol Metab. 2008;4(7):394–405.
48. Kong WM, Sheikh MH, Lumb PJ, Naoumova RP, Freedman DB, Crook M, et al. A 6-month randomized trial of thyroxine treatment in women with mild subclinical hypothyroidism. Am J Med. 2002;112(5):348–54.
49. Ittermann T, Völzke H, Baumeister SE, Appel K, Grabe HJ. Diagnosed thyroid disorders are associated with depression and anxiety. Soc Psychiatry Psychiatr Epidemiol. 2015;50(9):1417–25.
50. Hage MP, Azar ST. The link between thyroid function and depression. J Thyroid Res. 2012;2012:590–648.
51. Degner D, Haust M, Meller J, Rüther E, Reulbach U. Association between autoimmune thyroiditis and depressive disorder in psychiatric outpatients. Eur Arch Psychiatry Clin Neurosci. 2015;265(1):67–72.
52. Hall RCW, Hall RC. Anxiety and endocrine disease. Semin Clin Neuropsychiatry. 1999;4(2):72–83.
53. Aslan S, Ersoy R, Kuruoglu AC, Karakoc A, Cakir N. Psychiatric symptoms and diagnoses in thyroid disorders: a cross-sectional study. Int J Psychiatry Clin Pract. 2005;9(3):187–92.
54. Constant EL, Adam S, Seron X, Bruyer R, Seghers A, Daumerie C. Hypothyroidism and major depression: a common executive dysfunction? J Clin Exp Neuropsychol. 2006;28(5):790–807.
55. Bianchi GP, Zaccheroni V, Solaroli E, Vescini F, Cerutti R, Zoli M, et al. Health-related quality of life in patients with thyroid disorders. Qual Life Res. 2004;13(1):45–54.
56. Gulseren S, Gulseren L, Hekimsoy Z, Cetinay P, Ozen C, Tokatlioglu B. Depression, anxiety, health-related quality of life, and disability in patients with overt and subclinical thyroid dysfunction. Arch Med Res. 2006;37(1):133–9.
57. Fountoulakis KN, Iacovides A, Grammaticos P. Thyroid function in clinical subtypes of major depression. BMC Psychiatry. 2004;4(6):100968559.
58. Carta MG, Hardoy MC, Boi MF, Mariotti S, Carpiniello B, Usai P. Association between panic disorder, major depressive disorder and celiac disease. A possible role of thyroid autoimmunity. J Psychosom Res. 2002;53:789–93.
59. Marangell LB, Callahan AM. Mood disorders and the thyroid axis. Curr Opin Psychiatry. 1998;11(1):67–70.
60. Hendrick V, Altshuler L, Whybrow P. Psychoneuro-endocrinology of mood disorders: the hypothalamic-pituitary-thyroid axis. Psychiatr Clin North Am. 1998;21(2):277–92.

61. Müssig K, Leyhe T. Kognitive und affektive störungen bei autoimmunthyreoiditis. Der Nuklearmediziner. 2013;36(4):250–5.
62. Shojaie M, Eshraghian A. Primary hypothyroidism presenting with torsades de pointes type tachycardia: a case report. Cases J. 2008;1(1):298–301.
63. Schenck JB, Rizvi AA, Lin T. Severe primary hypothyroidism manifesting with torsades de pointes. Am J Med Sci. 2006;331(3):154–6.
64. Fernández-Lamo I, Montero-Pedrazuela A, Delgado-García JM, Guadaño-Ferraz A, Gruart A. Effects of thyroid hormone replacement on associative learning and hippocampal synaptic plasticity in adult hypothyroid rats. Eur J Neurosci. 2009;30(4):679–92.
65. Koibuchi N, Fukuda H, Chin WW. Promoter-specific regulation of the brain-derived neurotropic factor gene by thyroid hormone in the developing rat cerebellum. Endocrinology. 1999;140(9):3955–61.
66. Neveu I, Arenas E. Neurotrophins promote the survival and development of neurons in the cerebellum of hypothyroid rats in vivo. J Cell Biol. 1996;133(3):631–46.
67. Sui L, Ren WW, Li BM. Administration of thyroid hormone increases reelin and brain-derived neurotrophic factor expression in rat hippocampus in vivo. Brain Res. 2010;1313:9–24.
68. Monopoli MP, Raghnaill MN, Loscher JS, O'Sullivan NC, Pangalos MN, Ring RH, et al. Temporal proteomic profile of memory consolidation in the rat hippocampal dentate gyrus. Proteomics. 2011;11(21):4189–201.
69. Chen C, Zhou Z, Zhong M, Zhang Y, Li M, Zhang L, et al. Thyroid hormone promotes neuronal differentiation of embryonic neural stem cells by inhibiting STAT3 signaling through TRα1. Stem Cell Dev. 2012;21(14):2667–81.
70. Singh R, Upadhyay G, Kumar S, Kapoor A, Kumar A, Tiwari M, et al. Hypothyroidism alters the expression of Bcl-2 family genes to induce enhanced apoptosis in the developing cerebellum. J Endocrinol. 2003;176(1):39–46.
71. Beydoun MA, Beydoun HA, Kitner-Triolo MH, Kaufman JS, Evans MK, Zonderman AB. Thyroid hormones are associated with cognitive function: moderation by sex, race, and depressive symptoms. J Clin Endocrinol Metab. 2013;98(8):3470–81.
72. Churilov LP, Stroev YI, Serdyuk IY, Kaminova-Mudzhikova OM, Belyaeva V, Gvozdetsky AN, et al. Autoimmune thyroiditis: centennial jubilee of a social disease and its comorbidity. Pathophysiology. 2014;21(2):135–45.
73. Ralli M, De Virgilio A, Artico M, Longo L, de Vincentiis M, Greco A. New insights into the etiopathogenesis of Hashimoto's thyroiditis: the role of genetics and epigenetics. Autoimmun Rev. 2018;17(10):1065–6.
74. Dersch R, Tebartz van Elst L, Hochstuhl B, Fiebich BL, Stich O, Robinson T, et al. Anti-thyroid peroxidase and anti-thyroglobulin autoantibodies in the cerebrospinal fluid of patients with unipolar depression. J Clin Med. 2020;9(8):2391.
75. Aydin E, Bingöl Aydin D, Çarkaxhiu Bulut G, İşgüven ŞP. Psychopathological analysis of adolescent girls with autoimmune thyroiditis. Cureus. 2023;15(12):e50418.
76. Krysiak R, Drosdzol-Cop A, Skrzypulec-Plinta V, Okopien B. Sexual function and depressive symptoms in young women with thyroid autoimmunity and subclinical hypothyroidism. Clin Endocrinol. 2016;84(6):925–31.
77. Vasovic O, Nikolic-Djurovic M, Djukic V. Quality of life and mood disorders in patients with Hashimoto thyroiditis. BRAIN Broad Res Artif Intell Neurosci. 2020;11(1Sup2):67–74.
78. Jin C, Tiantian L, Qin X, Hao Y, Defa Z. Anxiety and depression in Hashimoto's thyroiditis. World Latest Med Inf. 2020;20(68):43–5.
79. Yali Y, Jinhua Z, Juan Q, Rongli S, Jing L, Zhongyan S, et al. Self-evaluation of anxiety and depression and their related factors in patients with autoimmune thyroiditis. J China Med Univ. 2019;48(10):887–890+909.
80. Jingyao L. Chronic autoimmune thyroiditis preliminary analysis of the relationship with depression. Master thesis, Dalian Medical University; 2014.
81. Wang B, Huang J, Chen L. Association between depression and anxiety disorders with euthyroid Hashimoto's thyroiditis: a systematic review and meta-analysis. Compr Psychoneuroendocrinol. 2024;20:100279.

82. Zettinig G, Asenbaum S, Fueger BJ, Hofmann A, Diemling M, Mittlboeck M, et al. Increased prevalence of sublinical brain perfusion abnormalities in patients with autoimmune thyroiditis: evidence of Hashimoto's encephalitis? Clin Endocrinol. 2003;59(5):637–43.
83. Haggerty JJ, Prange AJ. Borderline hypothyroidism and depression. Annu Rev Med. 1995;46:37–46.
84. Harris B, Oretti L, Lazarus J, Parkes A, John R, Richards C, et al. Randomised trial of thyroxine to prevent postnatal depression in thyroid antibody positive women. Br J Psychiatry. 2002;180:327–30.
85. Engum A, Bjero T, Myketun A, Dahl AA. An association between depression, anxiety and thyroid function a clinical fact or an artifact? Acta Psychiatr Scand. 2002;106:27–34.
86. Elenkov IJ, Chrousos GP. Stress hormones, proinflammatory and anti-inflammatory cytokines, and autoimmunity. Ann N Y Acad Sci. 2002;966:290–303.
87. Elenkov IJ, Wilder RL, Bakalov VK, Dimitrov MA, Fisher S, Crane M, et al. IL-12, TNF-alpha, and hormonal changes during late pregnancy and early postpartum: implications for autoimmune disease activity during these times. J Clin Endocrinol Metab. 2001;86:4033–8.
88. Biondi M, Zannino LG. Psychological stress, neuro-immunomodulation, and susceptibility to infectious diseases in animals and man: a review. Psychother Psychosom. 1997;66(1):3–26.
89. Hall RC, Stickney S, Beresford TP. Endocrine disease and behaviour. Integr Psychiatry. 1986;4:122–35.
90. Popkin MK, Mackenzie TB. Psychiatric presentations of endocrine dysfunction. In: Hall RC, editor. Psychiatric presentations of medical illness. New York: Spectrum Books; 1980. p. 142–3.
91. Haug TT, Mykletun A, Dahl AA. The association between anxiety, depression, and somatic symptoms in a large population: the Hunt-II study. Psychosom Med. 2004;66:845–51.
92. Hall RC. Psychiatric effects of thyroid hormone disturbance. Psychosomatics. 1983;24:7–22.
93. Whybrow PC, Prange AJ Jr, Treadway CR. Mental changes accompanying thyroid gland dysfunction. A reappraisal using objective psychological measurement. Arch Gen Psychiatry. 1969;20:48–63.
94. Haggerty JJ Jr, Garbutt JC, Evans DL, Golden RN, Pedersen C, Simon JS, et al. Subclinical hypothyroidism: a review of neuropsychiatric aspects. Int J Psychiatry Med. 1990;20:193–208.
95. Davidoff F, Gill J. Myxedema madness: psychosis as an early manifestation of hypothyroidism. Conn Med. 1977;41:618–21.
96. Gold MS, Pottash AL, Extein I. Hypothyroidism and depression. Evidence from complete thyroid function evaluation. JAMA. 1981;245:1919–22.
97. Davis JD, Tremont G. Neuropsychiatric aspects of hypothyroidism and treatment reversibility. Minerva Endocrinol. 2007;32:49–65.
98. Kessler RC. The costs of depression. Psychiatr Clin North Am. 2012;35(1):1–14.
99. Lépine J-P. The epidemiology of anxiety disorders: prevalence and societal costs. J Clin Psychiatry. 2002;63(suppl 14):4–8.
100. Singer PA, Cooper DS, Levy EG, Ladenson PW, Braverman LE, Daniels G, et al. Treatment guidelines for patients with hyperthyroidism and hypothyroidism: Standards of Care Committee, American Thyroid Association. JAMA. 1995;273(10):808–12.
101. Maier SF, Seligman ME. Learned helplessness: theory and evidence. J Exp Psychol Gen. 1976;105(1):3–46.
102. Lissek S, Powers AS, McClure EB, Phelps EA, Woldehawariat G, Grillon C, et al. Classical fear conditioning in the anxiety disorders: a meta-analysis. Behav Res Ther. 2005;43(11):1391–424.
103. Chiovato L, Vitti P, Santini F, Lopez G, Mammoli C, Bassi P, et al. Incidence of antibodies blocking thyrotropin effect in vitro in patients with euthyroid or hypothyroid autoimmune thyroiditis. J Clin Endocrinol Metab. 1990;71(1):40–5.
104. Pisanu A, Piu S, Cois A, Uccheddu A. Coexisting Hashimoto's thyroiditis with differentiated thyroid cancer and benign thyroid diseases: indications for thyroidectomy. Chir Ital. 2003;55(3):365–72.

105. Toulis KA, Anastasilakis AD, Tzellos TG, Goulis DG, Kouvelas D. Selenium supplementation in the treatment of Hashimoto's thyroiditis: a systematic review and a meta-analysis. Thyroid. 2010;20(10):1163–73.
106. deCarvalho GA, Bahls SC, Boeving A, Graf H. Effects of selective serotonin reuptake inhibitors on thyroid function in depressed patients with primary hypothyroidism or normal thyroid function. Thyroid. 2009;19(7):691–7.
107. Bathla M, Singh M, Relan P. Prevalence of anxiety and depressive symptoms among patients with hypothyroidism. Indian J Endocrinol Metab. 2016;20(4):468–74.
108. Shinkov A, Borissova A, Vlahov J, Dakovska L, Blajeva E. Male gender differences in the thyroid ultrasound features, thyroid peroxidase antibodies and thyroid hormone levels: a large population-based study. J Endocrinol Investig. 2014;37(3):269–76.
109. Weir K. APA offers new guidance for treating depression. APA. 2019;50(8):34.
110. Garber CE, Blissmer BP, Deschenes MR, Franklin BA, Lamonte MJ, Lee I, et al. Quantity and quality of exercise for developing and maintaining cardiorespiratory, musculoskeletal, and neuromotor fitness in apparently healthy adults: guidance for prescribing exercise. Med Sci Sports Exerc. 2011;43(7):1334–59.
111. McNeil JK, LeBlanc EM, Joyner M. The effect of exercise on depressive symptoms in the moderately depressed elderly. Psychol Aging. 1991;6:487–8.
112. Craft LL, Perna FM. The benefits of exercise for the clinically depressed. Prim Care Companion J Clin Psychiatry. 2004;6:104–11.
113. Del Toro-Barbosa M, Hurtado-Romero A, Garcia-Amezquita LE, García-Cayuela T. Psychobiotics: mechanisms of action, evaluation methods and effectiveness in applications with food products. Nutrients. 2020;12(12):3896.
114. Wani AL, Bhat SA, Ara A. Omega-3 fatty acids and the treatment of depression: a review of scientific evidence. Integr Med Res. 2015;4(3):132–41.
115. Menon V, Kar SK, Suthar N, Nebhinani N. Vitamin D and depression: a critical appraisal of the evidence and future directions. Indian J Psychol Med. 2020;42(1):11–21.
116. Eby GA, Eby KL. Rapid recovery from major depression using magnesium treatment. Med Hypotheses. 2006;67:362–70.
117. Hausenblas HA, Heekin K, Mutchie HL, Anton S. A systematic review of randomized controlled trials examining the effectiveness of saffron (*Crocus sativus* L.) on psychological and behavioral outcomes. J Integr Med. 2015;13:231–40.

Hashimoto's Thyroiditis: Association with Papillary Thyroid Carcinoma

14

14.1 Overview

Hashimoto's thyroiditis (chronic lymphocytic thyroiditis) is the most common autoimmune thyroid disease, which causes the immune system to attack and destroy the thyroid gland [1]. No consensus exists on the association between Hashimoto's thyroiditis and papillary thyroid carcinoma (PTC), which is the most prevalent form of thyroid cancer, comprising about 80–90% of all diagnosed thyroid cancers. Hashimoto's thyroiditis is a well-defined clinico-pathological entity, and its incidence has increased over the past 50 years [2]. It is characterized by hypothyroidism, the presence of serum anti-thyroglobulin and anti-peroxidase antibodies, and widespread lymphocytic infiltration with depletion of follicular cells. In addition to the classical Hashimoto's thyroiditis, recent studies have proposed that IgG4-related thyroiditis may be considered as a variant of the disease [3].

Dailey et al. were the first to propose an association between Hashimoto's thyroiditis and PTC in 1955, linking chronic inflammation to neoplastic changes [4]. However, whether Hashimoto's thyroiditis predisposes patients to the development of PTC has been a subject of long and ongoing debate [2, 3]. Some studies have revealed a higher risk of PTC in patients with HT [5–22], while others did not demonstrate the increased risk [23–25]. Lee et al. (2013) published a meta-analysis that included 38 eligible studies and found that PTC is significantly associated with pathologically confirmed Hashimoto's thyroiditis [26]. They reported that Hashimoto's thyroiditis showed a wide range of occurrence from 5% to 85% in thyroid specimens resected for PTC [9, 12, 14, 27–59], and added that the clinicopathological characteristics of PTC with concomitant Hashimoto's thyroiditis have not been definitively proposed [9, 12, 14, 27–59].

On the other hand, Jankovic et al. (2013) reported that there was no statistically significant correlation between Hashimoto's thyroiditis and PTC based on eight fine-needle aspiration (FNA) studies and eight thyroidectomy studies [60]. Because inconsistent results have been reported regarding the association between Hashimoto's thyroiditis and PTC risk, Lai et al. (2017) conducted a comprehensive

M. Sakr, *Thyroiditis*, https://doi.org/10.1007/978-3-032-19513-5_14

meta-analysis to investigate the possible associations of Hashimoto's thyroiditis and PTC; they confirmed that Hashimoto's thyroiditis predisposed patients to the development of PTC [61].

This chapter aims at clarifying the relationship between Hashimoto's thyroiditis (histologically proven) and PTC and identifying the clinico-pathological features of PTC with co-existent Hashimoto's thyroiditis.

14.2 Meta-analysis Studies

A total of 38 articles satisfied the eligibility criteria [9, 12, 14, 27–59] for the meta-analysis conducted by Lee et al. (2013) [26]. The number of patients in each study ranged from 6 to 1788, for a total of 10,648 PTC patients. Among the PTC patients, Hashimoto's thyroiditis was present in 2471 cases (23.2%) [26].

The meta-analysis conducted by Lai et al. (2017) that included 27 studies showed that the rate of PTC in patients with Hashimoto's thyroiditis from the 18 archival thyroidectomy studies (47,235 patients) ranged from 9.46% to 96.67%, with a mean rate of 40.11% [5, 7, 9, 11–17, 19–22, 27, 33, 35, 62]. The rate of PTC among patients with Hashimoto's thyroiditis from seven FNA studies (25,777 patients) ranged from 0.12% to 20.87%, with a mean rate of 6.46% [6, 10, 23, 25, 62–64], while the rate of PTC among patients with Hashimoto's thyroiditis from the three selective FNA (11,793 patients) ranged from 0.67% to 1.77%, with a mean rate of 1.12% [8, 18, 24].

14.2.1 Hashimoto's Thyroiditis in PTC Versus Benign Lesions

Eleven studies compared the occurrences of Hashimoto's thyroiditis in PTCs and in benign thyroid diseases such as nodular hyperplasia and follicular adenoma [9, 12, 14, 27–33]. Hashimoto's thyroiditis was found in 938 of 2317 PTC patients (40.5%), whereas it was found in 634 of 3019 benign thyroid diseases (21%). Thus, the co-existence of Hashimoto's thyroiditis was significantly associated with PTCs than benign lesions ($p = 0.001$).

14.2.2 Hashimoto's Thyroiditis in PTC Versus Other Carcinomas

Sixteen studies investigated the frequencies of Hashimoto's thyroiditis in PTCs and in other carcinomas such as follicular thyroid carcinoma (FTC) and medullary thyroid carcinoma (FTC) [12, 27, 28, 30, 31, 33–43]. Hashimoto's thyroiditis was present in 797 of 4664 PTC patients (17.1%) as compared to 57 of 725 other carcinoma patients (7.9%). The co-existence of Hashimoto's thyroiditis was thus significantly more related to PTCs than other thyroid carcinomas ($p = 0.001$).

14.2.3 Clinico-pathological Characteristics of PTCs with Hashimoto's Thyroiditis

14.2.3.1 Gender

The incidence of Hashimoto's thyroiditis in PTCs according to gender was compared in 23 studies [9, 12, 14, 27, 65, 34, 35, 39, 44–58]. Hashimoto's thyroiditis in PTCs was observed in 1677 of 7346 (23%) female patients as compared to 180 of 573 (11%) male patients. On the basis of this finding, there was a highly significant association of Hashimoto's thyroiditis in PTCs with females but not with males ($p = 0.001$).

14.2.3.2 Age

Fourteen studies addressed the frequency of Hashimoto's thyroiditis in PTCs according to patients' mean age [9, 12, 27, 31–44]. The mean age of PTC patients with Hashimoto's thyroiditis ranged from 39.5 to 69.0 years, whereas the mean age of PTC patients without Hashimoto's thyroiditis ranged from 38.2 to 56.3 years. There was no association between the mean age of PTC patients and the incidence of Hashimoto's thyroiditis in PTC.

14.2.3.3 Tumor Size

Eleven studies identified the prevalence of Hashimoto's thyroiditis in PTCs according to average tumor size [9, 12, 14, 24, 31, 32, 35–38, 65]. The mean tumor size of PTCs with Hashimoto's thyroiditis ranged from 0.6 to 4.8 cm, whereas those of PTCs without Hashimoto's thyroiditis ranged from 0.6 to 3.0 cm. Thus, the tumor size was not related to the frequency of Hashimoto's thyroiditis in PTC.

14.2.3.4 Tumor Extension

Eleven studies presented 4128 PTCs *without* extra-thyroidal extension and 2897 PTCs with extra-thyroidal involvement [11, 12, 34, 39, 44, 47–49, 55, 58, 59]. Hashimoto's thyroiditis was found in 722 (17.5%) of 4128 PTCs without extra-thyroidal extension and in 500 (17.2%) of 2897 PTCs with extra-thyroidal extension. The coexistence of Hashimoto's thyroiditis in PTCs was not thus associated with extra-thyroidal involvement of PTC.

14.2.3.5 Lymph Node Metastasis

Sixteen studies reported 4185 PTC patients without lymph node metastasis and 3462 patients with lymph node metastasis [5, 6, 9, 14, 16, 19, 24, 25, 27–29, 34, 36–38, 65]. Hashimoto's thyroiditis was seen in 746 (17.8%) of 4185 PTC cases without lymph node metastasis as compared to 622 (17.9%) of 3462 cases with lymph node metastasis. The difference between both groups was statistically significant ($p = 0.012$). It is thus conceivable that PTCs with Hashimoto's thyroiditis are related to the absence of lymph node metastasis.

14.2.3.6 Multi-focality

Twelve studies addressed the frequencies of Hashimoto's thyroiditis in single and multi-focal PTCs [9, 11, 12, 14, 44, 46, 48, 53, 54, 56, 57, 59]. The studies included 1378 patients with multi-focal PTC and 2549 with single PTC. Hashimoto's thyroiditis was present in 359 (26%) of 1378 multi-focal PTCs and in 541 (21%) of 2549 single PTCs. Hashimoto's thyroiditis was significantly more often observed in multi-focal PTCs than in single PTCs ($p = 0.015$).

14.2.3.7 Nodularity

Anil et al. (2010) [23] prospectively compared the prevalence of thyroid carcinoma between 164 patients with Hashimoto's thyroiditis and 551 patients without Hashimoto's thyroiditis and found that thyroid nodules in patients with Hashimoto's thyroiditis were no more likely to be malignant than those in patients without Hashimoto's thyroiditis. However, they included only patients with nodules ≥10 mm. In addition, only 4.9% of their Hashimoto's thyroiditis group and 10% of the control group underwent thyroidectomy for thyroid nodules [23].

14.2.4 Analysis of Survival

Four studies including 616 patients of PTC with Hashimoto's thyroiditis and 4241 of PTC without Hashimoto's thyroiditis reported that Hashimoto's thyroiditis in PTCs was significantly associated with a long duration of recurrence-free survival ($p = 0.001$) [34, 48, 55, 58].

14.3 Significance of Hashimoto's Thyroiditis in Papillary Thyroid Carcinoma

In the meta-analysis by Lee et al. (2013), the frequency of Hashimoto's thyroiditis in PTCs was about 23% (range 5–85%) [26]. The varying incidence rates of Hashimoto's thyroiditis in PTC may be due to several factors such as different diagnostic criteria for the disease, various surgical procedures, and heterogeneous patient characteristics. Most studies presented the incidence of Hashimoto's thyroiditis in surgically resected PTC cases. In cytology specimens of Hashimoto's thyroiditis patients, follicular cells often exhibit nuclear elongation, nuclear grooves, and even intra-nuclear inclusions, leading to a mis-diagnosis of PTC [66, 67].

In the meta-analysis by Lai et al. (2017), PTC was more often found in patients with Hashimoto's thyroiditis; however, there was also significant heterogeneity among the studies owing to variations in study methods, different patient inclusion criteria, and heterogeneous diagnostic criteria for HT and PTC [61]. In this meta-analysis [61], 3 types of studies were analyzed, namely, 3 selective FNA studies, 6 FNA studies, and 18 thyroidectomy studies. In the selective FNA studies, only selected patients underwent FNA or thyroidectomy; therefore, the rate of PTC among patients with Hashimoto's thyroiditis (1.12%) was lower than that in the FNA studies (3.58%) and thyroidectomy studies (33.28%).

The occurrence rate of Hashimoto's thyroiditis in PTC patients is 2.8 times higher than Hashimoto's thyroiditis patients in benign thyroid diseases. In addition, the incidence of Hashimoto's thyroiditis in patients with PTC is 2.4 times higher than in those patients with other types of thyroid carcinoma. Some studies supported the tight association between Hashimoto's thyroiditis and PTC, based on the fact that RET/PTC rearrangements were found in about 90% of Hashimoto's thyroiditis cases [68] and transgenic mice expressing RET/PTC developed Hashimoto's thyroiditis and PTCs [69].

Interestingly, PTC patients with co-existing Hashimoto's thyroiditis have distinctive clinico-pathological characteristics such as female gender, multi-focality, no extra-thyroidal extension, no lymph node metastasis, and long recurrence-free survival. In a study by Cipolla et al. (2005), PTC was present in 11 (57.9%) of 19 patients with nodular Hashimoto's thyroiditis [29]. The association with PTC was found in 40.2% nodular variant of Hashimoto's thyroiditis cases and in 8.1% of diffuse variant of Hashimoto's thyroiditis in another recent study by Graceffa et al. (2019) [70].

Recently, Danis et al. (2022) [71] reported the results of their retrospective study on 469 patients who underwent thyroidectomy during 7 consecutive years in a single institute (Dokuz Eylül University Hospital, Turkey). They found that 122 (26%) of patients had PTC, while 182 (38.8%) were diagnosed with Hashimoto's thyroiditis. The prevalence of Hashimoto's thyroiditis was 54.9% in patients with PTC and 33.1% in patients without ($p < 0.001$). Younger age and the presence of Hashimoto's thyroiditis were independently associated with PTC. The presence of Hashimoto's thyroiditis was associated with increased risk of development of PTC ($p < 0.001$) but not with TNM stage or recurrence. Lymph node metastasis at presentation was the strongest predictor of recurrence in their series after a median follow-up of 119.5 months ($p < 0.001$) [71]. The authors recommended that patients with (particularly the nodular variant) should be observed carefully and that thyroid FNAB should be encouraged if necessary [71].

Recently, Danis et al. (2022) [71] reported that Hashimoto's thyroiditis patients with PTC were younger than those without PTC. Similarly, Repplinger et al. (2008) found that the mean age of Hashimoto's thyroiditis patients with PTC was 44 years, whereas in the non-PTC group, the mean age of patients was 47 years [35].

Considerable controversy exists concerning the prognostic significance of Hashimoto's thyroiditis in PTC patients. Loh et al. (1999) [38] and Yoon et al. (2012) [44] reported that PTC with Hashimoto's thyroiditis was significantly associated with female gender and a lower incidence of extra-thyroidal invasion and lymph node metastasis. Although more recent data provided by Kim et al. (2018) suggested that PTC with Hashimoto's thyroiditis had a better prognosis than that without [72], it was also shown by Qu et al. (2016) that Hashimoto's thyroiditis did not affect the prognosis of PTC [73]. Several studies reported that PTC with

Hashimoto's thyroiditis had a tendency for multi-focal involvement [9, 12, 46, 54]. On the contrary, other studies have failed to present any significant clinicopathological characteristics in PTC with Hashimoto's thyroiditis [11, 27, 45].

The relationship between inflammation and PTC is complex and still not completely understood [74]. There may be a possible tight link between Hashimoto's thyroiditis and the development of PTC rather than a chance occurrence of two relatively common diseases. Paradoxically, Hashimoto's thyroiditis in PTC patients appears to play a role in impeding cancer progression. Therefore, the cross-link of these two conditions may represent a cause-and-effect relationship or a predisposing factor. It is hypothesized that PTC is induced or facilitated by a pre-existing lymphocytic infiltration. Conversely, lymphocytic infiltration of Hashimoto's thyroiditis may be due to autoimmune thyroiditis and/or immune reaction to tumor-specific antigens from a pre-existing PTC [2].

Tamimi et al. (2002) reported a significantly higher rate of lymphocytic infiltrate in patients with PTC, and that the activated inflammatory response present in Hashimoto's thyroiditis may create a favorable setting for malignant transformation [30]. The inflammatory response may cause DNA damage through the formation of reactive oxygen species, resulting in mutations that eventually lead to the development of PTC [60]. Several studies suggested that the association of Hashimoto's thyroiditis with PTC is antibody-specific [6, 75, 76]. However, the mechanism underlying this association is not known. Paradoxically, the lymphocytic infiltrate of Hashimoto's thyroiditis may be an immunological response with a cancer-retarding effect, contributing to a favorable outcome of PTC [34, 48, 58]. The relatively high prevalence of PTC in autopsy series may represent host immune control [7].

14.4 Molecular Basis of the Relationship Between Hashimoto's Thyroiditis and PTC

14.4.1 Relationship Between Hashimoto's Thyroiditis and PTC: Overview

Most of the studies evaluating the possible association between Hashimoto's thyroiditis and differentiated thyroid cancer (DTC) have found that Hashimoto's thyroiditis significantly increases the risk of DTC (especially PTC); however, other studies have not found this association [61].

In general, these studies have reported the following: (1) The findings based on thyroid FNA samples show a prevalence of PTC of 1.2%, reaching 27.5% in thyroidectomy samples. (2) The risk of documenting a PTC increases in surgical specimens in which changes consistent with Hashimoto's thyroiditis are observed. (3) The majority of cases in patients with Hashimoto's thyroiditis correspond to PTC (micro-carcinoma). (4) PTC in individuals with Hashimoto's thyroiditis is more frequent in women than in men. (5) The possible association between HT and FTC is not well established. (6) A histological subtype of oncocytic PTC (Warthin-type variant) is associated with Hashimoto's thyroiditis. (7) A higher PTC frequency has been proven in individuals with Hashimoto's thyroiditis and thyroid nodules (together with an elevated TSH value) [61].

14.4.2 Relationship Between Hashimoto's Thyroiditis and PTC: Molecular Mechanisms

Several mechanisms have been linked between Hashimoto's thyroiditis and DTC (most commonly PTC); these include inflammation, direct effect of TSH, increased expression of certain oncogenes, and altered cell-signaling pathways.

14.4.2.1 Inflammation (Thyroiditis)

The inflammatory response is capable of inducing a favorable environment for malignant transformation, as cytokines and some growth factors directed toward stromal cells can transform epithelial cells to malignant cells [74]. In an inflammatory setting, DNA methyltransferase-1 is affected by reactive oxygen species (ROS) and other pro-inflammatory factors, consequently increasing the DNA methylation of tumor suppressor genes and micro-RNAs, thus increasing the risk of cancer [74, 77, 78].

Moreover, Danis et al. (2022) [71] reported that the mean anti-thyroglobulin (anti-Tg) antibody and anti-thyroid peroxidase antibody (anti-TPO) titers were higher in the group with PTC diagnosis, but this was not statistically significant. Liu et al. (2017) found that anti-Tg and anti-TPO positivity significantly increased PTC risk [79]. This may lead to a hypothesis that when inflammation is severe, the risk of cancer development may be greater as a result of DNA damage due to free oxygen radicals.

14.4.2.2 Direct Effect of TSH

In general, TSH plays an important role in regulating thyroid function, in addition to increasing the number, size, and secretory activity of the gland, as well as increasing thyroid blood flow. The direct effect of TSH as a thyroid growth factor represents the second possible mechanism of increasing the risk of cancer [80–82]. Classical TSH actions are mainly mediated through the Gαs-adenylyl cyclase-protein kinase A-cyclic adenosine monophosphate pathway, which is associated with T4 and T3 production and thyrocyte proliferation. Several meta-analyses reported associated higher serum TSH concentration [82–84]. Thus, a constant tissue stimulation by TSH is capable of producing follicular epithelial hyperplasia; consequently, its elevation could be considered a promoter of thyroid cancer.

In the recent study by Danis et al. (2022) [71], the mean serum TSH was significantly higher in the PTC group than in the non-PTC group ($p = 0.018$). This may suggest that TSH can accelerate tumor formation as it enlarges the thyroid gland as a growth factor. Fiore et al. (2011) also hypothesized that TSH plays a role in PTC development in nodular Hashimoto's thyroiditis patients and claimed that hypothyroidism plays a key role in PTC development. Thus, the researchers gave L-T4 treatment to nodular Hashimoto's thyroiditis patients and reduced the risk of thyroid cancer development in nodular Hashimoto's thyroiditis patients [10].

14.4.2.3 Increased Expression of Certain Oncogenes

An increased suspicion that the relationship between Hashimoto's thyroiditis and PTC might be molecular has been recently raised. Thus, the third possible mechanism increasing the risk of cancer refers to the increased expression of certain oncogenes.

RET/PTC Gene Re-arrangement

In 1999, Wirtschafter et al. detected messenger RNA (mRNA) expression of RET/PTC1 and RET/PTC3 oncogenes in 95% of patients with Hashimoto's thyroiditis using reverse transcriptase polymerase chain reaction (RT-PCR) method with high sensitivity and specificity. The authors thus stated that all patients with Hashimoto's thyroiditis had molecular genetic evidence [68]. However, this study has been criticized as having highly false positive results due to its methodology [85]. Nikiforova et al. (2002) could *not* detect RET/PTC genetic rearrangement in Hashimoto's thyroiditis and Hashimoto's thyroiditis-based PTC using standard sensitive PCR [86].

As is known, RET/PTC1 and RET/PTC3 are the most common types of genetic re-arrangement in cancers, especially of the thyroid. This fusion causes activation of tyrosine kinase fragment of the RET gene and signaling to MAPK pathway. It is believed that RET/PTC activation is oncogenic for healthy thyroid follicular cells because thyroid tumor formation through this pathway has been shown in-vivo in transgenic mice [85].

In this aspect, the inflammatory process present in Hashimoto's thyroiditis may favor the appearance of genetic re-arrangement; additionally, the greater predisposition of thyrocytes to *RET* recombination could be explained by the arrangement of chromatin in the interphase nuclei [87]. Hence, an inflammatory phenomenon in which a scenario with an increased synthesis of free radicals, greater secretion of cytokines, and increased cell proliferation (among others) can promote the appearance of re-arrangement in the thyroid follicle cell predisposed to it by alterations in chromatin conformation. An induced state in which the thyrocytes are in a modified environment (loop-mediated with autocrine and paracrine patterns) in the presence of chemokines and cytokines could promote autonomous thyrocyte proliferation [88–90].

The p53 Family Mutations

The members of the p53 family include p53, p63, and p73, and mutations in *p63* have been proposed to have a role in the interface between Hashimoto's thyroiditis and PTC; in fact, a high expression of p63 has been found in both as reported by Unger et al. (2003) [91] and Burstein et al. (2004) [92]. These results have increased the debate regarding the possibility of p63 having a patho-biological link; however, these findings need to be clarified and reproduced [91, 92].

BRAF Mutation (BRAFV600E)

BRAF mutation (BRAFV600E) is the most frequently observed genetic abnormality in PTC, which is capable of inducing excessive proliferation and differentiation of tumor cells in its initial stages. It is also involved in tumorigenesis and in the conversion to a more aggressive undifferentiated phenotype [93–95]. Thus, individuals in whom PTC co-exists with Hashimoto's thyroiditis have been observed to be at lower risk of extra-thyroidal extension of the PTC, and additionally, it has been suggested that Hashimoto's thyroiditis antagonizes PTC progression in the presence of *BRAF*V600E. Therefore, the *BRAF*V600E mutation is less frequent in individuals in whom Hashimoto's thyroiditis co-exists with PTC, probably because Hashimoto's thyroiditis and the *BRAF*V600E mutation operate independently in the formation and progression of PTC [91–97].

Altered Cell-Signaling Pathways

Finally, some altered cell-signaling pathways with loss of cell cycle control mechanisms have been implicated in neoplastic transformation. For instance, phosphatidylinositol 3-kinase (PI3K), which plays a key role in the balance between cell survival and apoptosis, is also important in the inflammatory response, as it can activate chemokine receptors and leukocyte migration [96–99]. This may be the reason increased PI3K activation has been identified in various neoplasms, including thyroid cancer (activation of PI3K, in turn, phosphorylates Akt, which acts on downstream proteins to suppress pro-apoptotic signals contributing to tumorigenesis) [99, 100]. An increase in the expression of PI3K/Akt in individuals with HT and DTC has been found in some studies, suggesting a possible role in the molecular mechanism for thyroid carcinogenesis [15, 101].

The most frequently associated genetic alterations between Hashimoto's thyroiditis and DTC are summarized in Table 14.1 [15, 88–102]. Briefly, in Hashimoto's thyroiditis, the constant and sustained stimulation of TSH, together with the inflammatory process and the expression of oncogenes, has been shown to be the most "consistent" mechanisms, which can potentially induce a phenomenon of tumorigenesis and tumor progression, increasing the risk of DTC (Fig. 14.1).

Table 14.1 Summary of genetic alterations in Hashimoto's thyroiditis and thyroid cancer

Genetic alterations	Outcomes in Hashimoto's thyroiditis and DTC
RET/PTC re-arrangements	In experimental models in mice, designed to express RET/PTC, they more frequently develop thyroid hyperplasia, solid tumor variants of PTC and metastatic cancer, and findings of chronic thyroiditis. Between 3% and 60% of patients with PTC and around 90% of individuals with Hashimoto's thyroiditis have this genetic alteration
p63 Protein	It is commonly expressed in PTC and in Hashimoto's thyroiditis
*BRAF*V600E	*BRAF*V600E mutation is less frequent in individuals where Hashimoto's thyroiditis co-exists with PTC
PI3K/Akt pathway	Elevated expression of PI3K/Akt in individuals with Hashimoto's thyroiditis and DTC

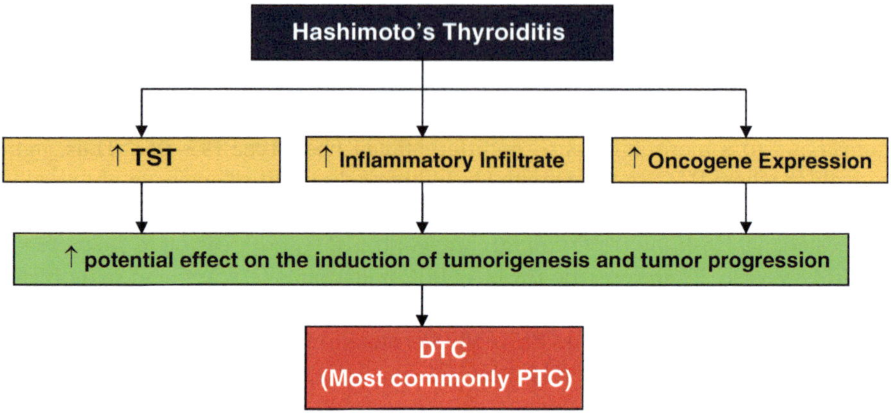

Fig. 14.1 Possible mechanism of tumorigenesis in Hashimoto's thyroiditis co-existing with differentiated thyroid cancer. TSH: thyroid-stimulating hormone, DTC: differentiated thyroid cancer, PTC: papillary thyroid cancer

Despite the several mechanisms that have been proposed to verify the relationship between Hashimoto's thyroiditis and DTC (most commonly PTC), it is still difficult to establish "causality" in the continuum of the pathogenesis between Hashimoto's thyroiditis and DTC. The relationship could be argued to be "non-causal," and that what really happens is the co-existence between two independent and highly prevalent entities, with enormous ease of early identification through laboratory tests, thyroid ultrasound, and thyroid cytology [103–105].

14.5 Conclusions

In conclusion, there is a close relationship between Hashimoto's thyroiditis and PTC. As the incidence of Hashimoto's thyroiditis is increased in PTC patients, careful clinical monitoring of the patients with Hashimoto's thyroiditis and meticulous histopathological examination of surgical specimens from these patients are required.

The pathophysiological link between Hashimoto's thyroiditis and DTC is intriguing. Observational studies have found a possible association between Hashimoto's thyroiditis and the risk of DTC (especially for PTC); however, the design of these studies does not allow the establishment of causality. On the other hand, the biological plausibility between Hashimoto's thyroiditis and thyroid cancer has been described; in this sense, the common denominator (biological and molecular) is inflammation; however, at the interface between thyroid autoimmunity and DTC, the interaction between genetic, epigenetic, and environmental factors, among others, is necessary [106].

The PTCs with Hashimoto's thyroiditis are characterized by female predominance, multi-focality, no extra-thyroidal extension, no lymph node metastasis, and better recurrence-free survival outcomes. Occurrence of Hashimoto's thyroiditis with PTC is not related to the age of the patient or the size of the tumor [26].

References

1. Dayan CM, Daniels GH. Chronic autoimmune thyroiditis. N Engl J Med. 1996;2:99–107.
2. Antonaci A, Consorti F, Mardente S, Giovannone G. Clinical and biological relationship between chronic lymphocytic thyroiditis and papillary thyroid carcinoma. Oncol Res. 2009;17:495–503.
3. Ahmed R, Al-Shaikh S, Akhtar M. Hashimoto's thyroiditis: a century later. Adv Anat Pathol. 2012;19:181–6.
4. Dailey ME, Lindsay S, Skahen R. Relation of thyroid neoplasms to Hashimoto disease of the thyroid gland. AMA Arch Surg. 1955;2:291–7.
5. Ahn D, Heo SJ, Park JH, Kim JH, Sohn JH, Park JY, et al. Clinical relationship between Hashimoto's thyroiditis and papillary thyroid cancer. Acta Oncol. 2011;8:1228–34.
6. Azizi G, Keller JM, Lewis M, Piper K, Puett D, Rivenbark KM, et al. Association of Hashimoto's thyroiditis with thyroid cancer. Endocr Relat Cancer. 2014;6:845–52.
7. Bradly DP, Reddy V, Prinz RA, Gattuso P. Incidental papillary carcinoma in patients treated surgically for benign thyroid diseases. Surgery. 2009;6:1099–104.
8. Chen YK, Lin CL, Cheng FT, Sung FC, Kao CH. Cancer risk in patients with Hashimoto's thyroiditis: a nationwide cohort study. Br J Cancer. 2013;9:2496–501.
9. Consorti F, Loponte M, Milazzo F, Potasso L, Antonaci A. Risk of malignancy from thyroid nodular disease as an element of clinical management of patients with Hashimoto's thyroiditis. Eur Surg Res. 2010;3-4:333–7.
10. Fiore E, Rago T, Latrofa F, Provenzale MA, Piaggi P, Delitala A, et al. Hashimoto's thyroiditis is associated with papillary thyroid carcinoma: role of TSH and of treatment with L-thyroxine. Endocr Relat Cancer. 2011;4:429–37.
11. Gul K, Dirikoc A, Kiyak G, Ersoy PE, Ugras NS, Ersoy R, et al. The association between thyroid carcinoma and Hashimoto's thyroiditis: the ultrasonographic and histopathologic characteristics of malignant nodules. Thyroid. 2010;8:873–8.
12. Kim KW, Park YJ, Kim EH, Park SY, Park DJ, Ahn SH, et al. Elevated risk of papillary thyroid cancer in Korean patients with Hashimoto's thyroiditis. Head Neck. 2011;5:691–5.
13. Konturek A, Barczynski M, Wierzchowski W, Stopa M, Nowak W. Coexistence of papillary thyroid cancer with Hashimoto thyroiditis. Langenbecks Arch Surg. 2013;3:389–94.
14. Kurukahvecioglu O, Taneri F, Yuksel O, Aydin A, Tezel E, Onuk E. Total thyroidectomy for the treatment of Hashimoto's thyroiditis coexisting with papillary thyroid carcinoma. Adv Ther. 2007;3:510–6.
15. Larson SD, Jackson LN, Riall TS, Uchida T, Thomas RP, Qiu S, et al. Increased incidence of well-differentiated thyroid cancer associated with Hashimoto thyroiditis and the role of the PI3k/Akt pathway. J Am Coll Surg. 2007;5:764–73.
16. Liu X, Zhu L, Cui D, Wang Z, Chen H, Duan Y, et al. Coexistence of histologically confirmed Hashimoto's thyroiditis with different stages of papillary thyroid carcinoma in a consecutive Chinese cohort. Int J Endocrinol. 2014;2014:769294.
17. Lun Y, Wu X, Xia Q, Han Y, Zhang X, Liu Z, et al. Hashimoto's thyroiditis as a risk factor of papillary thyroid cancer may improve cancer prognosis. Otolaryngol Head Neck Surg. 2013;3:396–402.
18. Mukasa K, Noh JY, Kunii Y, Matsumoto M, Sato S, Yasuda S, et al. Prevalence of malignant tumors and adenomatous lesions detected by ultrasonographic screening in patients with autoimmune thyroid diseases. Thyroid. 2011;1:37–41.

19. Paparodis R, Imam S, Todorova-Koteva K, Staii A, Jaume JC. Hashimoto's thyroiditis pathology and risk for thyroid cancer. Thyroid. 2014;7:1107–14.
20. Siriweera EH, Ratnatunga NV. Profile of Hashimoto's thyroiditis in Sri Lankans: is there an increased risk of ancillary pathologies in Hashimoto's thyroiditis? J Thyroid Res. 2010;2010:124264.
21. Zhang L, Li H, Ji QH, Zhu YX, Wang ZY, Wang Y, et al. The clinical features of papillary thyroid cancer in Hashimoto's thyroiditis patients from an area with a high prevalence of Hashimoto's disease. BMC Cancer. 2012;12:610.
22. Zhang Y, Dai J, Wu T, Yang N, Yin Z. The study of the coexistence of Hashimoto's thyroiditis with papillary thyroid carcinoma. J Cancer Res Clin Oncol. 2014;6:1021–6.
23. Anil C, Goksel S, Gursoy A. Hashimoto's thyroiditis is not associated with increased risk of thyroid cancer in patients with thyroid nodules: a single-center prospective study. Thyroid. 2010;6:601–6.
24. Isik S, Gokay F, Ozuguz U, Topaloglu O, Tutuncu Y, Berker D, et al. Comparison of the prevalence and sonographic features of thyroid nodules accompanying autoimmune thyroid diseases. Endokrynol Pol. 2010;6:658–64.
25. Matesa-Anic D, Matesa N, Dabelic N, Kusic Z. Coexistence of papillary carcinoma and Hashimoto's thyroiditis. Acta Clin Croat. 2009;1:9–12.
26. Lee JH, Kim Y, Choi JW, Kim YS. The association between papillary thyroid carcinoma and histologically proven Hashimoto's thyroiditis: a meta-analysis. Eur J Endocrinol. 2013;3:343–9.
27. Mazokopakis EE, Tzortzinis AA, Dalieraki-Ott EI, Tsartsalis AN, Syros PK, Karefilakis CM, et al. Coexistence of Hashimoto's thyroiditis with papillary thyroid carcinoma. A retrospective study. Hormones (Athens). 2010;9:312–7.
28. Matsumoto F, Fujii H, Abe M, Kajino K, Kobayashi T, Matsumoto T, et al. A novel tumor marker, Niban, is expressed in subsets of thyroid tumors and Hashimoto's thyroiditis. Hum Pathol. 2006;37:1592–600.
29. Cipolla C, Sandonato L, Graceffa G, Fricano S, Torcivia A, Vieni S, et al. Hashimoto's thyroiditis coexistent with papillary thyroid carcinoma. Am Surg. 2005;71:874–8.
30. Tamimi DM. The association between chronic lymphocytic thyroiditis and thyroid tumors. Int J Surg Pathol. 2002;10:141–6.
31. O'Hanlon DM, Little MP, Given HF, Quill DS. Thyroid disease in the west of Ireland: an atypical incidence of neoplasia. Ir Med J. 1997;90:70–1.
32. Okayasu I, Fujiwara M, Hara Y, Tanaka Y, Rose NR. Association of chronic lymphocytic thyroiditis and thyroid papillary carcinoma. A study of surgical cases among Japanese, and white and African Americans. Cancer. 1995;76:2312–8.
33. McLeod MK, East ME, Burney RE, Harness JK, Thompson NW. Hashimoto's thyroiditis revisited: the association with thyroid cancer remains obscure. World J Surg. 1988;12:509–16.
34. Huang BY, Hseuh C, Chao TC, Lin KJ, Lin JD. Well-differentiated thyroid carcinoma with concomitant Hashimoto's thyroiditis present with less aggressive clinical stage and low recurrence. Endocr Pathol. 2011;22:144–9.
35. Repplinger D, Bargren A, Zhang YW, Adler JT, Haymart M, Chen H. Is Hashimoto's thyroiditis a risk factor for papillary thyroid cancer? J Surg Res. 2008;150:49–52.
36. Van Savell H Jr, Hughes SM, Bower C, Parham DM. Lymphocytic infiltration in pediatric thyroid carcinomas. Pediatr Dev Pathol. 2004;7:487–92.
37. Harach HR, Escalante DA, Day ES. Thyroid cancer and thyroiditis in Salta, Argentina: a 40-yr study in relation to iodine prophylaxis. Endocr Pathol. 2002;13:175–81.
38. Loh KC, Greenspan FS, Dong F, Miller TR, Yeo PP. Influence of lymphocytic thyroiditis on the prognostic outcome of patients with papillary thyroid carcinoma. J Clin Endocrinol Metab. 1999;84:458463.
39. Singh B, Shaha AR, Trivedi H, Carew JF, Poluri A, Shah JP. Coexistent Hashimoto's thyroiditis with papillary thyroid carcinoma: impact on presentation, management, and outcome. Surgery. 1999;126:1070–6.

40. Schaffler A, Palitzsch KD, Seiffarth C, Hohne HM, Riedhammer FJ, Hofstadter F, et al. Coexistent thyroiditis is associated with lower tumour stage in thyroid carcinoma. Eur J Clin Investig. 1998;28:838–44.
41. Mancini A, Rabitti C, Conte G, Gullotta G, De Marinis L. Lymphocytic infiltration in thyroid neoplasms. Preliminary prognostic assessments. Minerva Chir. 1993;48:1283–8.
42. Baroni CD, Manente L, Maccallini V, Di Matteo G. Primary malignant tumors of the thyroid gland. Histology, age and sex distribution and pathologic correlations in 139 cases. Tumori. 1983;69:205–13.
43. Peterson CA. Lymphocytic thyroiditis in 757 thyroid operations. Am J Surg. 1957;94:223–8.
44. Yoon YH, Kim HJ, Lee JW, Kim JM, Koo BS. The clinicopathologic differences in papillary thyroid carcinoma with or without co-existing chronic lymphocytic thyroiditis. Eur Arch Otorrinolaringol. 2012;269:1013–7.
45. Muzza M, Degl'Innocenti D, Colombo C, Perrino M, Ravasi E, Rossi S, et al. The tight relationship between papillary thyroid cancer, autoimmunity and inflammation: clinical and molecular studies. Clin Endocrinol. 2010;72:702–8.
46. Kim HS, Choi YJ, Yun JS. Features of papillary thyroid microcarcinoma in the presence and absence of lymphocytic thyroiditis. Endocr Pathol. 2010;21:149–53.
47. French JD, Weber ZJ, Fretwell DL, Said S, Klopper JP, Haugen BR. Tumor-associated lymphocytes and increased FoxP3C regulatory T cell frequency correlate with more aggressive papillary thyroid cancer. J Clin Endocrinol Metab. 2010;95:2325–33.
48. Kim EY, Kim WG, Kim WB, Kim TY, Kim JM, Ryu JS, et al. Coexistence of chronic lymphocytic thyroiditis is associated with lower recurrence rates in patients with papillary thyroid carcinoma. Clin Endocrinol. 2009;71:581–6.
49. Kim SK, Song KH, Lim SD, Lim YC, Yoo YB, Kim JS, et al. Clinical and pathological features and the BRAF (V600E) mutation. Thyroid. 2009;19:137–41.
50. Bruland O, Fluge O, Akslen LA, Eiken HG, Lillehaug JR, Varhaug JE, et al. Inverse correlation between PDGFC expression and lymphocyte infiltration in human papillary thyroid carcinomas. BMC Cancer. 2009;9:425–9.
51. Onak Kandemir N, Barut F, Keser S, Karadayi N, Bektas S, Dogan Gun BB, et al. Chronic lymphocytic thyroiditis and tumor-infiltrating lymphocytes combined in thyroid papillary carcinoma. Turk Onkoloji Dergisi. 2009;24:172–6.
52. Ohmori N, Miyakawa M, Ohmori K, Takano K. Ultrasonographic findings of papillary thyroid carcinoma with Hashimoto's thyroiditis. Intern Med. 2007;46:547–50.
53. Neuhold N, Kaiser H, Kaserer K. Latent carcinoma of the thyroid in Austria: a systematic autopsy study. Endocr Pathol. 2001;12:23–31.
54. Kebebew E, Treseler PA, Ituarte PH, Clark OH. Coexisting chronic lymphocytic thyroiditis and papillary thyroid cancer revisited. World J Surg. 2001;25:632–7.
55. Kashima K, Yokoyama S, Noguchi S, Murakami N, Yamashita H, Watanabe S, et al. Chronic thyroiditis as a favorable prognostic factor in papillary thyroid carcinoma. Thyroid. 1998;8:197–202.
56. Asanuma K, Sugenoya A, Kasuga Y, Itoh N, Kobayashi S, Amano J. The relationship between multiple intrathyroidal involvement in papillary thyroid carcinoma and chronic non-specific thyroiditis. Cancer Lett. 1998;122:177–80.
57. Gomez Saez JM, Gomez Arnaiz N, Sahun de la Vega M, Soler Ramon J. Prevalence and significance of lymphocyte infiltration in papillary carcinoma of the thyroid gland. An Med Interna. 1997;14:403–5.
58. Matsubayashi S, Kawai K, Matsumoto Y, Mukuta T, Morita T, Hirai K, et al. The correlation between papillary thyroid carcinoma and lymphocytic infiltration in the thyroid gland. J Clin Endocrinol Metab. 1995;80:3421–4.
59. Del Rio P, Cataldo S, Sommaruga L, Concione L, Arcuri MF, Sianesi M. The association between papillary carcinoma and chronic lymphocytic thyroiditis: does it modify the prognosis of cancer? Minerva Endocrinol. 2008;33:1–5.
60. Jankovic B, Le KT, Hershman JM. Hashimoto's thyroiditis and papillary thyroid carcinoma: is there a correlation? J Clin Endocrinol Metab. 2013;2:474–82.

61. Lai X, Xia Y, Zhang B, Li J, Jiang Y. A meta-analysis of Hashimoto's thyroiditis and papillary thyroid carcinoma risk. Oncotarget. 2017;8(37):62414–24.
62. Buyukasik O, Hasdemir AO, Yalcin E, Celep B, Sengul S, Yandakci K, et al. The association between thyroid malignancy and chronic lymphocytic thyroiditis: should it alter the surgical approach? Endokrynol Pol. 2011;4:303–8.
63. Holm LE, Blomgren H, Lowhagen T. Cancer risks in patients with chronic lymphocytic thyroiditis. N Engl J Med. 1985;10:601–4.
64. de Alcantara-Jones DM, de Alcantara-Nunes TF, Rocha BO, de Oliveira RD, Santana AC, de Alcantara FT, et al. Is there any association between Hashimoto's thyroiditis and thyroid cancer? A retrospective data analysis. Radiol Bras. 2015;3:148–53.
65. Fiore E, Rago T, Scutari M, Ugolini C, Proietti A, Di Coscio G, et al. Papillary thyroid cancer, although strongly associated with lymphocytic infiltration on histology, is only weakly predicted by serum thyroid autoantibodies in patients with nodular thyroid diseases. J Endocrinol Investig. 2009;32:344–51.
66. Feldt-Rasmussen U, Rasmussen AK. Autoimmunity in differentiated thyroid cancer: significance and related clinical problems. Hormones. 2010;9:109–17.
67. Haberal AN, Toru S, Ozen O, Arat Z, Bilezikci B. Diagnostic pitfalls in the evaluation of fine needle aspiration cytology of the thyroid: correlation with histopathology in 260 cases. Cytopathology. 2009;20:103–8.
68. Wirtschafter A, Schmidt R, Rosen D, Kundu N, Santoro M, Fusco A, et al. Expression of the RET/PTC fusion gene as a marker for papillary carcinoma in Hashimoto's thyroiditis. Laryngoscope. 1997;107:95–100.
69. Powell DJ Jr, Russell J, Nibu K, Li G, Rhee E, Liao M, et al. The RET/PTC3 oncogene: metastatic solid-type papillary carcinomas in murine thyroids. Cancer Res. 1998;58:5523–8.
70. Graceffa G, Patrone R, Vieni S, Campanella S, Calamia S, Laise I, et al. Association between Hashimoto's thyroiditis and papillary thyroid carcinoma: a retrospective analysis of 305 patients. BMC Endocr Disord. 2019;19(Suppl 1):19–0351.
71. Danis N, Comlekci A, Yener S, Durak M, Calan M, Solmaz D, et al. Association between Hashimoto's thyroiditis and papillary thyroid cancer: a single center experience. Acta Endocrinol (Buchar). 2022;18(1):74–8.
72. Kim J, Chung HS, Choi MK, Roh YK, Yoo HJ, Park JH, et al. Associations between Hashimoto thyroiditis and clinical outcomes of papillary thyroid cancer: a meta-analysis of observational studies. Endocrinol Metab (Seoul). 2018;33(4):473–84.
73. Qu N, Zhang L, Lin DZ, Ji QH, Zhu YX, Wang Y. The impact of coexistent Hashimoto's thyroiditis on lymph node metastasis and prognosis in papillary thyroid microcarcinoma. Tumour Biol. 2016;37(6):7685–92.
74. Guarino V, Castellone MD, Avilla E, Melillo RM. Thyroid cancer and inflammation. Mol Cell Endocrinol. 2010;1:94–102.
75. Azizi G, Malchoff CD. Autoimmune thyroid disease: a risk factor for thyroid cancer. Endocr Pract. 2011;2:201–9.
76. Kim ES, Lim DJ, Baek KH, Lee JM, Kim MK, Kwon HS, et al. Thyroglobulin antibody is associated with increased cancer risk in thyroid nodules. Thyroid. 2010;8:885–91.
77. Menicali E, Guzzetti M, Morelli S, Moretti S, Puxeddu E. Immune landscape of thyroid cancers: new insights. Front Endocrinol (Lausanne). 2020;11:637826.
78. Pagano L, Mele C, Sama MT, Zavattaro M, Caputo M, De Marchi L, Paggi S, et al. Thyroid cancer phenotypes in relation to inflammation and autoimmunity. Front Biosci (Landmark Ed). 2018;23(12):2267–82.
79. Liu Y, Li C, Zhao W, Wang Y. Hashimoto's thyroiditis is an important risk factor of papillary thyroid microcarcinoma in younger adults. Horm Metab Res. 2017;49(10):732–8.
80. Frohlich E, Wahl R. The forgotten effects of thyrotropin-releasing hormone: metabolic functions and medical applications. Front Neuroendocrinol. 2019;52:29–43.
81. Pirahanchi Y, Toro F, Jialal I. Physiology, thyroid stimulating hormone. In: StatPearls [Internet]. Treasure Island: StatPearls Publishing; 2023.

82. Huang H, Rusiecki J, Zhao N, Chen Y, Ma S, Yu H, et al. Thyroid-stimulating hormone, thyroid hormones, and risk of papillary thyroid cancer: a nested case-control study. Cancer Epidemiol Biomarkers Prev. 2017;26(8):1209–18.
83. McLeod DS, Watters KF, Carpenter AD, Ladenson PW, Cooper DS, Ding EL. Thyrotropin and thyroid cancer diagnosis: a systematic review and dose-response meta-analysis. J Clin Endocrinol Metab. 2012;97(8):2682–92.
84. Wang Z, Lin Y, Jiang Y, Fu R, Wang Y, Zhang Q. The associations between thyroid-related hormones and the risk of thyroid cancer: an overall and dose-response meta-analysis. Front Endocrinol (Lausanne). 2022;13:992566.
85. Nikiforov YE. RET/PTC rearrangement-a link between Hashimoto's thyroiditis and thyroid cancer ... or not. J Clin Endocrinol Metab. 2006;91(6):2040–2.
86. Nikiforova MN, Caudill CM, Biddinger P, Nikiforov YE. Prevalence of RET/PTC rearrangements in Hashimoto's thyroiditis and papillary thyroid carcinomas. Int J Surg Pathol. 2002;10(1):15–22.
87. Melillo RM, Castellone MD, Guarino V, De Falco V, Cirafici AM, Salvatore G, et al. The RET/PTC-RAS-BRAF linear signaling cascade mediates the motile and mitogenic phenotype of thyroid cancer cells. J Clin Invest. 2005;115(4):1068–81.
88. Rhoden KJ, Unger K, Salvatore G, Yilmaz Y, Vovk V, Chiappetta G, et al. RET/papillary thyroid cancer rearrangement in nonneoplastic thyrocytes: follicular cells of Hashimoto's thyroiditis share low-level recombination events with a subset of papillary carcinoma. J Clin Endocrinol Metab. 2006;91(6):2414–23.
89. Ferrari SM, Fallahi P, Elia G, Ragusa F, Ruffilli I, Paparo SR, et al. Thyroid autoimmune disorders and cancer. Semin Cancer Biol. 2020;64:135–46.
90. Regua AT, Najjar M, Lo HW. RET signaling pathway and RET inhibitors in human cancer. Front Oncol. 2022;12:932353.
91. Unger P, Ewart M, Wang BY, Gan L, Kohtz DS, Burstein DE. Expression of p63 in papillary thyroid carcinoma and in Hashimoto's thyroiditis: a pathobiologic link? Hum Pathol. 2003;34(8):764–9.
92. Burstein DE, Nagi C, Wang BY, Unger P. Immunohistochemical detection of p53 homolog p63 in solid cell nests, papillary thyroid carcinoma, and Hashimoto's thyroiditis: a stem cell hypothesis of papillary carcinoma oncogenesis. Hum Pathol. 2004;35(4):465–73.
93. Scheffel RS, Dora JM, Maia AL. BRAF mutations in thyroid cancer. Curr Opin Oncol. 2022;34(1):9–18.
94. Cuccurullo V, Di Stasio GD, Cascini GL. PET/CT in thyroid cancer – the importance of BRAF mutations. Nucl Med Rev Cent East Eur. 2020;23(2):97–102.
95. Haroon Al Rasheed MR, Xu B. Molecular alterations in thyroid carcinoma. Surg Pathol Clin. 2019;12(4):921–30.
96. Kim WW, Ha TK, Bae SK. Clinical implications of the BRAF mutation in papillary thyroid carcinoma and chronic lymphocytic thyroiditis. J Otolaryngol Head Neck Surg. 2018;47(1):4.
97. Kim SK, Woo JW, Lee JH, Park I, Choe JH, Kim JH, et al. Chronic lymphocytic thyroiditis and BRAF V600E in papillary thyroid carcinoma. Endocr Relat Cancer. 2016;23(1):27–34.
98. Nozhat Z, Hedayati M. PI3K/AKT pathway and its mediators in thyroid carcinomas. Mol Diagn Ther. 2016;20(1):13–26.
99. Chu CA, Wang YW, Chen YL, Chen HW, Chuang JJ, Chang HY, et al. The role of phosphatidylinositol 3-kinase catalytic subunit type 3 in the pathogenesis of human cancer. Int J Mol Sci. 2021;22(20):10964.
100. Blume-Jensen P, Hunter T. Oncogenic kinase signalling. Nature. 2001;411(6835):355–65.
101. Singh A, Ham J, Po JW, Niles N, Roberts T, Lee CS. The genomic landscape of thyroid cancer tumourigenesis and implications for immunotherapy. Cells. 2021;10(5):1082.
102. Robbins HL, Hague A. The PI3K/Akt pathway in tumors of endocrine tissues. Front Endocrinol (Lausanne). 2015;6:188.
103. Dal Maso L, Panato C, De Paoli A, Mattioli V, Serraino D, Elisei R, et al. Trends in thyroid function testing, neck ultrasound, thyroid fine needle aspiration, and thyroidectomies in North-Eastern Italy. J Endocrinol Invest. 2021;44(8):1679–88.

104. Li M, Dal Maso L, Vaccarella S. Global trends in thyroid cancer incidence and the impact of overdiagnosis. Lancet Diabetes Endocrinol. 2020;8(6):468–70.
105. Gupta P, Gupta M, Koul N. Overdiagnosis and overtreatment; how to deal with too much medicine. J Family Med Prim Care. 2020;9(8):3815–9.
106. Vargas-Uricoechea H. Autoimmune thyroid disease and differentiated thyroid carcinoma: a review of the mechanisms that explain an intriguing and exciting relationship. World J Oncol. 2024;15(1):14–27.

Chronic Thyroiditis: Rare Inflammatory or Infiltrative Diseases

15

15.1 Focal Lymphocytic Thyroiditis (FLT)

15.1.1 Definition

Focal lymphocytic thyroiditis (FLT), also known as focal autoimmune thyroiditis, is a low-grade autoimmune thyroiditis (AIT) characterized by focal lymphocytic infiltrates of <5% of the thyroid gland, low levels of anti-thyroid antibodies, and lack of clinical symptoms. It is usually an incidental finding and is found coincidentally in 50% of women's and 25% of men's autopsies, without clinical relevance.

15.1.2 Prevalence

Thyroid nodules are common worldwide, and the prevalence of palpable thyroid nodules is 4–7% among adult populations [1, 2]. With the increased usage of ultrasound (US) in medical practice, an increasing number of non-palpable thyroid nodules are detected in 20–67% of the general population [3, 4]. Approximately, 5% of thyroid nodules may have malignancy [5, 6]. Many studies have suggested US criteria that could be used to differentiate malignancy from benign lesions [7, 8], although none of them have shown a significant impact on clinical practice, despite the wide acceptance and usefulness of the suggested criteria [9].

15.1.3 Microscopic (Histological) Description

Histologically, lymphocytic thyroiditis is characterized by the presence of lymphocytic aggregates with germinal centers, oncocytic (Hürthle, oxyphil) cells, and a variable degree of follicular atrophy and inter- or intra-lobular fibrosis [10–13], most likely reflecting the phase and severity of the disease process. Some patients have a diffusely heterogeneous, hypoechoic gland, an appearance that is not specific

M. Sakr, *Thyroiditis*, https://doi.org/10.1007/978-3-032-19513-5_15

for lymphocytic thyroiditis and that may be seen in multinodular goiter, Graves' disease, and subacute thyroiditis [10, 14, 15].

Although non-specific, a diffuse hypoechoic pattern in a patient with lymphocytic thyroiditis has been shown to correlate with diffuse replacement of the gland by lymphocytes and fibrosis and is highly predictive of either the existence or the future development of hypothyroidism [10].

Focal lymphocytic thyroiditis (FLT) is characterized by (1) the presence of focal aggregates of lymphocytes in inter- or intra-lobular fibrous tissue, (2) absence of oxyphilic metaplasia, (3) absence of follicular atrophy, and (4) absence of follicular disruption. In addition, it may be associated with other thyroid diseases [5].

15.1.4 Fine-Needle Aspiration (FNA)

Fine-needle aspiration biopsy (FNAB) is considered to be the best diagnostic tool for differentiating malignant from benign nodules. However, FNAB has a relatively high false-negative rate, ranging from 0.7% to 21% [16–18]. This often leads to a question of whether a repeat aspiration or follow-up with US should be performed for suspicious thyroid nodules [19, 20].

Although lymphocytic thyroiditis was originally described as the presence of a firm, diffusely enlarged gland, a large number of patients with lymphocytic thyroiditis have "nodular" enlargement of their thyroids and are often referred for FNA [10, 11, 21]. In up to 60% of these patients, biopsy of the focal palpable nodule will yield changes consistent with lymphocytic thyroiditis without evidence of malignancy [11, 14, 21, 22].

15.1.5 Ultrasonography (US)

The classic US appearance of Hashimoto's thyroiditis (chronic lymphocytic thyroiditis) is that of diffusely coarse and heterogeneous hypo-echogenicity [10, 14, 15, 23, 24] or appears as a fine micro-nodular pattern [25, 26]. However, lymphocytic thyroiditis can be observed as a "focal" thyroid nodule that usually appears to be "hypoechoic" with ill-defined margins: an appearance that is indistinguishable from that of a malignant nodule [5, 11, 21, 22, 26] (Fig. 15.1).

The US appearance of the thyroiditis nodules may be "hyper-echoic" an appearance causing less concern for malignancy [13, 27]. Additionally, partial cystic change, calcifications, and incomplete halo may be noted [13], but their appearance was not specifically described in the literature. Unfortunately, specific US features of focal lymphocytic thyroiditis (FLT) are not yet well established.

Langer et al. (2001) [5] reviewed the sonographic features of focal nodules that on FNA proved to be thyroiditis in 21 of 394 (5.3%) nodules in 20 patients without known chronic lymphocytic thyroiditis. The diagnosis of lymphocytic thyroiditis was made when the FNA smears satisfied the following criteria: (1) the smears were cellular and showed a mixture of follicular cells and Hürthle cells in a background

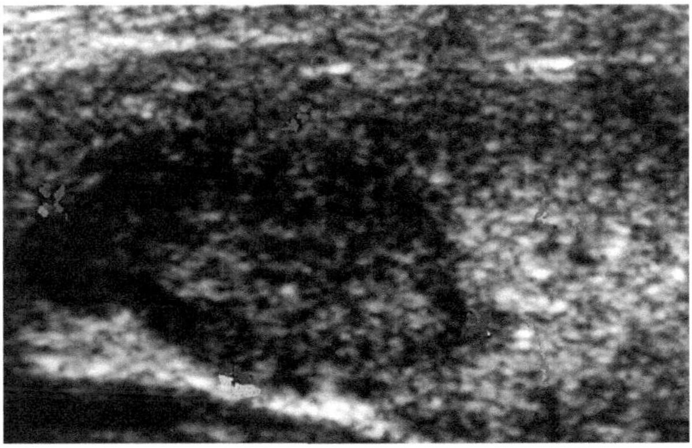

Fig. 15.1 Ultrasonography of a 35-year-old-woman with a 3-cm left-sided hypoechoic, poorly marginated nodule that proved to be papillary thyroid carcinoma. Sonographically guided fine-needle aspiration of this nodule was consistent with focal lymphocytic thyroiditis

of small mature lymphocytes, (2) the colloid was scant and mainly consisted of thick eosinophilic colloid, (3) the follicular and Hürthle cells were present as follicular groups, monolayer sheets, and scattered cells, (4) the lymphocytes were present in aggregates and were also scattered among the follicular and Hürthle cells groups, and (5) the follicular cells focally displayed nuclear atypia with nuclear enlargement and clearing but without nuclear grooves or inclusions.

The authors reported that the predominant echogenicity of the nodules that proved to be thyroiditis was hyper-echoic relative to parenchyma in 10 nodules (47.6%), hypoechoic in five (23.8%), iso-echoic in three (14.3%), and of mixed echogenicity in two (9.5%). The echogenicity of the nodules could not be assessed because of calcifications in one nodule (4.8%). Additionally, 18 nodules (85.7%) were completely solid, 1 (4.8%) contained minute cystic-appearing regions, and 2 (9.5%) were mixed cystic and solid in appearance. The margins of the nodule were irregular in 17 nodules (80.9%) and regular in 4 (19%). A partial surrounding halo was noted in 7 nodules (33.3%) and was absent in 14 (66.7%). Calcifications were noted in only five nodules (23.8%). They concluded that in a patient population undergoing sonography for palpable nodular disease without known thyroiditis, focal nodules of thyroiditis have a wide variety of appearances. Biopsy of these lesions is still necessary because there are no sonographic features that can reliably diagnose these lesions as thyroiditis and differentiate them from other lesions, particularly thyroid carcinoma.

More recently, Hwang et al. (2015) [28] sought to identify clinical and biochemical findings, in addition to US features, that could be used to differentiate FLT from thyroid malignancy in order to reduce the need for repetitive FNABs. They evaluated 214 patients who underwent FNAB and had shown thyroid nodules with suspicious US features. Papillary thyroid carcinoma (PTC) was confirmed by surgical pathology, while FLT and adenomatous hyperplasia (AH) were confirmed through more than two separate FNABs. Clinical, biochemical findings, and US features were all evaluated. Of 214 patients, 100 patients were diagnosed with PTC, 55 patients with FLT, and 59 with AH. The proportion of elevated thyroid-stimulating hormone (TSH) levels ($p = 0.014$) and thyroglobulin antibody (Tg-Ab) or thyroid peroxidase antibody (TPO-Ab) positivity ($p < 0.001$) in the FLT group was significantly higher than that in the PTC group. Regarding US features, absence of calcification ($p = 0.006$) and "diffuse thyroid disease" (DTD) pattern on US ($p < 0.001$) were frequently seen in the FLT group.

On multivariate analysis, Tg-Ab positivity, presence of a DTD pattern on US, and absence of calcification in nodules were associated with FLT, with the best specificity of 99% and positive predictive value of 96%. In contrast, a taller than wide shape of nodules was the only variable significant for differentiating AH from PTC [28]. This result is also consistent with previous studies that a taller-than-wide shape is the best predictor for malignancy [29, 30]. The authors [28] concluded that suspicious thyroid nodules with cytological benign results could be followed up with US rather than repeat FNAB, if patients exhibit Tg-Ab positivity, no calcifications in nodules, and a DTD pattern on US.

15.2 Post-partum Thyroiditis

Post-partum thyroiditis occurs in 2–16% of women within 6–12 months after delivery (or abortion) [31, 32]. It represents an exacerbation of a preceding (undiagnosed) autoimmune thyroiditis and is classically linked to the haplotypes HLA-DR3, -DR4, and -DR5. Most patients (85%) develop auto-antibodies against thyroid peroxidase (TPO) and thyroglobulin (Tg), which may disappear with time. Women with a known autoimmune thyroiditis prior to pregnancy and an elevated titer of auto-antibodies against Tg during pregnancy nearly always suffer from a post-partum exacerbation of their autoimmune thyroiditis. Clinically, patients may show a transient hyperthyroid state, which rapidly converts to hypothyroidism, and then to euthyroidism within 12 months. Treatment consists of thyroid hormone replacement when required.

15.3 Sarcoidosis

Sarcoidosis is a multiple systemic granulomatous disease [33]. Its main pathological feature is a non-caseous necrotic epithelial granuloma, which affects the lung, lymph nodes, and other organs. At present, the pathogenesis of sarcoidosis is unclear, and the existing research supports that individuals with genetic susceptibility have granulomatous reactions due to immune dysfunction caused by special antigens [34, 35]. The clinical manifestations of sarcoidosis are complex, diverse, and non-specific. The common symptoms of sarcoidosis patients are bilateral hilar lymphadenopathy, with (or without) diffuse changes in the pulmonary interstitium. Other symptoms are often manifested in the skin, eyes, heart, liver, spleen, and lymph nodes. Some patients are diagnosed in the physical examination without obvious clinical symptoms [36].

The first case of sarcoidosis and thyroid disease was reported back in 1938 [37]. Recently, studies about the relationship between sarcoidosis and thyroid disease have increased. Several studies have revealed a high prevalence of thyroid disease in sarcoidosis patients [38–44]. However, most of these studies were cross-sectional surveys and lacked clinical evidence. The lesions of sarcoid may appear in the thyroid gland of 1–4% of patients with systemic sarcoidosis [45]. Multinodular goiter (MNG) has been described as an initial presenting manifestation in a woman eventually diagnosed with systemic sarcoidosis [45]. This case illustrates the difficulty in diagnosing the cause of supine dyspnea in patients with sarcoidosis, illustrating the potential of a thyroid contribution to the overall clinical picture [45].

As reported by Anolik et al. (2012), thyroid dysfunction was found very infrequently (1–3%) in systemic sarcoidosis, but reached 26% in patients with cutaneous sarcoidosis [46]. Most thyroid dysfunction was mild, a male:female ratio of abnormal thyroid function of 1:1 was noted, Caucasians were more frequently affected than African Americans, and 20% of those with abnormal TSH were eventually classified as hypothyroid [46]. Infiltration of the thyroid with sarcoidosis is reported to occur in approximately 5% of patients with sarcoidosis [47].

Most recently, the systematic review and meta-analysis conducted by Xin et al. (2023) [48] included 6 articles, which involved 2044 sarcoidosis patients and 5652 controls [49–54] (Table 15.1). The studies found that the incidence of thyroid disease in patients with sarcoidosis was significantly increased compared to the controls suggesting that sarcoidosis patients should be screened for thyroid disease. In addition, the prevalence of clinical thyroid disease and thyroid antibodies was higher in patients with sarcoidosis than in controls.

The prevalence of sarcoidosis is related to age, gender, race, and region (country). It is reported that Afro-Caribbeans and African Americans are the two ethnic groups most affected by Sarcoidosis [55]. The prevalence of sarcoidosis in African Americans is 141/100,000 people as compared to only 49.8/100,000 people in Caucasians in the same region [56].

Whether sarcoidosis can be classified as an autoimmune disease has always been controversial. Some researchers believe that the gender orientation of sarcoidosis is not strong, specific auto-antibodies have not been found, and it is most common in

Table 15.1 Characteristics of the selected studies of acceptable quality

Study [Ref]	Year	Country	Cases (*n*)	Controls (*n*)	Tg-Ab positive		TPO-Ab positive	
					Case	Control	Case	Control
Nakamura et al. [49]	1997	Japan	45	170	17	15	15	14
Ilias et al. [50]	1998	Greece	26	26	3	0	3	0
Antonelli et al. [51]	2005	Italy	111	333	46	95	11	46
Malli et al. [52]	2012	Greece	68	75	42	13	4	3
Nowiński et al. [53]	2015	Poland	557	100	73	4	–	–
Wu et al. [54]	2016	China	123	4948	143	359	–	–

Ref reference, *Tg-Ab* thyroglobulin antibody, *TPO-Ab* thyroid peroxidase antibody

the lungs and thoracic lymph nodes (LNs) rather than common autoimmune diseases such as skin and joints involving organs. Therefore, it cannot be certainly classified as an autoimmune disease [57]. On the other hand, there is also a lot of evidence that suggests similarities between sarcoidosis and autoimmune diseases, such as systemic lupus erythematosus (SLE), rheumatoid arthritis, Sjogren's syndrome, and other autoimmune diseases [58].

HLA genotypes are also related to disease susceptibility and prognosis. In a national-level questionnaire-based study conducted on 3835 self-reported sarcoidosis patients, they reported that hypothyroidism is a co-existing disease in sarcoidosis patients and that such patients have more multiple organ presentations, such as skin, joints, eyes, liver, and lacrimal glands showing sarcoid presentations than the typical pulmonary sarcoidosis [59].

Both sarcoidosis and thyroid disease have been associated with HLA genes. Brewerton et al. (1977) first reported an HLA-88 association between thyroid disease and acute sarcoidosis [60]. Several other studies showed HLA-B and HLA-DRB1 association with both sarcoidosis and thyroid disease [61–63]. In 2006, Papi et al. demonstrated that class-I HLA and class-II might play complementary roles in promoting both thyroid disease and sarcoidosis through a common immunopathogenic pathway [64]. The association between Hashimoto's thyroiditis and sarcoidosis could be due to increased thyroid-specific T-cell activation caused by increased expression of Th1/Th17 cells in both diseases as reported by Semiz et al. (2018) [65].

15.4 Amyloidosis

15.4.1 Introduction

Amyloidosis is a group of heterogeneous diseases resulting from the pathological deposition of an insoluble protein known as amyloid [66, 67]. Amyloid is derived from soluble precursors that undergo a conformational change resulting in a protein of a beta pleated sheet configuration [66–68]. It deposits in the extra-cellular space of various organs compromising function and creating a mass effect. It is a diverse disease with many subtypes, each with a specific organ predilection. Therefore, it can present with a wide spectrum of signs and symptoms.

15.4.2 Definitions

"Amyloidosis" is defined as the accumulation of amorphous, proteinaceous material (amyloid) in different parts of the body.

"Amyloid goiter" is the deposition of amyloid in the glandular parenchyma of the thyroid gland in such quantities to cause a clinically apparent enlargement of the gland [69–71]. Although this rare entity was first reported by von Rokitansky in 1855 in the context of systemic amyloidosis, clinically apparent thyroid enlargement due to large amounts of amyloid deposition was first recognized 3 years later by Beckmann. In 1904, von Eisenberg coined the term "amyloid goiter" to describe the latter [72].

15.4.3 Prevalence

Amyloid goiter is a rare presentation of thyroid swelling, which occurs with either primary or secondary amyloidosis. Deposition of amyloid in the thyroid gland occurs in 15% of primary amyloidosis and 20% in secondary amyloidosis [73]. Even though involvement of the thyroid gland by amyloid is quite common, clinically significant enlargement of the thyroid due to amyloid deposition is extremely rare, and most cases are not diagnosed prior to surgery [74].

15.4.4 Sub-types of Amyloidosis in Amyloid Goiter

The two main subtypes of amyloidosis implicated in amyloid goiter are primary (AL amyloidosis) and secondary amyloidosis (AA amyloidosis) [66, 67]. In developed countries, the most common cause of amyloid goiter is primary amyloidosis [75, 76]; however, in the developing world, secondary amyloidosis is a more common cause. Overall, amyloid goiter occurs more often in patients with primary compared to those with secondary amyloidosis [77].

15.4.4.1 Primary Amyloidosis (AL Amyloidosis)

Primary amyloidosis is linked to disorders of plasma cells collectively known as "plasma cell dyscrasia," in which there is over-production of plasma cells, antibodies, and misshapen light chains. Light chains deposit in tissues in the form of AL amyloid [66, 67]. The deposition can either be in a single organ (localized primary amyloidosis) or in multiple organs (systemic primary amyloidosis). Localized primary amyloidosis presenting with an isolated amyloid goiter is extremely rare [78, 79].

15.4.4.2 Secondary Amyloidosis (AA Amyloidosis)

Secondary amyloidosis is associated with chronic inflammatory conditions [66, 67]. The acute phase reactant, serum amyloid A, is produced in excess and deposits in various organs in the form of amyloid A [66, 67]. In secondary amyloidosis, amyloid goiter has been described to occur as a sequela of long-standing Familial Mediterranean Fever (FMF) [74, 80, 81]. inflammatory bowel disease (IBD) [82, 83], rheumatoid arthritis (RA) [82, 84], tuberculosis (TB) [71, 78], and bronchiectasis [85].

15.4.5 Clinical Presentation

Clinically, patients with an amyloid goiter will usually present with a firm, non-tender, rapidly growing swelling over weeks to years [66]. The swelling can be unilateral or bilateral, diffuse or nodular [66], and can be accompanied by compressive symptoms such as dysphagia, dysphonia, or dyspnea [67, 77–79, 81, 86]. With such clinical course, malignancy, especially anaplastic thyroid cancer, should be the most important differential diagnosis, and initial investigations should aim to rule out malignancy. In addition to the focal deposition of amyloid in thyroid tissues associated with most cases of medullary thyroid carcinoma (MTC) [87, 88], several cases of papillary thyroid carcinoma (PTC) have been reported in association of amyloid goiter [89–92].

Even though the thyroid is extensively involved by amyloid deposition, patients with amyloid goiter are usually euthyroid; however, this is not the rule, as some patients may present with a hyperthyroid [93] or hypothyroid state [74, 80, 87, 94–97].

It is noteworthy that, in patients with amyloid goiter, it is exceedingly rare to have clinically evident parathyroid gland enlargement due to amyloid deposition [77]. Four previous cases were described in the literature [77, 98–100]. In all four cases, the pre-operative laboratory investigations, including parathyroid hormone (PTH) levels, were all normal. An enlarged parathyroid gland was only seen intra-operatively. This stresses the importance of examining the size of the parathyroid glands during surgery for amyloid goiter.

15.4.6 Investigations/Diagnosis

15.4.6.1 Imaging

Ultrasonography (US), computerized tomography (CT) scan, and magnetic resonance imaging scans (MRI) have been used to investigate goiters [101]. Imaging patterns in amyloid goiter may vary according to the proportion of adipose tissue relative to amyloid [101]. Thus, complex or hypoechoic masses may be seen on ultrasonography [101]. In cases in which adipose tissue predominates, diffuse fat-equivalent hypo-density with or without calcifications can be seen on CT scan [101]. Proteinaceous substances within the nodule can cause high intensity on T1-weighted images, and fibrillar amyloid structures can lead to increased intensity on T2-weighted images [101]. Thus, on MRI, increased signal intensity will be seen on T1 and T2 weighted images [101].

15.4.6.2 Fine-Needle Aspirate Cytology (FNAC)

Fine-needle aspirate cytology (FNAC) is usually performed as part of the work-up of thyroid nodules. In amyloid goiter, FNAC will show abundant irregular fragments of a pink amorphous material [66], and has been reported in conjunction with infiltration of other endocrine organs such as the pituitary gland [102]. It is estimated that 10–40% FNAs performed on amyloid goiters will only show atypical follicular cells [66]. Unfortunately, this may limit the ability of FNAC to distinguish between amyloid goiter and medullary thyroid carcinoma (MTC) [70, 79]. Therefore, obtaining a precise diagnosis of amyloid goiter requires histopathology [79].

15.4.6.3 Histopathology

Histopathology usually reveals diffuse infiltration by mature adipose tissue, with attenuated scattered thyroid follicles and an extra-cellular eosinophilic amorphous substance (amyloid) deposited in the hyalinized stroma (Fig. 15.2). The extra-cellular substance is positive by the Congo red stain (Fig. 15.3), resulting in an apple-green green birefringence under polarized light microscopy [66, 67, 78]. The exact mechanism responsible for fatty metaplasia in amyloid goiter is unknown. A theory suggests that amyloid deposition compromises capillary function resulting in relative ischemia; this triggers stromal fibroblasts to undergo metaplasia [94, 95].

The presence of amyloid in a thyroid specimen, along with its clinical course, should raise the suspicion of medullary thyroid cancer (MTC), which should be ruled out. In MTC, using a calcitonin immune-stain, amyloid will be limited to an intra tumoral distribution as opposed to a wide distribution in amyloid goiter and the absence of tumor cells [77]. Subsequently, immunohistochemistry (IHC) can then be used to differentiate between types of amyloid [93].

Although microscopic amyloid deposition in the thyroid gland is common in patients with certain conditions, amyloid deposition resulting in an "overt goiter" is a rare event [67, 87, 94, 103]. Evidence of thyroid micro-deposits is seen in more than 80% of MTCs [104, 105], and in 30–80% of patients with amyloidosis [89]. Those are typically incidental findings not leading to amyloid goiter [77].

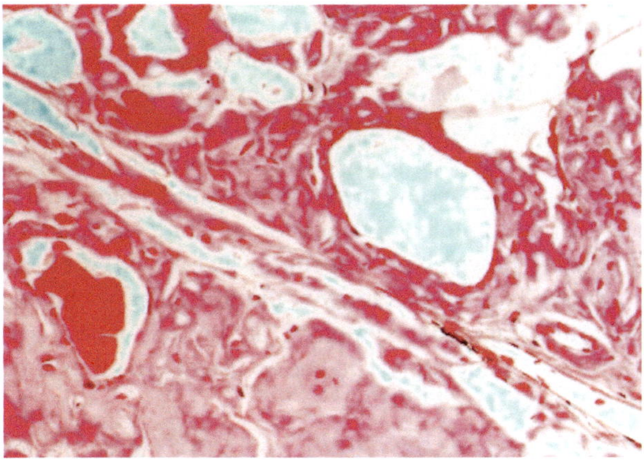

Fig. 15.2 Microscopy of thyroid lesion showing deposition of acellular amorphous eosinophilic material (amyloid). Hematoxylin and Eosin stain

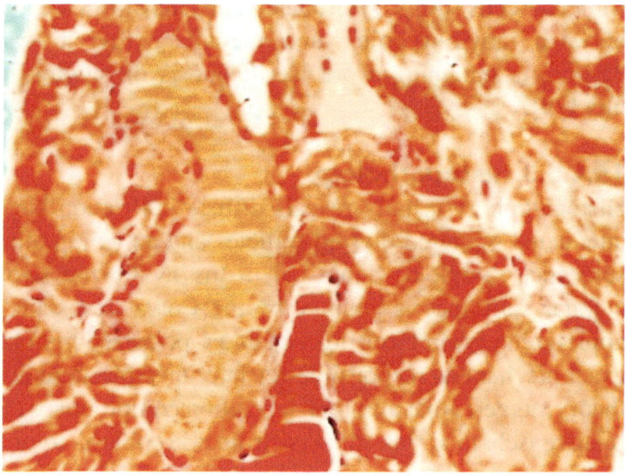

Fig. 15.3 Microscopy of thyroid lesion showing amyloid deposits rendered "salmon pink" by Congo Red staining

15.4.7 Differential Diagnosis

As mentioned before, definite diagnosis of amyloid goiter is generally only possible post-operatively by histopathological examination, but a high index of suspicion is required in patients with an enlarging thyroid gland and a concomitant history of chronic inflammatory processes or plasma cell dyscrasia, and should be maintained whenever amyloid deposits are seen on FNAC. Every effort should be made to delineate the extent of the disease [79].

Amyloid goiter must be differentiated from other types of goiters or malignancies, particularly MTC. In patients who were previously healthy, plasma cell dyscrasia should be excluded.

15.4.8 Treatment

Once the diagnosis of amyloid goiter is established, the extent of the disease has to be delineated. Whether AL or AA amyloidosis is diagnosed, the patient should also be screened for predisposing conditions, as amyloid goiter can be the first presentation of a long-standing disease [66, 77, 79, 82, 106]. This was seen in a case by Orrego et al. [66]. Their previously healthy patient presented with a thyroid swelling and was diagnosed with amyloid goiter AL type. Post-operative investigations revealed long-standing monoclonal gammopathy of undetermined significance with no other systemic involvement of amyloid. Hill et al. [77] presented a case of amyloid goiter in which post-operative investigations revealed multiple myeloma.

Typically, thyroidectomy is the treatment of choice in patients with an amyloid goiter if compressive symptoms are present or concerns of malignancy are present. However, the definitive diagnosis usually requires a thorough histological evaluation of the thyroid [79].

15.4.9 Summary

Amyloid goiter is a rare entity; a high index of suspicion is required in patients with an enlarging thyroid gland and a concomitant history of chronic inflammatory processes or plasma cell dyscrasia. FNA biopsy should be performed to exclude the top differential of primary thyroid malignancy. Definitive diagnosis typically occurs after thyroidectomy and histological examination. Thyroidectomy may also be for relief of compression symptom. Systemic work-up required to delineate the extent of the disease, and in previously healthy individuals, plasma cell dyscrasia should be excluded [107].

15.5 Drug-Induced Thyroiditis

Certain drugs have been reported to cause thyroiditis, such as chronic I_2 therapy, long-term lithium therapy, and anti-convulsants (e.g., phenytoin, carbamazepine). Moreover, patients with chronic hepatitis or cancer treated with interferon-alpha (IFN)-α will develop a painless thyroiditis in about 1–5% of cases [108]. Elevated anti-thyroid antibodies are noted in a higher percentage of these patients, and permanent hypothyroidism or Graves' disease may appear. Thus, TSH should be measured prior to initiation of IFN-α therapy and periodically during treatment [109].

A painless thyroiditis has been reported in about 2% of the patients treated with interleukin-2 (IL-2), which is used for immune-modulation in malignant melanoma, renal cell carcinoma, and leukemia, alone or in combination with chemotherapy. Finally, the anti-arrhythmic drug amiodarone contains 35% I_2 and may cause a thyrotoxic crisis or, conversely, hypothyroidism. Amiodarone decreases the conversion of T4 to the biologically active T3. If amiodarone therapy is stopped, it is not eliminated for months due to its very long half-life [110].

References

1. Mortensen JD, Woolner LB, Bennett WA. Gross and microscopic findings in clinically normal thyroid glands. J Clin Endocrinol Metab. 1955;15:1270–80.
2. Singer PA. Evaluation and management of the solitary thyroid nodule. Otolaryngol Clin N Am. 1996;29:577–91.
3. Mazzaferri EL. Management of a solitary thyroid nodule. N Engl J Med. 1993;328:553–9.
4. Ross DS. Nonpalpable thyroid nodules--managing an epidemic. J Clin Endocrinol Metab. 2002;87:1938–40.
5. Langer JE, Khan A, Nisenbaum HL, Baloch ZW, Horii SC, Coleman BG, et al. Sonographic appearance of focal thyroiditis. AJR Am J Roentgenol. 2001;176:751–4.
6. Hegedüs L. Clinical practice. The thyroid nodule. N Engl J Med. 2004;351:1764–71.
7. Kim EK, Park CS, Chung WY, Oh KK, Kim DI, Lee JT, et al. New sonographic criteria for recommending fine-needle aspiration biopsy of nonpalpable solid nodules of the thyroid. AJR Am J Roentgenol. 2002;178:687–91.

8. Peccin S, de Castsro JA, Furlanetto TW, Furtado AP, Brasil BA, Czepielewski MA. Ultrasonography: is it useful in the diagnosis of cancer in thyroid nodules? J Endocrinol Investig. 2002;25:39–43.
9. Hegedüs L. Thyroid ultrasonography as a screening tool for thyroid disease. Thyroid. 2004;14:879–80.
10. Marcocci C, Vitti P, Cetani F, Catalano F, Concetti R, Pinchera A. Thyroid ultrasonography helps to identify patients with diffuse lymphocytic thyroiditis who are prone to develop hypothyroidism. J Clin Endocrinol Metab. 1991;72:209–13.
11. Friedman M, Shimaoka K, Rao U, et al. Diagnosis of chronic lymphocytic thyroiditis (nodular presentation) by needle aspiration. Acta Cytol. 1981;25:513–22.
12. Jayaram G, Marwaha RK, Gupta RK, Sharma SK. Cytomorphologic aspects of thyroiditis: a study of 51 cases with functional, immunologic and ultrasonographic data. Acta Cytol. 1987;31:687–93.
13. Takashima S, Fukuda H, Nomura N, et al. Thyroid nodules: re-evaluation with ultrasound. J Clin Ultrasound. 1995;23:179–84.
14. Gutekunst R, Hafermann W, Mansky T, Scriba PC. Ultrasonography related to clinical and laboratory findings in lymphocytic thyroiditis. Acta Endocrinol. 1989;121:129–35.
15. Hayashi N, Tamaki N, Konishi J, et al. Sonography of Hashimoto's thyroiditis. J Clin Ultrasound. 1986;14:123–6.
16. Ylagan LR, Farkas T, Dehner LP. Fine needle aspiration of the thyroid: a cytohistologic correlation and study of discrepant cases. Thyroid. 2004;14:35–41.
17. Sangalli G, Serio G, Zampatti C, Bellotti M, Lomuscio G. Fine needle aspiration cytology of the thyroid: a comparison of 5469 cytological and final histological diagnoses. Cytopathology. 2006;17:245–50.
18. Raab SS, Vrbin CM, Grzybicki DM, Sudilovsky D, Balassanian R, Zarbo RJ, et al. Errors in thyroid gland fine-needle aspiration. Am J Clin Pathol. 2006;125:873–82.
19. Shin JH, Han BK, Ko K, Choe YH, Oh YL. Value of repeat ultrasound-guided fine-needle aspiration in nodules with benign cytological diagnosis. Acta Radiol. 2006;47:469–73.
20. Chernyavsky VS, Shanker BA, Davidov T, Crystal JS, Eng O, Ibrahim K, et al. Is one benign fine needle aspiration enough? Ann Surg Oncol. 2012;19:1472–6.
21. Pollock WF, Sprong DH Jr. Surgical aspects of thyroiditis. Arch Surg. 1960;80:720–32.
22. Takashima S, Matsuzuka F, Nagareda T, et al. Thyroid nodules associated with Hashimoto thyroiditis: assessment with US. Radiology. 1992;185:125–30.
23. Pedersen OM, Aardal NP, Larssen TB, Varhaug JE, Myking O, Vik-Mo H. The value of ultrasonography in predicting autoimmune thyroid disease. Thyroid. 2000;10:251–9.
24. Raber W, Gessl A, Nowotny P, Vierhapper H. Thyroid ultrasound versus antithyroid peroxidase antibody determination: a cohort study of four hundred fifty-one subjects. Thyroid. 2002;12:725–31.
25. Set PAK, Oleszczuk-Raschke K, VonLengerke JH, Brämswig J. Sonographic features of Hashimoto thyroiditis in childhood. Clin Radiol. 1996;51:167–9.
26. Yeh HC, Futterweit W, Gilbert P. Micronodulation: ultrasonographic sign of Hashimoto thyroiditis. J Ultrasound Med. 1996;15:813–9.
27. Lin JD, Huang BY, Wend HF, Hsueh C. Thyroid ultrasonography with fine-needle aspiration cytology for the diagnosis of thyroid cancer. J Clin Ultrasound. 1997;25:111–8.
28. Hwang S, Shin DY, Kim EK, Yang WI, Byun JW, Lee SJ, et al. Focal lymphocytic thyroiditis nodules share the features of papillary thyroid cancer on ultrasound. Yonsei Med J. 2015;56(5):1338–44.
29. Cappelli C, Castellano M, Pirola I, Gandossi E, De Martino E, Cumetti D, et al. Thyroid nodule shape suggests malignancy. Eur J Endocrinol. 2006;155:27–31.
30. Cappelli C, Pirola I, Cumetti D, Micheletti L, Tironi A, Gandossi E, et al. Is the anteroposterior and transverse diameter ratio of nonpalpable thyroid nodules a sonographic criteria for recommending fine-needle aspiration cytology? Clin Endocrinol. 2005;63:689–93.
31. Amino N, Tada H, Hidaka Y. Postpartum autoimmune thyroid syndrome: a model of aggravation of autoimmune disease. Thyroid. 1999;9:705–13.

32. Stagnaro-Green A. Clinical review: postpartum thyroiditis. J Clin Endocrinol Metab. 2002;87:4042–7.
33. Baughman RP, Culver DA, Judson MA. A concise review of pulmonary sarcoidosis. Am J Respir Crit Care Med. 2011;183(5):573–81.
34. Dempsey OJ, Paterson EW, Kerr KM, Denison AR. Sarcoidosis. BMJ. 2009;339:b3206.
35. Baughman RP, Lower EE, Gibson K. Pulmonary manifestations of sarcoidosis. Presse Med. 2012;41(6 Pt 2):e289–302.
36. Chen ES, Moller DR. Sarcoidosis-scientific progress and clinical challenges. Nat Rev Rheumatol. 2011;7:457–67.
37. Spencer J, Warren S. Boeck's sarcoid: report of a case, with clinical diagnosis confirmed at autopsy. Arch Intern Med. 1938;62:285–96.
38. Leppard B. Sarcoidosis and hyperthyroidism. Proc R Soc Med. 1971;64:396.
39. Christianson HB, Mitchell WT. Sarcoidosis and myxedema. South Med J. 1972;65:749–52.
40. Cohen JD, Clarke SW. Sarcoidosis and thyrotoxicosis. Proc R Soc Med. 1974;667:220–1.
41. Lender M, Dollberg L. Coincidence of sarcoidosis and Hashimoto's thyroiditis. Am Rev Respir Dis. 1975;112:113–7.
42. Sasaki H, Harada T, Eimoto T, Matsuoka Y, Okumura M. Concomitant association of thyroid sarcoidosis and Hashimoto's thyroiditis. Am J Med Sci. 1987;294:441–3.
43. Bell NH. Endocrine complications of sarcoidosis. Endocrinol Metab Clin N Am. 1991;20:645–54.
44. Fazzi P, Fallahi P, Ferrari SM. Sarcoidosis and thyroid autoimmunity. Front Endocrinol. 2017;8:177.
45. Hoang TD, Mai VQ, Clyde PW, Glister BC, Shakir MK. Multinodular goiter as the initial presentation of systemic sarcoidosis: limitation of fine-needle biopsy. Respir Care. 2011;56(7):1029–32.
46. Anolik RB, Schaffer A, Kim EJ, Rosenbach M. Thyroid dysfunction and cutaneous sarcoidosis. J Am Acad Dermatol. 2012;66(1):167–8.
47. Vailati A, Marena C, Aristia L, Sozze E, Barosi G, Inglese V, Luisetti M, Bossolo PA. Sarcoidosis of the thyroid: report of a case and a review of the literature. Sarcoidosis. 1993;10(1):66–8.
48. Xin C, Niu L, Fan H, Xie J, Sun X. Increased incidence of thyroid disease in patients with sarcoidosis: a systematic review and meta-analysis. Endocr Connect. 2023;12(9):e230157.
49. Nakmura H, Mikami T, Kitahara A, Andoh S, Nagasawa S, Nishiyama K, et al. High incidence of positive autoantibodies against thyroid peroxidase and thyroglobulin in patients with sarcoidosis. Clin Endocrinol. 1997;46:467–72.
50. Ilias I, Panoutsopoulos G, Batsakis C, Nikolakakou D, Filippou N, Christakopoulou I. Thyroid function and autoimmunity in sarcoidosis: a case-control study. Croat Med J. 1998;39(4):404–6.
51. Antonelli A, Fazzi P, Fallahi P, Ferrari SM, Ferrannini E. Prevalence of hypothyroidism and Graves disease in sarcoidosis. Chest. 2006;130:526–32.
52. Malli F, Bargiota A, Theodoridou K, Florou Z, Bardaka F, Koukoulis GN, Gourgoulianis KI, Daniil Z. Increased primary autoimmune thyroid diseases and thyroid antibodies in sarcoidosis: evidence for an under-recognised extrathoracic involvement in sarcoidosis? Hormones (Athens). 2012;11(4):436–43.
53. Nowiński A, Puścińska E, Goljan A, Peradzynska J, Bednarek M, Korzybski D, et al. The influence of comorbidities on mortality in sarcoidosis: a observational prospective cohort study. Clin Respir J. 2017;11(5):648–56.
54. Wu CH, Chung PI, Wu CY, Chen YT, Chiu YW, Chang YT, et al. Comorbid autoimmune diseases in patients with sarcoidosis: a nationwide case-control study in Taiwan. J Dermatol. 2017;44(4):423–30.
55. Spagnolo P. Sarcoidosis: a critical review of history and milestones. Clin Rev Allergy Immunol. 2015;49:1–5.
56. Baughman RP, Field S, Costabel U, Crystal RG, Culver DA, Drent M, et al. Sarcoidosis in America. Analysis based on health care use. Ann Am Thorac Soc. 2016;13(8):1244–52.

57. Sharma OP. Sarcoidosis and other autoimmune disorders. Curr Opin Pulm Med. 2002;8:452–6.
58. Starshinova AA, Malkova AM, Basantsova NY, Zinchenko YS, Kudryavtsev IV, Ershov GA, et al. Sarcoidosis as an autoimmune disease. Front Immunol. 2020;10:2933.
59. Alzghoul BN, Amer FN, Barb D, Innabi A, Mardini MT, Bai C, et al. Prevalence and characteristics of self-reported hypothyroidism and its association with nonorgan-specific manifestations in US sarcoidosis patients: a nationwide registry study. ERJ Open Res. 2021;7(1):00754-2020.
60. Brewerton DA, Cockburn C, James DC, James DG, Neville E. HLA antigens in sarcoidosis. Clin Exp Immunol. 1977;27:227–9.
61. Grunewald J, Eklund A, Olerup O. Human leukocyte antigen class I alleles and the disease course in sarcoidosis patients. Am J Respir Crit Care Med. 2004;169:696–702.
62. Petrone A, Giorgi G, Galgani A, Alemanno I, Corsello SM, Signore A, et al. CT60 single nucleotide polymorphisms of the cytotoxic T-lymphocyte-associated antigen-4 gene region is associated with Graves' disease in an Italian population. Thyroid. 2005;15:232–8.
63. Marga M, Denisova A, Sochnev A, Pirags V, Farid NR. Two HLA DRB 1 alleles confer independent genetic susceptibility to Graves disease: relevance of cross-population studies. Am J Med Genet. 2001;102(2):188–91.
64. Papi G, Briganti F, Artioli F, Cavazza A, Carapezzi C, Roggeri A, et al. Sarcoidosis of the thyroid gland associated with hyperthyroidism: review of the literature and report of two peculiar cases. J Endocrinol Investig. 2006;29:834–9.
65. Semiz H, Yalcin M, Kobak S. Coexistence of sarcoidosis and Hashimoto thyroiditis. Reumatismo. 2018;70:106–10.
66. Orrego J, Chorny J. Amyloid goiter as the first recognizable manifestation OF immunoglobulin light chain amyloidosis. AACE Clin Case Rep. 2019;5(5):e326–9.
67. Cannizzaro M, Lo Bianco S, Saliba W, D'Errico S, Pennetti Pennella F, Buttafuoco G. A rare case of primary thyroid amyloidosis. Int J Surg Case Rep. 2018;53:179–81.
68. Schönland SO, Hegenbart U, Bochtler T. Immunohistochemistry in the classification of systemic forms of amyloidosis: a systematic investigation of 117 patients. Blood. 2012;119:488–93.
69. Ibrahimov M, Yilmaz M, Kilic E, Akil F, Rasidov R, Karaman E. Rapidly progressive thyroid mass: amyloid goiter. J Craniofac Surg. 2012;23(16):e555–6.
70. Ozdemir BH, Uyar P, Ozdemir FN. Diagnosing amyloid goitre with thyroid aspiration biopsy. Cytopathology. 2006;17(5):262–6.
71. Villa F, Dionigi G, Tanda ML, Rovera F, Boni L. Amyloid goiter. Int J Surg. 2008;6(suppl 1):S16–8.
72. Arean VM, Klein RE. Amyloid goiter. Review of the literature and report of a case. Am J Clin Pathol. 1961;36:341–55.
73. Battaglia S. Results of a statistical investigation on amyloidosis. Pathobiology. 1964;27:792–808.
74. Yidiz L, Kefeli M, Kose B, Baris S. Amyloid goiter: two cases and a review of the literature. Ann Saudi Med. 2009;29:138–41.
75. Falk RH, Comenzo RL, Skinner M. The systemic amyloidoses. N Engl J Med. 1997;337:898–909.
76. Hirota S, Miyamoto M, Kasugai T, Kitamura Y, Morimura Y. Crystalline light-chain deposition and amyloidosis in the thyroid gland and kidneys of a patient with myeloma. Arch Pathol Lab Med. 1990;114:429–31.
77. Hill K, Diaz J, Hagemann I, Chernock R. Multiple myeloma presenting as massive amyloid deposition in a parathyroid gland associated with amyloid goiter: a medullary thyroid carcinoma mimic on intra-operative frozen section. Head Neck Pathol. 2017;12(2):269–73.
78. Sethi Y, Gulati A, Singh I, Rao S, Singh N. Amyloid goiter: a case of primary thyroid amyloid disease. Laryngoscope. 2011;121:961–4.
79. Joung K, Park J, Kim K, Koo B. Primary amyloid goiter mimicking rapid growing thyroid malignancy. Eur Arch Otorrinolaringol. 2013;271(2):417–20.

80. Altiparmak MR, Pamuk ON, Pamuk GE, Apaydin S, Ataman R, Serdengecti K. Amyloid goitre in familial Mediterranean fever: report on three patients and review of the literature. Clin Rheumatol. 2002;21(6):497–500.
81. Vergneault H, Terre A, Buob D, Buffet C, Dumont A, Ardois S, et al. Amyloid goiter in familial Mediterranean fever: description of 42 cases from a French cohort and from literature review. J Clin Med. 2021;10(9):1983.
82. Kazdaghli Lagha E, M'sakni I, Bougrine F, Laabidi B, Ben Ghachem D, Bouziani A. Amyloid goiter: first manifestation of systemic amyloidosis. Eur Ann Otorhinolaryngol Head Neck Dis. 2010;127:108–10.
83. Aydin B, Koca YS, Koca T, Yildiz I, Gerek Celikden S, Ciris M. Amyloid goiter secondary to ulcerative colitis. Case Rep Endocrinol. 2016;2016:3240585.
84. Seker A, Erkinuresin T, Demirci H. Amyloid goiter in a patient with rheumatoid arthritis and end-stage renal disease. Indian J Nephrol. 2020;30(2):125–8.
85. Goldsmith JD, Lai ML, Daniele GM, Tomaszewski JE, LiVolsi VA. Amyloid goiter: report of two cases and review of the literature. Endocr Pract. 2000;6:318–23.
86. Jakubović-Čičkušić A, Hasukić B, Sulejmanović M, Čičkušić A, Hasukić Š. Amyloid goiter: a case report and review of the literature. Saudi J Med Med Sci. 2020;8:151–5.
87. Hamed G, Heffess CS, Shmookler BM, Wenig BM. Amyloid goiter. A clinicopathologic study of 14 cases and review of the literature. Am J Clin Pathol. 1995;104(3):306–12.
88. Pinto A, Nose V. Localized amyloid in thyroid: are we missing it? Adv Anat Pathol. 2013;20(1):61–7.
89. Ozdemir D, Dagdelen S, Erbas T. Endocrine involvement in systemic amyloidosis. Endocr Pract. 2010;16(6):1056–63.
90. Coca-Pelaz A, Vivanco-Allende B, Alvarez-Marcos C, Suarez-Nieto C. Multifocal papillary thyroid carcinoma associated with primary amyloid goiter. Auris Nasus Larynx. 2012;39(5):549–51.
91. Nessim S, Tamilia M. Papillary thyroid carcinoma associated with amyloid goiter. Thyroid. 2005;15(4):382–5.
92. Coli A, Bigotti G, Zucchetti F, Negro F, Massi G. Papillary carcinoma in amyloid goitre. J Exp Clin Cancer Res. 2000;19(3):391–4.
93. Tokyol C, Demir S, Yilmaz S, Topak N, Paşali T, Polat C. Amyloid goiter with hyperthyroidism. Endocr Pathol. 2004;15:89–90.
94. Law JH, Dean DS, Scheithauer B, Earnest F 4th, Sebo TJ, Fatourechi V. Symptomatic amyloid goiters: report of 5 cases. Thyroid. 2013;23:1490–5.
95. Schroder BW. Lipomatous lesions of the thyroid gland: a review. Appl Pathol Int. 2007;57:449–53.
96. Jacques TA, Stearns MPJ. Diffuse lipomatosis of the thyroid with amyloid deposition. J Laryngol Otol. 2013;127(Supplement 04):426–8.
97. Siddiqui MA, Gertz M, Dean D. Amyloid goiter as a manifestation of primary systemic amyloidosis. Thyroid. 2007;17(1):77–80.
98. Ori Y, Halpern M, Sadov R, Feinmesser R, Ramadan R, Korzets A. Familial Mediterranean fever, an amyloid thyroid goiter and an enlarged parathyroid gland. Isr Med Assoc J. 2012;14:232–3.
99. Villamil CF, Massimi G, D'Avella J, Cole SR. Amyloid goiter with parathyroid involvement: a case report and review of the literature. Arch Pathol Lab Med. 2000;124:281–3.
100. Abdou AG, Kandil MA. A case of amyloid goiter associated with intrathyroid parathyroid and lymphoepithelial cyst. Endocr Pathol. 2009;20:243–8.
101. Aksu AO, Ozmen MN, Oguz KK, Akinci D, Yasavun U, Firat P. Diffuse fatty infiltration of the thyroid gland in amyloidosis: sonographic, computed tomographic, and magnetic resonance imaging findings. J Ultrasound Med. 2010;29:1251–5.
102. Ozdemir D, Dagdelen S, Erbas T, Sokmensuer C, Erbas B, Cila A. Amyloid goiter and hypopituitarism in a patient with systemic amyloidosis. Amyloid. 2011;18(1):32–4.

103. Di Crescenzo V, Garzi A, Petruzziello F, Cinelli M, Catalano L, Zeppa P. Nodular goiter with amyloid deposition in an elderly patient: fine-needle cytology diagnosis and review of the literature. BMC Surg. 2013;13(Suppl 2):S43.
104. Hazard JB. The C cells (parafollicular cells) of the thyroid gland and medullary thyroid carcinoma. A review. Am J Pathol. 1977;88:213–50.
105. Franc B, Rosenberg-Bourgin M, Caillou B, Dutrieux-Berger N, Floquet J, Houcke-Lecomte M. Medullary thyroid carcinoma: search for histological predictors of survival (109 proband cases analysis). Hum Pathol. 1998;29:1078–84.
106. Aparna C, Renuka I, Bala G, Vijayasri M. Primary amyloid goitre. Int J Otolaryngol Head Neck Surg. 2014;03(1):29–31.
107. Lari E, Burhamah W, Lari A, Alsafran S, Ismail A. Amyloid goiter – a rare case report and literature review. Ann Med Surg (Lond). 2020;57:295–8.
108. Preziati D, La Rosa L, Covini G, Marcelli R, Rescalli S, Persani L, et al. Autoimmunity and thyroid function in patients with chronic active hepatitis treated with recombinant interferon alpha-2a. Eur J Endocrinol. 1995;132:587–93.
109. Roti E, Minelli R, Giuberti T, archelli S, Schianchi C, Gardini E, et al. Multiple changes in thyroid function in patients with chronic active HCV hepatitis treated with recombinant interferon-alpha. Am J Med. 1996;172:482–7.
110. Harjai KJ, Licata AA. Effects of amiodarone on thyroid function. Ann Intern Med. 1997;126:63–73.

Surgical Intervention in Thyroiditis

16

16.1 Introduction

Thyroiditis is a common thyroid disorder affecting many individuals worldwide. Its commonest variant is Hashimoto's thyroiditis (chronic lymphocytic thyroiditis). The usual presenting symptom at the time of diagnosis is hypothyroidism. Most patients are asymptomatic. A few cases may experience neck pain, neck tightness, diffuse goiter, or even more obvious symptoms, such as dysphagia, shortness of breath, and solitary or multinodular goiter (MNG) that may harbor malignancy [1].

In general, the standard treatment of thyroiditis is medical in the form of replacing thyroid hormone in cases of hypothyroidism, antibiotics in patients with acute suppurative thyroiditis, and corticosteroids for some cases of Riedel thyroiditis. Surgical interventions for the treatment of thyroiditis are exceptionally indicated, accounting for <1% of all thyroid procedures [2]. The most frequent surgical indications are abscess for drainage, compressive symptoms, and the presence or suspicion of malignancy. However, surgeries in cases of thyroiditis carry the risk of intra-operative and post-operative complications. It is conceivable that each case should be individualized in deciding whether to operate or not by assessing the benefit-risk ratio [1].

Many reports in the literature cover the medical management of thyroiditis; however, only a few discuss the surgical part in the form of surgery indications, surgery type, and post-operative complications, in comparison to non-thyroiditis cases.

16.2 Factors That Positively Influence the Decision of Surgery in Thyroiditis

16.2.1 Surgical Indications

The reported indications of surgery in thyroiditis include compressive symptoms such as dysphagia, dyspnea, or shortness of breath with impact on daily activities,

M. Sakr, *Thyroiditis*, https://doi.org/10.1007/978-3-032-19513-5_16

and voice change. Other indications are pain, cosmetic deformity, toxic multinodular goiter (MNG), nodular variant of Hashimoto's thyroiditis, lack of response to medical therapy, retro-sternal extension (TSE), and more seriously, presence or suspicion of malignancy in the thyroid gland [2–7]. In cases of acute suppurative thyroiditis (AST), surgery is indicated for the treatment of an abscess and/or fistula [8].

16.2.2 Risk of Malignancy

The risk of cancer in patients with thyroiditis exists mainly in the case of a solitary or cold nodule, a positive family history of thyroid cancer, and a rapidly growing goiter. The prevalence of thyroid cancer in Hashimoto's thyroiditis ranges from 0.4% [9] to 28% [10]. Several studies looked at the thyroid cancer association with thyroiditis [3, 6, 11–14]. Some researchers reported an increased risk [3, 14], while others did not [6, 12]. Moreover, Abbasgholizadeh et al. [15] published a meta-analysis study in 2021, reporting that Hashimoto's thyroiditis is associated with all types of thyroid malignancies, except follicular and anaplastic thyroid cancer. The authors concluded that there are inconsistent findings regarding the risk of cancer co-existence with thyroiditis, except for the well-known risk of lymphoma in patients with long-standing Hashimoto's thyroiditis [15]. Yet, this risk should be borne in mind by the surgeon managing thyroiditis patients. Bage and Kalatharan [11] (2021) concluded that the risk of malignant transformation in long-standing cases of Hashimoto's thyroiditis is prevented due to total thyroidectomy.

16.2.3 Improvement of Pre-operative Local Symptoms After Thyroidectomy

Hashimoto's thyroiditis has been reported to be linked with diminished quality of life (QOL) [16, 17]. Several authors reported that patients with thyroiditis showed a significant improvement in pre-operative symptoms as well as enhancement of the QOL after thyroidectomy [6, 11, 18–20]. It was also reported that compressive symptoms, such as difficulty in swallowing and neck tightness, are relieved after surgery [11, 18, 20]. This is an encouraging outcome of thyroidectomy for both patients and surgeons. However, surgical intervention is recommended in only severely symptomatic cases, such as compression symptoms in which the risks of the thyroid disease exceed those of the operation [19].

Patients with Hashimoto's thyroiditis may benefit after thyroidectomy in terms of QOL; specifically, physical, emotional, mental, and social functioning. The QOL, with domains of physical, mental, and sexual life, of both Hashimoto's thyroiditis and benign goiter patients is diminished and significantly improves post-operatively [20].

16.3 Factors That Negatively Influence the Decision of Surgery in Thyroiditis

16.3.1 Impact of Thyroiditis on Surgery

Thyroidectomy for thyroiditis is technically more difficult than non-thyroiditis cases, requiring more operative time and longer hospitalization [21]. Due to the intra-operative difficulties encountered during thyroidectomy in thyroiditis cases, surgery is not generally recommended [22]. These difficulties result in a higher risk of post-operative complications. Another issue is the intra-operative differentiation in inexperienced hands between chronic level VI cervical lymphadenopathy in patients with Hashimoto's thyroiditis and metastatic lymph nodes from a co-existing thyroid cancer or even a parathyroid gland (PTG) [3]. Therefore, surgery on thyroiditis cases should be performed by a senior, specialized surgeon who has a long experience with difficult thyroidectomies and can manage intra-operative challenges, such as bleeding and difficulty in identification of RLN and/or PTG. This will hopefully reduce post-operative complications [1].

16.3.2 Risk of Post-operative Complications

Transient or permanent post-operative complications are the usual concerns of surgeons. The risk of temporary or permanent hypocalcemia and/or RLN palsy may occur after any total thyroidectomy (TT). However, the incidence of temporary hypocalcemia and transient RLN palsy was found to be higher in thyroiditis patients [4]. Several studies reported a low incidence of permanent hypocalcemia and RLN palsy post-operatively, albeit with a higher incidence of temporary hypocalcemia [6, 23, 24]. In 2021, Gan et al. [23] published a meta-analysis study, which revealed that the rate of transient hypocalcemia was significantly higher in the Hashimoto's thyroiditis group (16.9%) compared with the benign nodular group (13.2%) ($p < 0.001$). However, there was no significant difference in the risk of permanent hypoparathyroidism between the two groups (1.17% and 0.99%, respectively) ($p = 0.431$). Moreover, there were no significant differences between the Hashimoto's thyroiditis group and the benign nodular group in the risk for transient RLN palsy (3.93% and 3.91%, respectively) ($p = 0.842$) and in the risk for permanent RLN palsy (1.15% and 0.78%, respectively) ($p = 0.234$) [23].

In the case of associated thyroid cancer, TT with level-VI lymph node dissection was found to be related to a higher risk of hypocalcemia [25, 26]. Meticulous intra-operative dissection can decrease the risk of post-operative hypocalcemia [27]. One study found a statistically significant difference regarding permanent hoarseness of voice in patients with Hashimoto's thyroiditis compared with those with non-Hashimoto's thyroiditis [22]. Other documented post-thyroidectomy complications in cases of thyroiditis are bleeding, neck hematoma, and surgical site infection (SSI). However, the risk is comparable with non-thyroiditis cases except for temporary hypocalcemia and transient RLN palsy, as they were found to occur more in thyroiditis cases [5, 6, 21, 23, 24]. Moreover, even when thyroid cancer patients were eliminated, post-operative complications were found to be higher in patients with Hashimoto's thyroiditis [22].

16.4 Surgery in the Different Types of Thyroiditis

16.4.1 Decision-Making

The different thyroiditis types or variants are usually treated medically, and surgery is rarely indicated. The treating surgeon should consider all the factors affecting the decision to operate on this special group of patients, including indications of surgery, symptomatic improvement post-operatively, risk of thyroid malignancy, intra-operative difficulty, and potential post-operative complications. Table 16.1 summarizes the characteristics of studies in the literature reporting surgical treatment of patients with different types (variants) of thyroiditis. It includes the indications of surgery, the type of surgery, and post-operative complications encountered.

16.4.2 Autoimmune Thyroiditis/Hashimoto's Thyroiditis

Patients with "autoimmune thyroiditis" are effectively managed with thyroid hormone replacement therapy, and surgical treatment is the exception. Technical difficulties are encountered by the surgeon as the glands are firm, rigid, and highly vascular, and the surrounding tissues are inflamed with lymphadenopathy, rendering the parathyroid glands (PTGs) and recurrent laryngeal nerves (RLNs) at risk. In the rare instance where a large Hashimoto's thyroiditis may develop and become symptomatic, total thyroidectomy (TT) is an option [2, 29, 30]. Moreover, as thyroiditis patients bear a higher risk of developing thyroid carcinoma, a cold nodule suspicious on fine-needle aspiration (FNA) may indicate a thyroid lobectomy. Similarly, the rapid growth of a chronic lymphocytic thyroid gland is suggestive of non-Hodgkin lymphoma (NHL). While TT may surgically cure a stage I lymphoma (confined to the thyroid), most thyroid lymphomas involve regional lymph nodes (LNs) and distant sites and require multi-modal systemic therapy. Open biopsy or thyroid lobectomy is sufficient in these cases to establish the definitive diagnosis.

16.4.3 Fibrotic Variant of Hashimoto's Thyroiditis

The fibrotic variant of Hashimoto's thyroiditis is characterized by a rapid enlargement of a pre-existing goiter, which causes suspicion of a thyroid malignancy and consequently total thyroidectomy.

Table 16.1 Characteristics of studies in the literature on surgical treatment of thyroiditis

Authors [Reference]	Year	Country	Methods	*N*	Type of thyroiditis	Indication of surgery	Type of surgery	Post-operative complications
Peterson [12]	1957	USA	Retrospective	757	HT	Nodular goiter, pressure symptoms, and suspicion of malignancy	Lobectomy, STT, isthmic-tomy	N/A
Lindem and Clark [5]	1969	USA	Retrospective	46	And Riedel's thyroiditis	Suspicious mass, pressure symptoms, hyperthyroidism, cosmesis, failed medical treatment	NTT	Wound seroma, transient hypocalcemia, and transient RLN paralysis
Clark et al. [13]	1980	USA	Retrospective	75	HT	Nodular goiter, diffuse goiter, STN	Lobectomy, STT, NTT ± neck dissection	Transient hypocalcemia, vocal cord palsy, and corneal abrasion
Pisanu et al. [3]	2003	Italy	Retrospective	44	HT	Result of FNA	TT	Morbidity not increased by HT
McManus et al. [18]	2011	USA	Retrospective	75	HT	Compressive symptoms and suspicion of malignancy	Lobectomy, STT, TT	Transient or permanent complications
Pradeep et al. [6]	2011	India	Retrospective	271	HT	Suspicion of malignancy, compression, pain, cosmesis	TT	Temporary hypo-calcemia
Seifman et al. [14]	2011	Australia	Retrospective	112	HT	Malignancy, risk of cancer, compression, thyrotoxicosis, patient request	TT	Permanent RLN palsy, hypoparathyroidism, and post-operative hemorrhage
Promberger et al. [19]	2014	Austria	Prospective cohort study	248	HT	Dysphagia and tightness in the neck	Lobectomy, TT, NTT	Hypocalcemia, RLN injury, postoperative bleeding, and SSI

(continued)

Table 16.1 (continued)

Authors [Reference]	Year	Country	Methods	*N*	Type of thyroiditis	Indication of surgery	Type of surgery	Post-operative complications
Zivaljevic et al. [20]	2015	Serbia	Prospective cohort study	143	HT	Toxic adenoma MNG, HT, and suspicious malignancy	TT, hemi-thyroidectomy	Transient and permanent complications
Ranganath et al. [28]	2016	USA	Retrospective	10	de Quervain's	Dysphagia, suspicious nodules	Lobectomy, TT, LN sampling	N/A
Ravikumar et al. [4]	2018	India	Retrospective	272	HT + nodular goiter	Compression, suspicious or proven cancer, RSE, toxic MNG, cosmesis	TT	Temporary hypocalcemia and transient RLN palsy
Thomusch et al. [24]	2018	Germany	Prospective multicenter European study	18,955	HT, GD, de Quervain's and Riedel thyroiditis	Suspicious or malignancy, hyperthyroidism compression, recurrence, and GD + ophthalmopathy	Lobectomy, STT, NTT, TT	Temporary and permanent hypocalcemia and RLN palsy, SSI, bleeding, cardio-vascular, pulm, and thrombo-embolic complications
Saadi et al. [21]	2019	USA		62	HT and GD	Symptomatic cases	TT/STT	Neck hematoma, RLN palsy, hypocalcemia, and SSI
Lafontaine et al. [8]	2021	Australia	Systematic review	200	AST	Failed aspiration and medical treatment, presence of abscess and/or fistula	I&D, TT, and partial thyroidectomy	IJV thrombo-phlebitis, mediastinitis, pericarditis, esophageal perforation, fistula, obstruction, severe laryngeal edema, Horner's syndrome, MSOF, and death
Gan et al. [23]	2021	China	Meta-analysis	1582	HT	N/A	Lobectomy, TT	Transient/permanent hypocalcemia, or RLN palsy

Bage and Kalatharan [11]	2021	India	Hospital-based descriptive study	30	HT	Painful cases, failed medical therapy	TT	N/A

USA United States of America, *HT* Hashimoto's thyroiditis, *STT* subtotal thyroidectomy, *N/A* not available, *RLN* recurrent laryngeal nerve, *MNG* multinodular goiter, *STN* solitary thyroid nodule, *NTT* near total thyroidectomy, *TT* total thyroidectomy, *FNA* fine-needle aspiration, *RSE* retro-sternal extension, *GD* Graves' disease, *AST* acute suppurative thyroiditis, *LN* lymph node, *I&D* incision and drainage, *SSI* surgical site infection, *IJV* internal jugular vein, *pulm* pulmonary

16.4.4 Subacute de Quervain's Thyroiditis

A subacute de Quervain's thyroiditis exceptionally deserves thyroidectomy as it carries a high risk of complications [28]. This indication is given when intractable neck pain is present in spite of a consequent analgesic treatment and L-thyroxin replacement therapy over a period of 6 months [2].

16.4.5 Riedel's Fibrosing Thyroiditis

Riedel's fibrosing thyroiditis often requires an open biopsy to confirm the diagnosis and rule out an anaplastic carcinoma. Isthmectomy and/or lobectomy is often required to decompress the trachea and esophagus [31–34]. Thyroidectomy can be highly demanding because of the dense fibrotic reaction extending beyond the thyroid, which puts the surrounding structures at risk of injury resulting in hypoparathyroidism and RLN injury even when limited surgery is performed by experienced surgical specialists as documented in a series from the Mayo clinic where 39% of patients with Riedel's thyroiditis suffered surgical complications [35]. Previous and contemporary experience therefore recommends that extensive surgical procedures be considered inappropriate [31, 33, 35, 36]. Microscopic surgery has recently been attempted by Jung (2017) to minimize complications [37].

16.4.6 Amiodarone-Induced Thyrotoxicosis

The anti-arrhythmic drug amiodarone contains 35% I_2 and may cause a thyrotoxic crisis or conversely, cause hypothyroidism. Amiodarone decreases the conversion of T4 to the biologically active T3. If amiodarone therapy is stopped, it is not eliminated for months due to its very long half-life [38]. Amiodarone-induced thyrotoxicosis in the setting of a rare patient with otherwise intractable arrhythmia is an indication for thyroidectomy.

16.4.7 Acute Suppurative Thyroiditis (AST)

The consequences of acute suppurative thyroiditis (AST) are known to be numerous, either from the disease process itself or from its treatment [8]. Thus, AST is a classical indication for surgical drainage followed by antibiotic therapy and rarely for lobectomy when the suppurative process is necrotizing.

References

1. Alnefaie SM. Surgical decision-making in thyroiditis: a review article. Cureus. 2023;15(9):e46055.

2. Roher HD, Schulte KM. Operative therapie bei thyreoiditis. In: Rothmund M, Harder F, Siewert JR, editors. Praxis der Viszeralchirurgie: Endokrine Chirurgie. Berlin, Heidelberg/ New York: Springer; 2000. p. 199–202.
3. Pisanu A, Piu S, Cois A, Uccheddu A. Coexisting Hashimoto's thyroiditis with differentiated thyroid cancer and benign thyroid diseases: indications for thyroidectomy. Chir Ital. 2003;55:365–72.
4. Ravikumar K, Muthukumar S, Sadacharan D, Suresh U, Sundarram T, Periyasamy S. The impact of thyroiditis on morbidity and safety in patients undergoing total thyroidectomy. Indian J Endocrinol Metab. 2018;22:494–8.
5. Lindem MC Jr, Clark JH. Indications for surgery in thyroiditis. Am J Surg. 1969;118:829–31.
6. Pradeep PV, Ragavan M, Ramakrishna BA, Jayasree B, Skandha SH. Surgery in Hashimoto's thyroiditis: indications, complications, and associated cancers. J Postgrad Med. 2011;57:120–2.
7. Nenkov R, Radev R, Khristozov K, Kuzmanov I, Kornovski S, Kuzmanov S, et al. Hashimoto's thyroiditis: indications for surgical treatment. Khirurgiia (Sofiia). 2005;3:28–32.
8. Lafontaine N, Learoyd D, Farrel S, Wong R. Suppurative thyroiditis: systematic review and clinical guidance. Clin Endocrinol. 2021;95:253–64.
9. Matesa-Anic D, Matesa N, Dabelic N, Kusic Z. Coexistence of papillary carcinoma and Hashimoto's thyroiditis. Acta Clin Croat. 2009;48:9–12.
10. Shih ML, Lee JA, Hsieh CB, Yu JC, Liu HD, Kebebew E, et al. Thyroidectomy for Hashimoto's thyroiditis: complications and associated cancers. Thyroid. 2008;18:729–34.
11. Bage AM, Kalatharan P. Role of total thyroidectomy in painful (symptomatic) Hashimoto's thyroiditis: descriptive study. Indian J Otolaryngol Head Neck Surg. 2021;73:296–303.
12. Peterson CA. Lymphocytic thyroiditis in 757 thyroid operations. Am J Surg. 1957;94:223–8.
13. Clark OH, Greenspan FS, Dunphy JE. Hashimoto's thyroiditis and thyroid cancer: indications for operation. Am J Surg. 1980;140:65–71.
14. Seifman MA, Grodski SF, Bailey M, Yeung MJ, Serpell JW. Surgery in the setting of Hashimoto's thyroiditis. ANZ J Surg. 2011;81:519–23.
15. Abbasgholizadeh P, Naseri A, Nasiri E, Sadra V. Is Hashimoto thyroiditis associated with increasing risk of thyroid malignancies? A systematic review and meta-analysis. Thyroid Res. 2021;14:26.
16. Bianchi GP, Zaccheroni V, Solaroli E, Vescini F, Cerutti R, Zoli M, et al. Health-related quality of life in patients with thyroid disorders – a study based on Short-Form 36 and Nottingham Health Profile Questionnaires. Qual Life Res. 2004;13:45–54.
17. Ott J, Promberger R, Kober F, Neuhold N, Tea M, Huber JC, et al. Hashimoto's thyroiditis affects symptom load and quality of life unrelated to hypothyroidism: a prospective case-control study in women undergoing thyroidectomy for benign goiter. Thyroid. 2011;21:161–7.
18. McManus C, Luo J, Sippel R, Chen H. Should patients with symptomatic Hashimoto's thyroiditis pursue surgery? J Surg Res. 2011;170:52–5.
19. Promberger R, Hermann M, Pallikunnel SJ, Seemann R, Meusel M, Ott J. Quality of life after thyroid surgery in women with benign euthyroid goiter: influencing factors including Hashimoto's thyroiditis. Am J Surg. 2014;207:974–9.
20. Zivaljevic VR, Bukvic Bacotic BR, Sipetic SB, Stanisavljevic DM, Maksimovic JM, Diklic AD, et al. Quality of life improvement in patients with Hashimoto thyroiditis and other goiters after surgery: a prospective cohort study. Int J Surg. 2015;21:150–5.
21. Saadi R, Brandt A, Kim Y, Cottrill E, Saunders B, Schaefer E, et al. Degree of technical difficulty of thyroidectomy for autoimmune thyroid disease. Head Neck. 2020;42:262–8.
22. McManus C, Luo J, Sippel R, Chen H. Is thyroidectomy in s with Hashimoto thyroiditis more risky? J Surg Res. 2012;178:529–32.
23. Gan X, Feng J, Deng X, Shen F, Lu J, Liu Q, et al. The significance of Hashimoto's thyroiditis for postoperative complications of thyroid surgery: a systematic review and meta-analysis. Ann R Coll Surg Engl. 2021;103:223–30.
24. Thomusch O, Sekulla C, Billmann F, Seifert G, Dralle H, Lorenz K. Risk profile analysis and complications after surgery for autoimmune thyroid disease. Br J Surg. 2018;105:677–85.

25. Chisholm EJ, Kulinskaya E, Tolley NS. Systematic review and meta-analysis of the adverse effects of thyroidectomy combined with central neck dissection as compared with thyroidectomy alone. Laryngoscope. 2009;119:1135–9.
26. Henry JF, Gramatica L, Denizot A, Kvachenyuk A, Puccini M, Defechereux T. Morbidity of prophylactic lymph node dissection in the central neck area in patients with papillary thyroid carcinoma. Langenbecks Arch Surg. 1998;383:167–9.
27. Nair CG, Babu MJ, Menon R, Jacob P. Hypocalcaemia following total thyroidectomy: an analysis of 806 patients. Indian J Endocrinol Metab. 2013;17:298–303.
28. Ranganath R, Shaha MA, Xu B, Migliacci J, Ghossein R, Shaha AR. de Quervain's thyroiditis: a review of experience with surgery. Am J Otolaryngol. 2016;37:534–7.
29. Khan A, Nosé V. Pathology of the thyroid gland. In: Lloyd RV, editor. Endocrine pathology. Totowa: Humana; 2004. p. 153–89.
30. Kon YC, DeGroot LJ. Painful Hashimoto's thyroiditis as an indication for thyroidectomy: clinical characteristics and outcome in seven patients. J Clin Endocrinol Metab. 2003;88:2667–72.
31. Singer PA. Thyroiditis. Acute, subacute, and chronic. Med Clin North Am. 1991;75(1):61–77.
32. Guimaraes VC. Subacute and Reidel's thyroiditis. In: Jameson JL, De Groot LJ, editors. Endocrinology: adult and pediatric. 6th ed. Philadelphia: Elsevier; 2010. p. 1600–3.
33. Marin F, Araujo R, Paramo C, Lucas T, Salto L. Riedel's thyroiditis associated with hypothyroidism and hypoparathyroidism. Postgrad Med J. 1989;65(764):381–3.
34. Pearce EN, Farwell AP, Braverman LE. Thyroiditis. N Engl J Med. 2003;348(26):2646–55.
35. Fatourechi MM, Hay ID, McIver B, Sebo TJ, Fatourechi V. Invasive fibrous thyroiditis (Riedel thyroiditis): the Mayo clinic experience, 1976-2008. Thyroid. 2011;21(7):765–72.
36. Lee SL, Ananthakrishnan S. Infiltrative thyroid disease. In: Rose BD, Mulder JE, editors. UpToDate. Wellesley: BDR, Inc.; 2011. p. 1–21.
37. Jung K-Y. Surgical treatment for Riedel's thyroiditis: a case report. Int J Thyroidol. 2017;10(1):66–9.
38. Harjai KJ, Licata AA. Effects of amiodarone on thyroid function. Ann Intern Med. 1997;126:63–73.